Contemporary Issues in Prostate Cancer: A Nursing Perspective

Contemporary Issues in Prostate Cancer: A Nursing Perspective

EDITED BY

JEANNE HELD-WARMKESSEL
MSN, RN, CS, AOCN

Fox Chase Cancer Center
Philadelphia, Pennsylvania

Jones and Bartlett Publishers
Sudbury, Massachusetts
BOSTON • TORONTO • LONDON • SINGAPORE

World Headquarters
Jones and Bartlett Publishers
40 Tall Pine Drive
Sudbury, MA 01776
978-443-5000
info@jbpub.com
www.jbpub.com

Jones and Bartlett Publishers Canada
2100 Bloor Street West
Suite 6-272
Toronto, ON M6S 5A5
CANADA

Jones and Bartlett Publishers International
Barb House, Barb Mews
London W6 7PA
UK

PRODUCTION CREDITS
Senior Acquisitions Editor: Greg Vis
Production Editor: Linda DeBruyn
Manufacturing Director: Therese Bräuer
Editorial and Production Service: Bookwrights
Cover Design: Dick Hannus
Text Design: Connie Leavitt
Printing and Binding: Malloy Lithographing

Library of Congress Cataloging-in-Publication Data
Contemporary issues in prostate cancer: a nursing perspective / edited by Jeanne Held-Warmkessel.
    p. ; cm. — (Jones and Bartlett series in oncology)
    Includes bibliographical references and index.
    ISBN 0-7637-1081-4 (pbk.)
    1. Prostate—Cancer. 2. Prostate—Cancer—Nursing. I. Held-Warmkessel, Jeanne. II. Series.
    [DNLM: 1. Prostatic Neoplasms—nursing. WJ 752 C761 2000]
    RC280.P7 C67 2000
    616.99'463–dc21   99-044509

Cover illustration by Stephanie Torta

Printed in the United States of America
03 02 01 00 99 10 9 8 7 6 5 4 3 2 1

This book is dedicated to
My husband, Brian Warmkessel,
My mother, Irene Held,
My parrot, Dolly "Bubbie,"
with thanks for their patience.

Contents

Preface   *xi*
Acknowledgments   *xii*
Contributors   *xiii*
Reviewers   *xiv*

1 EPIDEMIOLOGY, RISK FACTORS AND PREVENTION STRATEGIES   1
Peg Esper, MSN, RN, CS, AOCN
Epidemiology-Etiology • Risk Factors • Prevention • Nursing Implications • Summary

2 SCREENING AND EARLY DETECTION   24
Anne Robin Waldman, MSN, RN, C, AOCN
Introduction • Controversy Over Screening • High-Risk and Contributing Factors • Who Should Be Screened? • Factors Influencing Screening for Cancer • Barriers to Screening • Screening Tools • Cost Versus Benefit of Early Detection • Development of a Screening Program in Philadelphia • Conclusion

3 CELLULAR CHARACTERISTICS, PATHOPHYSIOLOGY, AND DISEASE MANIFESTATIONS   36
Jennifer Cash, MS, ARNP
Introduction • Carcinogenesis and Pathology • Grading and Prognostic Indicators of Prostate Cancer • Factors for Tumor Development, Progression and Metastasis • Clinical Manifestations • Conclusion

4 ASSESSMENT AND DIAGNOSIS   49
Cindy Jo Horrell, MS, CRNP, AOCN
Introduction • Clinical Presentation • History • Physical Examination • Laboratory • Imaging • Biopsy • Conclusion

5 STAGING OF PROSTATE CANCER   66
Mary Collins, RN, MSN, OCN
Introduction • Classification Systems • Clinical Staging • Significance of Tumor Staging • Pathologic Stage • Histologic Grade • Combining Clinical Factors to Predict Pathologic Stage • Conclusions

6 TREATMENT DECISION MAKING   81
William Tester, MD, FACP & Maria DeVito Brouch, MS, RN
Introduction • Patient Data Collection • Treatment Options • Common Complications of Treatment • Treatment Selection for the Individual Patient • Psychosocial Issues • Nursing Issues and Concerns

7 EXPECTANT MANAGEMENT: THE ART AND SCIENCE
OF WATCHFUL WAITING   102
Maureen E. O'Rourke, RN, PhD & Andrew S. Griffin, MD, FACS
Introduction • Rationale for Expectant Management • Rationale Against
Expectant Management • Therapeutic Goal of Expectant Management •
Patient Eligibility Criteria • Patient and Partner Views of the Expectant
Management Option • Protocol for Expectant Management • When Should
Treatment Be Pursued? • Nursing Management of Patients Choosing
the Expectant Management Option • Psychoeducational Interventions to
Minimize Uncertainty • Conclusion

8 SURGICAL CARE OF THE PATIENT WITH PROSTATE CANCER   117
Dawn M. Osborne, BSN, RN, C
Introduction • Transurethral Resection of the Prostate • Radical Retropubic
Prostatectomy • Cryoablation of the Prostate • Bilateral Orchiectomy •
Summary

9 A PATIENT'S PERSPECTIVE ON THE DIAGNOSIS AND TREATMENT OF
PROSTATE CANCER WITH RADIATION THERAPY   135
Edgar Herbert, Jr.

10 RADIATION THERAPY   137
Heidi M. Volpe, MSN, RN, CCRA
Introduction • Pretreatment Workup • Simulation-Treatment Planning •
External Beam Radiation • Three-Dimensional Conformal Radiation Therapy •
External Beam Side Effects • Interstitial Implantation (Brachytherapy) •
Combination Therapy • Psychosocial Issues • Conclusion

11 HORMONAL THERAPY   170
Laura Stempkowski, MS, CUNP, AOCN
Rationale for Hormonal Manipulation • Primary Hormonal Manipulation •
Indications for Hormonal Manipulation • Side Effect Management • Hormone-
Refractory Disease–Androgen Independence • Novel Approaches to Hormonal
Manipulation • Conclusion

12 CHEMOTHERAPY FOR PROSTATE CANCER   195
Jeanne Held-Warmkessel, MSN, RN, CS, AOCN
Introduction • Chemotherapy • Treatment Options After Chemotherapy Failure
• Chemotherapy Candidates • Patient Education • Nursing Management •
Psychosocial Issues • Conclusion

13 QUALITY OF LIFE AFTER TREATMENT FOR PROSTATE CANCER   227
Esther Muscari Lin, RN, MSN, ACNP, AOCN & Maria D. Kelly, MD
Quality of Life Definition • Reasons for QOL Research in Prostate Cancer •
Challenges to QOL Research in Prostate Cancer • HRQOL Instruments •
HRQOL in Localized Prostate Cancer • Treatment Options for Localized

Prostate Cancer • Urinary Incontinence • Sexual Dysfunction • Bowel Disturbances • HRQOL in Advanced Prostate Cancer • Conclusion

14 ADVANCED PROSTATE CANCER: SYMPTOM MANAGEMENT   254
Jeanne Held-Warmkessel, MSN, RN, CS, AOCN
Bladder Outlet Obstruction • Ureteral Obstruction • Leg Edema • Disseminated Intravascular Coagulation • Bone Pain • Spinal Cord Compression • Conclusion

15 PROSTATE CANCER RESOURCES FOR PATIENTS, FAMILIES, AND PROFESSIONALS   286
Carol Blecher, MS, RN, AOCN
Early Detection and Screening Information • Information Regarding Prostate Cancer Diagnosis and Treatment Options • Materials Dealing with Advanced Prostate Cancer • Psychosocial and Support Resources • Audiovisual Materials • Resources for Prostate Cancer Information • Books About Prostate Cancer • Personal Accounts • Worldwide Web Resources

Index   *307*

Preface

The issues of prostate cancer detection and management have undergone significant changes since the discovery of prostate-specific antigen (PSA). Yet there are no textbooks that specifically address nursing care and management of patients with prostate cancer. That is the purpose of *Contemporary Issues in Prostate Cancer: A Nursing Perspective.* Users of this book will find chapters devoted to risk factors, screening, diagnosis, and the different treatment modalities used in prostate cancer management. Additional topics include advanced disease symptom management, pathophysiology, and patient education resources. Oncology nurses and advanced practice nurses in general medical oncology, surgical oncology, and urologic oncology will find this text useful, as will both nursing and medical students.

Why *Contemporary Issues?* Nurses need to be aware of the recent trends in prostate cancer management such as the changing incidence of the disease. Prostate cancer is the most commonly diagnosed cancer among American males,[1] and disease rates vary based on race and ethnic group.[2] There is also variation in the incidence of prostate cancer in the United States. Between 1976 and 1994, the incidence of prostate cancer doubled.[3] Since then, however, the rate of prostate cancer diagnoses has declined.[4] It has been hypothesized that the increase is related to the use of PSA screening.[5] During the early use of this screening, men with elevated PSA levels were evaluated for the presence of prostate cancer. With the ongoing use of PSA screening, the pool of men with a potential prostate cancer diagnosis was minimized. Hence, the number of new potential cancer patients was reduced.[6] Another trend in prostate cancer management is the diagnosis of prostate cancer at an earlier stage, with lower grade tumors.[7]

Nurses need the most up-to-date information available to provide accurate patient education and competent nursing care to men with prostate cancer. Accurate information is the cornerstone of prevention, early detection, and treatment of prostate cancer. This book will help the nurse interpret confusing and contradictory information, and provide the most current information for use during patient education sessions. It is my goal to assist the nurse in all aspects of prostate cancer patient care. I would like to hear from readers and users of this book.

ACKNOWLEDGMENTS

A project of this size is not accomplished without the expertise of others. I thank the chapter contributors, without whom this text would not have been possible, the editorial staff at Jones and Bartlett including Greg Vis, Linda DeBruyn, Amy Austin, John Danielowich, and Christine Tridente; and the Nursing Department at Fox Chase Cancer Center, including Joanne Hambleton, MSN, RN, CNA; Andrea Barsevick, DNSc, RN, AOCN; Terry Cotteta, MSN, RN; Pam Kedziera, MSN, RN, AOCN; and Carolyn Weaver, MSN, RN, AOCN. I give special thanks to my mother, my husband, and my office-mate, Linda Schiech, MSN, RN, OCN, for their never ending patience

REFERENCES

1. Landis SH, Murray T, Bolden S, Wingo PA. Cancer statistics. *CA Cancer J Clin* 1999;49:8-31.
2. Haas GP, Sakr WA. Epidemiology of prostate cancer. *CA Cancer J Clin* 1997;47:273-287.
3. Ries LAG, Kosary CL, Hankey BF, et al (eds). *SEER Cancer Statistics Review,* 1973-1994. Bethesda, MD: National Cancer Institute, 1997.
4. Wingo PA, Landis S, Ries LAG. An adjustment to the 1997 estimate for new prostate cancer cases. *Cancer* 1997;80:1810-1813.
5. Potosky AL, Miller BA, Albertsen PC, Kramer BS. The role of increasing detection in the rising incidence of prostate cancer. *JAMA* 1995;273:548-552.
6. Gann PW. Interpreting recent trends in prostate cancer incidence and mortality. *Epidemiology* 1997;8:117-120.
7. Mettlin CJ, Murphy GP, Ho R, et al. The National Cancer Data Base report on longitudinal observations on prostate cancer. *Cancer* 1996;77:2162-2166.

Contributors

Carol Blecher, MS, RN, AOCN; *Oncology Clinical Nurse Specialist;* Valley Hospital, Ridgewood, New Jersey

Maria DeVito Brouch, MS, RN; *Oncology Clinical Liaison;* Albert Einstein Medical Center; Philadelphia, Pennsylvania; *Adjunct Faculty,* LaSalle University, Philadelphia, Pennsylvania

Jennifer Cash, MS, ARNP; *ARNP, Radiation Oncology;* University Community Hospital, Tampa, Florida

Mary Collins, RN, MSN, OCN; *Nurse Coordinator;* Breast and Prostate Cancer Center, Carle Cancer Center, Urbana, Illinois

Peg Esper, MSN, RN, CS, AOCN; *Nurse Practitioner, Medical Oncology;* University of Michigan Comprehensive Cancer Center, Ann Arbor, Michigan

Andrew S. Griffin, MD, FACS; *President, Medical Staff;* Medical Park Hospital, Winston-Salem, North Carolina

Jeanne Held-Warmkessel, MSN, RN, CS, AOCN; *Clinical Nurse Specialist;* Fox Chase Cancer Center, Philadelphia, Pennsylvania

Edgar Herbert, Jr., Lake Lure, North Carolina

Cindy Jo Horrell, MS, CRNP, AOCN; *Oncology Nurse Practitioner;* Clinical Associates, Regional Cancer Center, Erie, Pennsylvania

Maria D. Kelly, MD; *Associate Professor, Clinical Radiation Oncology;* The University of Virginia Health Sciences Center, Charlottesville, Virginia

Esther Muscari Lin, RN, MSN, ACNP, AOCN; *Oncology Clinical Nurse Specialist/Clinician;* The University of Virginia Cancer Center, Charlottesville, Virginia

Maureen E. O'Rourke, RN, PhD; *Assistant Professor of Nursing;* University of North Carolina, Greensboro, North Carolina; *Adjunct Assistant Professor of Medicine,* Hematology/Oncology, Wake Forest University School of Medicine, Winston-Salem, North Carolina

Dawn M. Osborne, BSN, RN, C; *Clinical Coordinator;* Department of Surgery, Albert Einstein Medical Center, Philadelphia, Pennsylvania

Laura Stempkowski, MS, CUNP, AOCN; *Nurse Practitioner,* Department of Urology, Dartmouth-Hitchcock Medical Center, Lebanon, New Hampshire

William Tester, MD, FACP; *Director;* Albert Einstein Cancer Center, Philadelphia, Pennsylvania

Heidi M. Volpe, MSN, RN, CCRA; *Research Coordinator;* Department of Radiation Oncology, Albert Einstein Medical Center, Philadelphia, Pennsylvania

Anne Robin Waldman, MSN, RN, C, AOCN; *Oncology Clinical Nurse Specialist;* Albert Einstein Cancer Center, Philadelphia, Pennsylvania; *Adjunct Faculty,* LaSalle University, Philadelphia, Pennsylvania

REVIEWERS

EPIDEMIOLOGY, RISK FACTORS, AND PREVENTION STRATEGIES

PEG ESPER

OVERVIEW

EPIDEMIOLOGY-ETIOLOGY
  Introduction
  Molecular Factors
RISK FACTORS
  Age
  Racial-Ethnic Factors
  Genetic Factors
  Smoking-Ethanol Use
  Occupation and Exposure History
  Hormonal-Steroid Factors

Sexuality Issues
Body Size and Energy Expenditure
Dietary-Nutritional Factors
PREVENTION
  Hormonal Approaches
  Miscellaneous Approaches
  Prevention Trials
NURSING IMPLICATIONS
SUMMARY

EPIDEMIOLOGY-ETIOLOGY

INTRODUCTION

Prostate cancer continues to be a serious public health problem. Incidence rates for American men exceed 179,300; approximately 37,000 deaths are attributed to this disease annually. At present, men in the United States have a one in five lifetime risk of being diagnosed with prostate cancer, and approximately 20% will have metastatic disease at diagnosis.[1] Prostate cancer is now the most frequently diagnosed cancer in American men and is the second leading cause of cancer-related deaths among males.[1]

One of the formidable characteristics of prostate cancer is its ability to span the continuum of aggressiveness. Prostate cancer can present as an indolent condition in which individuals are asymptomatic and may remain so indefinitely or as an aggressive malignancy that devastatingly impacts the individual's length and quality of life. Although new strategies for early diagnosis (see Chapters 2, 4) continue to be a major focus in prostate cancer research, its inherent nature has made prostate cancer screening a much-debated topic. The early diagnosis of indolent varieties of prostate cancer that otherwise might never be clinically detected continues to raise concern. At the same time, there is inconclusive evidence that early detection significantly reduces morbidity and mortality from prostate cancer.[2] Most researchers and those who provide clinical care for prostate cancer patients agree, however, that the consuming sequelae of advanced disease are sufficient causes for further exploration into the etiology, risk factors, and possible prevention of this all too common malignancy.

The majority of prostate cancers are adenocarcinomas; the preponderance of these occur in the peripheral zone of the gland (70%). Another 20% occur in the transitional zone and approximately 10% in the central zone of the prostate.[3] Still, the etiology of prostate cancer remains unclear. Although hormonal influences are deemed to be associated to varying degrees and are discussed in greater depth later, other factors, such as benign prostatic hypertrophy (BPH), have demonstrated no direct causative effect. The process in which normal prostate cells are transformed to malignant ones is believed to encompass several genetic events. In the development of cancer, the normal cell is believed to undergo first an initiative event followed by a promoting event that can lead to progression and the ability to invoke metastatic disease.[4] Considerable variation exists, however, in movement from the latent to the clinically progressive form of prostate cancer in different geographic populations.[5–7] The existence of variations in latent or histologic prostate cancer versus the clinically evident version is exemplified in several studies in which pathologic review of prostate autopsy specimens has been performed. Histologic prevalence (latent disease) has been found to be similar around the world, whereas the prevalence of clinically evident disease differs significantly from country to country.[8] Such data suggest that perhaps environmental factors play a role in prostate cancer development. Specific environmental factors as well as other perceived risk factors are discussed.

MOLECULAR FACTORS

Additional molecular and biologic etiologic factors in prostate cancer development have been identified in the literature. Although Helpap and colleagues[9] found no obvious relationship between the development of prostate cancer and atypical adenomatous hyperplasia (AAH), they did propose that prostatic intraepithelial neoplasia (PIN) was the most likely precursor of prostate cancer in the dorsoperipheral zone.[9] PIN as a precursor to the development of prostate cancer has been documented in several additional studies.[10, 11] More recently, the role of plasma insulin-like growth factor I (IGF-I) and vascular endothelial growth factor (VEGF) has been researched, both prospectively and in vivo. These studies indicate a role in the regulation of epithelial-stromal interactions in sex hormone–related prostate cancer and increased risk in individuals with higher plasma IGF-I levels.[12, 13]

Some of the most comprehensive population-based information available on prostate cancer comes from the Cancer Surveillance, Epidemiology, and End Results (SEER) program. This database includes information on cancers diagnosed in defined areas of the United States and has provided important leads in studying racial differences in prostate cancer occurrence.[14]

RISK FACTORS

A plethora of contradictory information exists in the literature regarding the causes of prostate cancer. There has been suggestion that such discrepancies may be related to differences based on patient age, resulting in a "two-disease" theory of prostate cancer.[15] This section explores some of the consistencies and inconsistencies in what are the most frequently cited "risk factors" for the development of prostate cancer.

AGE

Although prostate cancer has been detected as early as the third decade of life, it is primarily a malignancy seen in individuals over the age of 60. In fact, in individuals in the birth-to-39-year age range, the risk of developing prostate cancer is less than 1 in 10,000; this risk increases to one in six for those men between the ages of 60 and 79 (Figure 1-1).[1] After the age of 50, there is nearly an exponential increase in both the incidence and mortality from prostate cancer; the rate of increase after age 40 is higher than for any other cancer in men.[5, 16] The prevalence of prostate cancer in this age group has also been demonstrated in multiple autopsy studies in which, despite variations in clinically evident disease, histologic cancer is present in approximately 15 to 30% of men from a variety of countries.[5] Histologic tumors have been found in 70 to 90% of men by the age of 80 to 90 on autopsy without preference for national origin.[6, 7]

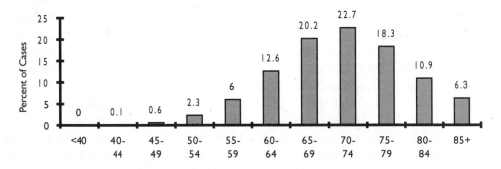

FIGURE 1-1. Prostate cancer distribution by age, SEER Program, 1973–1995
From Stanford JL, Stephenson RA, Coyle LM, et al. *Prostate Cancer Trends 1973–1995*. Bethesda, MD: Cancer Surveillance, Epidemiology, and End Results (SEER) Program, National Cancer Institute, 1998.

The exact etiology of increases in prostate cancer with age is believed to be multifactorial in nature. One theory has linked the relationship with increases in male life expectancy, particularly in the United States. Because men in the United States are living longer, the histologic version of the malignancy may have time to become clinically significant. This process appears to be multistep in nature and requires androgens. Dihydrotestosterone (DHT) is responsible for targeting specific androgen response elements that are involved in the regulation of cellular proliferation in the prostate. In the aging process, the steps that take place, including the irreversible transformation of testosterone to alpha-DHT by 5 α-reductase with resultant accumulation of DHT over time, may be involved in the eventual cellular transformation.[17]

RACIAL-ETHNIC FACTORS

Significant variation exists in the incidence of prostate cancer among men of different racial and ethnic backgrounds. An increasing body of literature has reported on incidence increases within the African-American population. The incidence of prostate cancer in African-American males is significantly higher than their Caucasian counterparts (180.6/100,000 compared with 134.7/100,000). From 1988 to 1992, the mortality from prostate cancer for African-American men was double that of Caucasian males. African-American males are also diagnosed with distant disease 18% of the time versus 10% for Caucasian males.[18]

An additional concern is whether or not a more aggressive form of prostate cancer exists in the African-American population.[19] In a study by Moul and colleagues,[20] after multivariate adjustment, black race was found to be a poor prognostic factor for recurrence after planned curative radical prostatectomy ($P = .019$).

Studies have suggested that the biology of prostate cancer in African-American men is different because they present with a significantly higher Gleason score than their age-matched Caucasian counterparts.[21] Others found this to be substantiated only in those aged 65 and younger.[19, 20] Younger African-American men have been found, stage for stage, to have a worse prognosis.[19–21] A retrospective study by the U.S. Department of Defense determined that in an equal-access medical care system (military personnel), African-Americans had a higher relative risk in younger groups, presented with higher stage, and demonstrated increased progression in distant metastatic disease but survived longer with metastatic disease than their Caucasian counterparts.[22] Powell[23] hypothesized that African-Americans have aggressive and nonaggressive forms of prostate cancer and that, although the nonaggressive form behaves much like that of Caucasian men, the aggressive form occurs at an earlier age and takes on more contentious behavior.

Several studies have attempted to link differences in serum testosterone levels with the racial differences seen in prostate cancer incidence. A 1994 study evaluated total testosterone and free testosterone levels in college-age men and found African-American men to have a 15% higher total testosterone level and 13% higher free testosterone level than Caucasians.[21] A 1992 study conducted by Ellis and Nyborg, however, included non-Hispanic whites, blacks, Hispanics, and several additional racial and ethnic groups of

TABLE 1-1. Prostate Cancer—SEER Incidence and Mortality 1988–1992

Ethnicity	Incidence	Mortality
Black	180.6	53.7
Chinese	46.0	6.6
Filipino	69.8	13.5
Hawaiian	57.2	19.9
Japanese	88.0	11.7
Native American*	52.5	16.2
White (Total)	134.7	24.1
White Hispanic	92.8	15.9
White non-Hispanic	137.9	24.4

Rates are per 100,000 and are age adjusted to the 1970 U.S. standard.

*Based only on data from New Mexico.

From Stanford JL, Stephenson RA, Coyle LM, et al. *Prostate Cancer Trends 1973–1995*. Bethesda, MD: Cancer Surveillance, Epidemiology, and End Results (SEER) Program, National Cancer Institute, 1998.

men aged 31 to 50 and noted only a 3.3% increase of testosterone levels over the African-American study population.[24] This was possibly attributed to age-related testosterone levels. It is believed that early differences in circulating testosterone levels may still contribute to observed racial disparity in prostate cancer risk. African-Americans with prostate cancer have also been shown to have higher prostate-specific antigen (PSA) and PSA density than other ethnic groups.[25]

In a study of 369 men in a single institution, Powell and colleagues found African-American men to have positive surgical margins 58% of the time as opposed to 40% of the time in Caucasian men, leading to more pathologically locally advanced prostate cancer.[26] This, too, is a factor that may be associated with the poorer survival rates among African-American men. Continued research efforts at the molecular and biologic level are needed in this population.

Mortality from prostate cancer in males of Chinese, Filipino, Hawaiian, Japanese, American Indian, and Hispanic origin is lower than in both African-American and Caucasian males (Table 1-1). Incidence rates were lowest for those of Korean ethnicity, at a rate of 24.2/100,000.[18] Figure 1-2 provides incidence rates within the United States, and Figure 1-3 displays international incidence rates.

Of interest is a report on the incidence of prostate cancer in two additional ethnic groups. Glover and colleagues[27] found the incidence of prostate cancer to be higher in Jamaican men compared with African-American or Caucasian men in the United States and associated with greater morbidity. The incidence and mortality rates of prostate cancer are also increasing for Native North American Indians. Although its incidence is lower in non-Hispanic Caucasians, prostate cancer has the highest ranking incidence and mortality for cancer in Native North American Indian men.[28] More in-depth and culturally sensitive screening efforts are important in both of these groups.

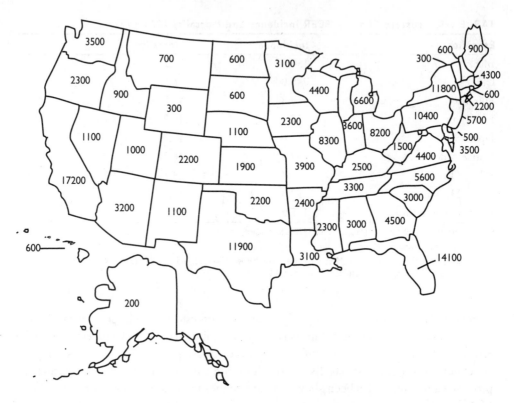

FIGURE 1-2. United States estimated prostate cancer rates—1998
From Stanford JL, Stephenson RA, Coyle LM, et al. *Prostate Cancer Trends 1973–1995*. Bethesda, MD: Cancer Surveillance, Epidemiology, and End Results (SEER) Program, National Cancer Institute, 1998.

Risk factors associated with race or ethnicity have often been linked to socioeconomic status. Past studies have attempted to link racial discrepancies in prostate cancer incidence with socioeconomic status (SES). This has been a difficult task because a large number of clinical trial participants are of a lower SES. However, those studies that have corrected for SES have, in general, not found SES to account for racial differences observed in incidence or mortality.[29] To date, no convincing data exist that substantiate correlation of prostate cancer risk with either increased or decreased SES.[30]

GENETIC FACTORS

Ongoing studies continue to provide evidence that supports a familial or hereditary component to prostate cancer development.[31–37] A clinical definition for hereditary prostate cancer has been suggested to include the following criteria: (1) three or more affected individuals within one nuclear family; (2) three successive generations of affected individuals, either maternal or paternal lineage; or (3) two or more relatives affected before age 55.[31] Ghadirian and colleagues[32] found an almost eightfold difference in the occurrence of prostate cancer among first-degree family members in a case-controlled study of 140 men with prostate cancer. This increase was also found in a study by Spitz and col-

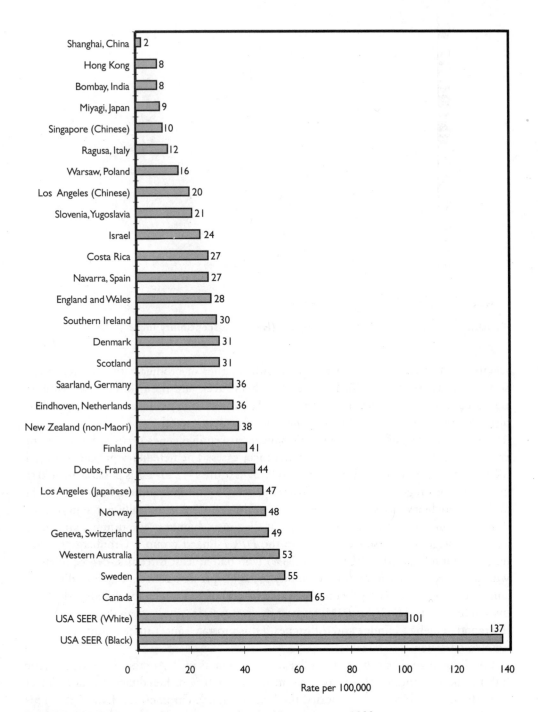

FIGURE 1-3. International prostate cancer incidence rates—1998

From Stanford JL, Stephenson RA, Coyle LM, et al. *Prostate Cancer Trends 1973–1995*. Bethesda, MD: Cancer Surveillance, Epidemiology, and End Results (SEER) Program, National Cancer Institute, 1998.

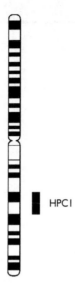

Possible location of HPC1 at 1q24-25 on Chromosome 1

FIGURE 1-4. Hereditary prostate cancer 1 (*HPC 1*) susceptibility locus

leagues.[33] In several other analyses, men with a father or brother with prostate cancer were found to be twice as likely to develop this cancer, and the risk increased with an increased number of affected relatives.[34–36] Male relatives of breast cancer patients have also been reported to have a higher incidence of prostate cancer.[37]

An inheritance of mutated prostate cancer–susceptible genes is suspected to be the cause in approximately 9% of all prostate cancer cases. The hereditary prostate cancer 1 locus (*HPC1*) is found on chromosome 1q24-25 (Figure 1-4). *HPC1* is possibly related to gene locus heterogeneity. A retrospective case study found that, although the hereditary and nonhereditary cases of prostate cancer evaluated were genetically not significantly different from each other, a younger age at diagnosis, higher grade tumors, and more advanced stage of disease were noted in the *HPC1*-linked group.[38] Gronberg and colleagues[39] found that 31 of 91 families (34%) who had at least three first-degree relatives with prostate cancer had this susceptibility locus for prostate cancer. These findings are similar to those reported by Cooney and others[40]; 20 of 59 families exhibited evidence of disease linkage to *HPC1* locus. More recently, however, in a linkage analysis of 49 families reported on by McIndoe and colleagues,[41] this prostate cancer susceptibility locus was not demonstrated.

Additional genetic causes are under investigation as well. Another potential genetic link has been identified that may account for up to 16% of hereditary prostate cancer cases. Jianfeng and others[42] identified the locus on the X chromosome (Xq27-28). This may help further the understanding of what has been proposed as an X-linked mode of inheritance in this malignancy.[42] The idea of an X-linked mode of inheritance in prostate cancer stems from studies such as that by Schaid and colleagues,[43] which demonstrated a significantly increased age-adjusted risk of prostate cancer among the brothers compared with the fathers of probands in a survey of 5,486 men who had undergone radical prostatectomy for localized prostate cancer between 1966 and 1995. This may be a potential factor in reports of a higher incidence of prostate cancer in male relatives of breast cancer patients.[37]

Gronberg and colleagues,[44] in studying potential genetic factors attributed to increased incidence of prostate cancer, evaluated 4,840 male twin pairs in Switzerland. Of the 458 identified cases of prostate cancer, 16 monozygotic and 6 dizygotic twin pairs were found in which both of the twins carried a prostate cancer diagnosis. The higher rate of monozygotic concordance may further indicate a potential genetic event in prostate cancer incidence.[44]

Although familial and genetic links seem to involve only a small percentage of the total prostate cancer population, it is recommended that measures to facilitate screening in men with familial risk should be instituted by the age of 40.[38] This is in keeping with the current American Cancer Society recommendations, which include annual PSA and digital rectal exam (DRE) beginning at age 50 as well as for younger men who are at high risk, such as African-Americans and those with strong familial predisposition.[45]

SMOKING-ETHANOL USE

Although a small number of older studies implicated cigarette smoking as a risk factor in the development of prostate cancer,[46, 47] more recent studies generally negate this.[48] In their study involving more than 1,000 men with diagnosed prostate cancer compared with matched controls, Lumey and colleagues[49] evaluated the association between lifetime cigarette smoking and prostate cancer risk. Findings failed to support any increased risk of prostate cancer with past and current use, pack-years, lifetime tar exposure, and other smoking-related factors.[49] Rohan and associates[50] reported similar findings in their case-control study in British Columbia and Ontario; they found no increased risk for prostate cancer regardless of pack-years, years since quitting, and use of filtered or nonfiltered cigarettes compared with nonsmokers. In addition, no race-based differences were found to be associated with smoking and prostate cancer risk.[51]

The questionable issue appears to be associated with incidence not in regard to smoking history but in relation to the adverse effect on survival. Data from four large prospective studies suggested that, although smoking did not adversely impact incidence, individuals who currently smoked experienced a significant negative impact on survival with decreased time to death than their nonsmoking counterparts.[52]

Past reviews have also implicated ethanol intake as a potential risk factor. At this time, no convincing data support a relationship between prostate cancer risk and ethanol use. Van der Gulden and associates[53] conducted a case-control study in the Netherlands in which 345 patients with primary prostate cancer and 1,346 controls with BPH were evaluated for both tobacco and ethanol histories. No significant correlations were found between smoking or alcohol consumption and the risk for prostate cancer.[53] However, a

National Cancer Institute of Uruguay study found that beer drinking slightly increased prostate cancer incidence. *N*-nitroso compounds found in beer were postulated to have a possible role in prostate carcinogenesis.[54] Similar links with *N*-nitroso compounds have been made in relation to stomach cancer incidence.

OCCUPATION AND EXPOSURE HISTORY

As part of the comprehensive look at factors contributing to increased prostate cancer risk, the issue of occupational and exposure hazards has been discussed. Men residing in rural areas have been reported to present with more advanced stages of prostate cancer than men living in urban areas.[55] One of the larger more recent studies was conducted in Montreal, Canada, in which, over a 7-year period, approximately 450 confirmed cases of prostate cancer along with 1,550 cancer controls and more than 500 population controls were interviewed using a somewhat exhaustive list of workplace chemicals. The results of this study found a suggestion of increased prostate cancer risk for aircraft fabricators, metal product fabricators, electric power workers, water transport workers, railway transport workers, and structural metal erectors.[56] Several chemicals have also been described as possessing a moderately strong link with the development of prostate cancer, including polyaromatic hydrocarbons from coal, liquid fuel combustion products, metallic dust, lubricating oils, and greases.[56]

Other chemical exposures that have been studied in relation to increased risk for prostate cancer include acetic acid and acetic anhydrate, which are essential in the synthesis of cellulose triacetate fiber found in silks and photographic films. Whorton and colleagues,[57] in their retrospective cohort mortality study, found an excess of prostate cancer in former chemical plant workers. This, however, was a small sample with questionable ability to generalize these findings.

Costantino and coworkers[58] described another occupational hazard in relation to coke oven workers. In their 30-year follow-up history of almost 16,000 workers, they found a significant excess in mortality from cancer of the respiratory system and prostate. Reported risk was as high as 1.93 in coke oven workers versus nonoven workers.[58]

In Kamradt and colleagues'[59] anecdotal report, the risk of prostate cancer was believed to be negatively affected in Vietnam War veterans who were exposed to the war pesticide chemical Agent Orange. Further investigation of this agent as a potential risk factor was indicated.[59] Earlier reviews suggested an increased risk for prostate cancer associated with cadmium exposure.[5] There are currently no studies to either support or dispute this.

An occupation frequently cited over the years as posing a higher risk for prostate cancer is that of farming. Keller-Byrne and colleagues,[60] in their meta-analysis of peer-reviewed articles published between January 1983 and June 1994, found a positive association between prostate cancer and farming both in their total review and in an analysis limited to retrospective studies. No association was found in the analysis limited to articles that reported a standard mortality ratio. This conclusion suggested that exposure to hormonally active agricultural chemicals was the most likely explanation for the positive association.[60] In a study of Illinois farmers, Keller and Howe[61] reported a positive association between hay and beef production and prostate cancer. In addition, Dich and Wiklund[62] reported a significantly increased risk associated with agrochemical exposure and prostate cancer. Van der Gulden and Vogelzang,[63] in their review of the literature, found a positive relationship between the use of pesticides and other agricultural chemicals and prostate cancer risk, placing farmers at only a slightly higher risk of being diagnosed with prostate cancer. Their review demonstrated that agricultural workers may have an increased risk of prostate cancer as a result of the specific types of farming in which they are involved. Differences in practice among counties and regions alter the types of exposures experienced. Meat and dairy farmers, those with a large number of acres to spray with fertilizer, differences in pesticide use, and grain elevator work all represent variation in exposures that may impact risk. Exposure to diesel exhaust fumes from tractors has been suggested as a potential risk factor as well. These variations may well account for inconsistencies seen in studies that deal with prostate cancer risk and agricultural work. Another emphasis of the analysis was that the studies reviewed tended to group farmers together whether or not they were the farm owners, the foremen, or the farmhands. Van der Gulden and Vogelzang[63] hypothesized that three separate groupings should be used in determining the degree of increased prostate cancer risk in this population.

HORMONAL-STEROID FACTORS

The effect of hormonal influences in the development of prostate cancer has been well documented but remains poorly understood. The growth of normal prostate endothelium is dependent on androgens.[64] It is thought that alteration in hormone metabolism may be involved in the disease progression, from the histologic to the clinically significant form of prostate cancer.[5]

Early studies suggested that low testosterone levels might have some protective effect against prostate cancer. Morgentaler and colleagues,[65] however, found that prostate cancer was present in 11 of the 77 males (14%) with low total or free testosterone levels, normal DREs, and PSA levels less than 4.0 ng/mL. Their findings suggested that DRE and PSA are not effective screening measures in this population and that prostatic biopsy may be indicated before initiation of hormonal supplementation.[65]

It has been postulated that pituitary hormones, sex steroid hormones, and sex hormone–binding globulin levels (SHBG) are involved in the development of prostate cancer. Results of multiple studies over the last 20 years have provided conflicting results. Andersson and colleagues,[66] in a case-control study, analyzed these hormones and SHBG in newly diagnosed prostate cancer patients and population controls of similar ages. Evaluation of luteinizing hormone (LH), follicle-stimulating hormone (FSH), estradiol, testosterone, androstenedione, albumin, SHBG, and free testosterone levels were compared using standard t tests. Using multivariate analysis, no significant associations could be found in any of the measured levels.[66] A similar study by Signorello and colleagues[67] also included measurement of DHT levels. Their findings suggest a significant inverse relationship between DHT and the risk of prostate cancer but did not find this to be true for estradiol or testosterone serum levels.[67]

Phytoestrogens are found in low-fat diets that include a high soy content. Soy is a rich source of isoflavonoids, which, broken down to biochanin A, have been shown to inhibit the growth of androgen-dependent and androgen-independent prostate cancer cells in culture. Anecdotal reports suggested that phytoestrogens may play a protective role in the development of prostate cancer.[68] No large controlled studies have been found in the literature to either support or deny this possibility.

The effect on hormonal levels in cases of pituitary dysfunction has also been reported in an anecdotal fashion. The androgen replacement therapy that these patients receive may lead to an increased risk for prostate cancer, and it has been recommended that these individuals be closely monitored for prostate cancer occurrence.[69] Still no large studies in the literature support this hypothesis.

As suggested by Giovannucci and colleagues,[70] a possible protective effect may be related to hormonal changes associated with diabetes. A history of adult-onset type II diabetes mellitus (more than 5 years from diagnosis) was found to be associated with a decreased relative risk (RR) of prostate cancer (RR = 0.75) in a retrospective study of more than 1,000 nonstage A1 prostate cancer patients.[70] Although the etiology of this process is unknown at present, it has been postulated that low testosterone levels in this population may contribute to the protective influence. Additional reviews may provide more insight into the potential basis for this relationship.

SEXUALITY ISSUES

Because of the inherent difficulties and biases in evaluating sexual activity, it is unclear whether frequency of sexual activity plays any role in prostate cancer risk.[5] Several studies, however, have assessed the role of human papillomavirus (HPV) and prostate cancer risk.[71–73] Strickler and colleagues[71] evaluated a sample of African-American and Italian men with known prostate cancer. In a case-control study, prostate cancer and BPH specimens were tested using polymerase chain reaction (PCR). No HPV DNA was detected in any of the specimens, and no differences between the prostate cancer cases and controls were identified in their response to HPV-16 or HPV-11 virus–like particles, suggesting no association of HPV with an increased risk of prostate cancer.[71] This confirmed results of an earlier review by Cuzick, who found it unlikely that anogenital papillomaviruses have a role in prostate carcinogenesis.[72]

In opposition, however, Dillner and colleagues[73] performed a nested case-control study (modification of a basic cohort study in which both cases and controls are drawn from the cohort population, allowing effects of potentially confounding variables to be reduced or eliminated) using serum bank samples of 165 cases of prostate cancer with two matched controls per sample. The researchers identified a 2.6-fold increased risk of prostate cancer when HPV-18 antibodies were detected to be present. HPV-16 was also believed to be associated with prostate cancer occurrence (RR = 2.4). The authors purported that, although infection with oncogenic HPV would only be found in a minority of prostate cancers, the widespread incidence of prostate cancer would make this finding of value if substantiated in the cancer prevention arena.[73]

Even more debated has been the relationship between vasectomy and prostate cancer risk. It has been suggested that the promotion of antisperm antibody may result from vasectomy, leading to an immunologic response that subsequently increases the risk for prostate cancer. After a review of five studies in 1993, the National Institute of Health issued a statement indicating there is insufficient evidence to establish a real association between vasectomy and prostate cancer.[74] Despite this, Sandlow and Kreder,[75] in a survey of 759 U.S. urologists, found that more than 25% reported alterations in their screening patterns, with 27% practicing earlier screening. Twenty percent were reluctant to recommend vasectomy to men with a strong family history of prostate cancer even though more than 90% responded that prior studies had little or no effect on practice patterns.[75]

Two subsequent studies in India and China have raised the argument for an association between vasectomy and prostate cancer risk.[76, 77] Hsing and colleagues[76] presented data suggesting an increased risk for prostate cancer in Chinese men with a history of vasectomy; China is a low-risk country but is experiencing an increase in the incidence of vasectomy. In a hospital-based case-control study, 10% of those with prostate cancer had undergone vasectomy at least 10 years before versus 3% of controls.[76] Similarly, a case-control study conducted in India found an overall risk of prostate cancer to be 1.48 in those men who had undergone vasectomy after controlling for multiple factors. Again, the risk was believed to be more significant in men who had undergone vasectomy at least two decades before their cancer diagnosis or were age 40 or older at the time of the procedure.[77]

Zhu and colleagues[78] did not find this in a case-control study conducted with members of a health maintenance organization. Their findings were not significant based on time since vasectomy or age at procedure, although the odds ratio estimate for prostate cancer was increased in men with a father or brother with prostate cancer.[78] Furthermore, Bernal-Delgado and colleagues,[79] in their meta-analysis, found no increased risk in individuals who have had a vasectomy. To date, data concerning vasectomy and prostate cancer risk continue to be equivocal.

BODY SIZE AND ENERGY EXPENDITURE

A somewhat surprising number of studies have focused on the areas of anthropometric measurements, body mass index (BMI), and total energy intake as potential indicators for prostate cancer risk. A criticism of these studies has been the lack of consistency in the methods used for eliciting these data. Anthropometric measurement has been as basic as height and weight measurement and as complex as the measurement of biacromial (between the acromia) breadth-height ratios.[80–83] A Duke University case-control study found that anthropometric variables such as a slight upper body skeleton may be associated with the development of prostate cancer.[80] Andersson and colleagues,[81] in a study of more than 2,000 Swedish construction workers diagnosed with prostate cancer participating in a 20-year follow-up study, found that increased weight, taller height, and increased BMI were all positively associated with prostate cancer risk. They did, however, find a stronger relationship to mortality than to incidence.

Obesity has been believed to be a contributing factor in prostate cancer risk as a normal conclusion of the endocrine changes associated with weight gain such as increased estrogen and decreased testosterone levels. Data have been somewhat difficult to interpret in this area. Cerhan and others[82] reported that obesity and weight gain in later life were associated with increased prostate cancer risk, whereas Giovannucci and colleagues[83] found that obesity before age 10 was prospectively associated with a lower risk of prostate cancer. This same study also reported that increased height ($\geq$ 74 inches) had a strong direct association with the risk of metastatic disease (RR = 2.29).[83]

Another difficult variable to interpret is that of energy expenditure or exercise. It has been assumed that increased activity might decrease the risk of prostate cancer. In Oliveria and Lee's[84] review of 17 studies evaluating the effect of exercise and prostate cancer risk, 9 were supportive of this concept, 5 reported inconclusive findings, and 3 actually presented data that demonstrated an increased risk of prostate cancer related to increased physical activity.

It appears that, until more uniform methods for evaluating these potential risk factors are identified, there will be many unanswered questions in regard to data interpretation. Considerable physiologic rationale attributable to variations of body stature, weight, and energy expenditure may be worthy of further investigation to expand the current body of knowledge related to prostate cancer etiology.

DIETARY-NUTRITIONAL FACTORS

The relationship between diet and risk of prostate cancer has been a topic of research for some time and continues to be considered an integral area for study. High-fat diets have demonstrated increases in prostate cancer relative risk with a factor of 1.6 to 1.9.[85] Dietary patterns can have a direct effect on circulating androgen levels. For instance, those men on high-fiber diets generally have lower circulating testosterone and estradiol levels. Sex steroids have been found to bind with feces and lower plasma levels as a result of greater excretion.[45] Although dietary fat intake has been recognized as contributing to prostate cancer risk, additional dietary constituents such as vitamins A, C, D, and E and calcium, fructose, and β-carotene have also become the subjects of more recent study in the literature.

It has been hypothesized that dietary fat intake may be partially responsible for the variations seen between histologic and clinically significant prostate cancer based on geographic location. For example, men in Asian countries where dietary fat intake is less have a lower incidence rate than American men.[5, 45, 86] Whittemore and colleagues[87] found a positive association between total fat intake and prostate cancer risk across ethnic groups residing within the United States and Canada. In their study, Asian-Americans were found to have higher prostate cancer risk associated with saturated fats than their African-American or Caucasian counterparts.[87] Much of the data linking dietary fat with prostate cancer risk were retrospective and came under censor for errors of recall bias.[86] Le Marchand and colleagues,[88] however, found, in a cohort of more than 20,000 men of various ethnicities interviewed over a 5-year period, a total of 198 incident cases of prostate cancer. Of those, the RR associated with intake of increased animal fat products was 1.6.[88] Several additional studies have reported similar findings.[89, 90]

Theories related to the association of fat intake and prostate cancer risk stem from animal models that have demonstrated carcinogenesis and tumor growth in the presence of polyunsaturated fats. In situations involving exposure to long-chain omega-3 fatty acids, inhibitory effects were seen.[91] It was suggested that specific dietary fatty acids be further evaluated in relation to their association with increased risk for prostate cancer development.[91, 92] Specifically, several authors[91–94] have recommended evaluating the role of polyunsaturated omega-6 and omega-3 fatty acids.

Another variation of this theme, involving total energy and prostate cancer risk, has been the subject of several reports.[95, 96] A population-based case-control study in Sweden identified a positive association between prostate cancer risk and total energy intake as well as total fat intake. In other words, a higher caloric intake was believed to be correlated with an increased prostate cancer risk. The hypothesized mechanism was an alteration of the sympathetic nervous system in which sympathetic innervation has been shown to influence the growth rate of the prostate.[95]

The role of vitamin A remains largely undecided. Studies conflict in relation to the promotion or protection abilities of vitamin A. This may be in part due to the fact that vitamin A comes from both animal (vitamin A) and plant (carotenoid) sources. Of the plant sources, lycopene, which is primarily found in tomato-based products, has been identified by several authors as exhibiting some protective benefit.[96–98] In contrast, retinol has been associated, although often weakly, as a possible promoting nutrient.[95, 99] The role of vitamin A and carotenoids in prostate cancer continues to remain uncertain.

In Heinonen and colleagues'[100] prospective study, vitamin E was found to have a positive benefit in decreasing the risk of prostate cancer incidence and mortality in male smokers. Participants were randomized to diets supplemented with α-tocopherol, β-carotene, both, or placebo over a period of 5 to 8 years. An increase in both incidence and mortality was seen in the β-carotene arm.[100] These results are intriguing; yet supportive data in the literature are limited.

It has also been suggested that vitamin D metabolites have a suppressive effect on prostate cancer development.[101] This is believed to be related in part to its antiproliferative cell growth and development modulating properties. This hypothesis was not supported, however, in a nested case-control study, in which no benefit was observed in the evaluation of plasma levels of the two major vitamin D metabolites when compared in affected and control patients.[102] Yet in Giovannucci and colleagues'[103] prospective study, in which calcium and fructose intake was measured, higher fructose ingestion was associated with a lower risk of advanced prostate cancer (RR = 0.51). Fructose ingestion lead to stimulation of vitamin D (1, 25(OH)$_2$D) production, which was purported to have a protective influence on prostate cancer development. In addition, higher calcium intake was associated with a higher risk of advanced prostate cancer (RR = 2.97).[103] The physiologic effects of vitamin D and calcium homeostasis were not considered in any of the literature reviewed, but this may be an area worthy of further exploration in the risk-benefit ratio analysis.

Additional micronutrients and dietary behaviors have been evaluated without significant findings. Measurement error may still be a factor. Additional exploration of the nutritional effects on prostate cancer development with larger prospective groups and blood sampling have been recommended for future studies.[104, 105]

PREVENTION

A logical progression from the previous review of risk factors is the discussion of prostate cancer prevention. Risk factors likely play a role in the initiation to promotion or promotion to progression phases of prostate cancer development. Prevention efforts seek to intercede just before the point at which histologic or latent prostate cancer becomes a clinically apparent entity.

HORMONAL APPROACHES

Prostate cancer prevention efforts have taken on a variety of forms over the last several years. The endocrinologic nature of prostate cancer has made an argument for prevention strategies that involve hormonal manipulations. Androgens are required for the functional activity, growth, and maintenance of the prostate gland. As discussed previously, androgens are also believed to play a role in prostate cancer development.[106] LH-releasing hormone is produced by the pituitary and stimulates the anterior pituitary production of LH and FSH. It is LH that stimulates the Leydig cells of the testicles to produce testosterone. Within the prostate, testosterone is converted by the enzyme 5-α-reductase to DHT, which is the primary intraprostatic androgen. DHT binds to androgen receptors on the nuclear matrix, and this combination is largely responsible for cell growth and replication.[16]

A reasonable conclusion is that, by blocking or inhibiting 5-α-reductase, prostate cancer prevention may be possible. This has been the basis for what is known as the Prostate Cancer Prevention Trial. The Southwest Oncology Group and the Eastern Cooperative Oncology Group, along with the Cancer and Leukemia Group B, are involved in a National Cancer Institute–sponsored double-blind, placebo-controlled trial in which 18,000 men have been randomized to receive either finasteride (5 mg/day) or placebo (matching capsule) for 7 years.[107– 109] Finasteride is a testosterone analogue and acts as a competitive inhibitor with 5-α-reductase. Side effects reported previously in men being treated for BPH were infrequently seen and included impotence, decreased libido, and decreased ejaculatory volume ($< 5\%$ of men). After all men have been in the trial for 7 years, the researchers will compare groups for the presence of prostate cancer. Each man will undergo a prostate biopsy at the end of 7 years. The results of this study will provide valuable data in regard not only to the potential of 5-α-reductase inhibitors to help prevent prostate cancer but also the overall epidemiology of prostate cancer. The growing interest in chemoprevention trials has led to the development of the National Cancer Institute's Prevention Trials Decision Network, which functions as the formal evaluation and approval body for large-scale chemoprevention trials and coordination of data management.[109]

The role of estrogens in prostatic neoplasia has been hypothesized with estrogen inhibition identified as a possible chemoprevention strategy. Kelloff and colleagues[110] postulated that the inhibition of aromatase, the enzyme that promotes the final step in estrogen biosynthesis, would accomplish this. Several aromatase inhibitors are already available for other uses or are currently in clinical trials, including: aminoglutethimide, liarozole hydrochloride, anastrozole, vorozole, and letrozole.[110]

MISCELLANEOUS APPROACHES

Another agent that has been evaluated in a small-scale study and is still being investigated is fenretinide (N-4-hydroxyphenylretinamide) (4HPR). In a chemoprevention trial for men at high risk for prostate cancer on the basis of elevated PSA levels, patients received an oral 4HPR preparation for twelve 28-day cycles. They were evaluated at 6 and 12 months with transrectal ultrasonography and at 12 months with prostate biopsy. The preliminary results of this study were inconclusive. There is still interest in pursuing this modulator of vitamin A; additional trials are ongoing.[111, 112]

A case-control study in New Zealand found a trend toward reduced rates of prostate cancer associated with regular use of nonsteroidal antiinflammatory drugs (NSAIDs) (RR = 0.73). This is believed to be somehow related to the role of cyclooxygenase activity in prostate cancer prevention. To date, little attention has been given to any potential role for NSAIDs in the chemoprevention of prostate cancer.[113]

The use of anti-angiogenesis agents in cancer prevention in general has been a focus of research interest. In vitro study of the angiogenic process in urologic tumors has shown that antiangiogenic agents affect urologic tumor models. Currently, several investigations are bringing these agents into the chemoprevention arena.[114]

PREVENTION TRIALS

The appropriate time to initiate chemoprevention studies in the population as well as the clinical endpoints to follow remain heavily debated topics. Although PSA is a biomarker frequently used as an endpoint in both chemoprevention and advanced prostate cancer clinical trials, there are few data regarding normal or the natural history of PSA in men younger than 40.[115] There is also limited knowledge on the effect of chemoprevention agents on PSA. As a result, it is suggested that the effect of these agents on PSA must be part of the evaluation process.[115] Histologic prostate cancer has been identified at much earlier ages than expected, and, as a result, disease initiation may also start sooner than anticipated. This also infers that the use of cancer incidence as an endpoint may be inappropriate in tumors that are identified as "slow growing" such as prostatic neoplasms.[116] Therefore, surrogate endpoint biomarkers (SEBs) have been suggested as a means to decrease the high costs associated with lengthy chemoprevention trials. These include

PSA, morphometric markers, ploidy, high-grade PIN, angiogenesis, proliferative markers, and oncogene c-*erb* B-2 expression.[110] The combination of several SEBs was advocated to gain data on sensitivity, specificity, and negative predictive value.[116, 117] Bostwick[118] also targeted five different populations that appear to be the best candidates for prostate cancer prevention trials. Among them are patients with known prostate cancer before surgery, men at increased risk for prostate cancer, men with normal risk for prostate cancer development, patients with high-grade PIN, and patients with early cancer treated with watchful waiting.[118]

NURSING IMPLICATIONS

Nurses and other health care providers play an integral role not only in identifying patients at risk for prostate cancer but also in counseling those patients on issues related to screening and follow-up care.

It is imperative to be able to identify individuals and populations at increased risk for prostate cancer. Individuals participating in screening activities, whether part of a regular physical exam or a large-scale screening initiative (i.e., Health O'Rama), are interested in knowing their risk for a specific type of malignancy.[119]

To provide risk information to individuals, the nurse needs to complete a comprehensive assessment of the patient's family history, health history, ethnicity, and personal lifestyle habits (including dietary and occupation information). Although few nurses possess advanced epidemiologic training, an understanding on common risk factors will allow for appropriate identification and direction for patients.

Information on prevention is another frequent request by individuals who exhibit a high-risk profile for prostate cancer as well as those who do not. Certainly, appropriate screening is critical to early detection and prevention. It is important to discuss with patients the benefits of early detection of prostate cancer. Screening evaluations based on risk level, age, and ethnicity should be recommended on the basis of the guidelines described here and in Chapter 2 in relation to DRE, transrectal ultrasonography, and PSA. The role of genetic testing in prostate cancer is yet to be determined and has not reached the level of scientific maturity seen in other malignancies such as breast and colon cancer. There does appear to be sufficient data to suggest that individuals may want to consider avoiding diets high in animal fat as a reasonable adjunct aimed at prevention.

Patients must be informed, however, that identification of risk factors is not a guarantee that they will or will not be affected by prostate cancer. For instance, Labrie and coworkers[120] reported that normal PSAs were found in approximately 25 to 33% of patients with prostate cancer at diagnosis. The concept of screening for prostate cancer, in general, poses many medical, ethical, and legal issues.[121] Nurses need to provide an opportunity for patients and their significant others to share concerns and fears related to risk factor identification and to make appropriate referrals to other members of the health care team as appropriate.

SUMMARY

The plethora of potential risk factors described in this chapter demonstrates the naïveté of basic science and the complexity of the pathogenesis of this disease. Although risk factors such as age, ethnicity, and genetics are beyond an individual's control, risks associated with diet and occupational hazards may benefit from additional focus, particularly in the design of chemoprevention strategies.

Chemoprevention is still in its infancy stages, and the results of trials such as the Prostate Cancer Prevention Trial discussed here will, it is hoped, lend valuable information regarding the feasibility of such trials in this population. Factors such as cultural sensitivity and access to care must be a matter of priority as these trials are being developed.

The dramatically high incidence of prostate cancer and the inability to find effective agents to treat metastatic disease clearly establish support for the modification of risk factors, early detection, and treatment of prostate cancer. The multiplicity of factors involved in these processes, however, speaks to the need for continued advancement of research in all facets of treating this malignancy.

REFERENCES

1. Landis SH, Murray T, Bolden S, Wingo PA. Cancer statistics, 1999. *CA Cancer J Clin* 1999;49:8–31.
2. Porter AT, Zimmerman J, Ruffin M, et al. Recommendations of the first Michigan conference on prostate cancer. *Urology* 1996;48:519–533.
3. Pienta KJ, Sandler H, Wilson TG. Prostate cancer. In: Pazdur R, Coia LR, Hoskins WJ (eds). *Cancer Management: A Multidisciplinary Approach.* New York: PRR, 1998:395–415.
4. Archer MC. Chemical carcinogenesis. In: Tannock IF, Hill RP (eds). *The Basic Science of Oncology,* 2nd ed. New York: McGraw-Hill, 1992:102–118.
5. Pienta KJ, Esper PS. Risk factors for prostate cancer. *Ann Intern Med* 1993;118:793–803.
6. Bassett MT, Levy LM, Chetsanga C, et al. Zimbabwe National Cancer Registry: Summary data 1986–1989. *Cent Afr J Med* 1992;38:91–94.
7. Sakr WA, Haas GP, Cassin BF, et al. The frequency of carcinoma and intraepithelial neoplasia of the prostate in young males. *J Urol* 1993;150:379–385.
8. Pienta KJ. The epidemiology of prostate cancer: Clues for chemoprevention. *In Vivo* 1994;8:419–422.
9. Helpap BG, Bostwick DG, Montironi R. The significance of atypical adenomatous hyperplasia and prostatic intraepithelial neoplasia for the development of prostate carcinoma: An update. *Virch Arch* 1995;426:425–434.
10. Davidson D, Bostwick DG, Qian J, et al. Prostatic intraepithelial neoplasia as a risk factor for adenocarcinoma: Predictive accuracy in needle biopsies. *J Urol* 1996;154:1295–1299.
11. Bostwick D. Evaluating prostate needle biopsy: Therapeutic and prognostic importance. *CA Cancer J Clin* 1997;47:297–319.
12. Wang YZ, Wong YC. Sex hormone-induced prostatic carcinogenesis in the noble rat: The role in insulin-like growth factor-I (IGF-I) and vascular endothelial growth factor (VEGF) in the development of prostate cancer. *Prostate* 1998;35:165–77.
13. Chan JM, Stampfer MJ, Giovannucci E, et al. Plasma insulin-like growth factor-I and prostate cancer risk: A prospective study. *Science* 1998;279 (5350):563–566.
14. Stanford JL, Stephenson RA, Coyle LM, et al. *Prostate Cancer Trends 1973–1995.* Bethesda, MD: SEER Program, National Cancer Institute, 1998.
15. Rowley KH, Mason MD. The aetiology and pathogenesis of prostate cancer. *Clin Oncol* 1997;9: 213–218.
16. Henderson BE, Bernstein L, Ross R. Etiology of cancer: Hormonal factors. In: DeVita VT, Hellman S, Rosenberg SA (eds). *Cancer—Principles & Practice of Oncology.* Philadelphia: Lippincott-Raven, 1997:219–229.

17. Oesterline J, Fuks Z, Lee CT, Scher HI. Cancer of the Prostate. In: DeVita VT, Hellman S, Rosenberg SA (eds). *Cancer—Principles & Practice of Oncology.* Philadelphia: Lippincott-Raven, 1997: 1322–1386.

18. Parker SL, Davis KJ, Wingo PA, et al. Cancer statistics by race and ethnicity. *CA Cancer J Clin* 1998; 48:31–38.

19. Pienta KJ, Demers R, Hoff M, et al. Effect of age and race on the survival of men with prostate cancer in the metropolitan Detroit tricounty area: 1973 to 1987. *Urology* 1993;150:797–802.

20. Moul JW, Douglas TH, McCarthy WF, McLeod DG. Black race is an adverse prognostic factor for prostate cancer recurrence following radical prostatectomy in an equal access health care setting. *J Urol* 1996;155:1667–1673.

21. Ross R, Bernstein L, Judd H, et al. Serum testosterone levels in healthy young black and white men. *JNCI* 1986;76:45–48.

22. Optenberg SA, Thompson IM, Friedrichs P, et al. Race, treatment and long-term survival from prostate cancer in an equal-access medical care delivery system. *JAMA* 1995;274:1599–1605.

23. Powell IJ. Prostate cancer in the African American: Is this a different disease? *Semin Urol Oncol* 1998; 16:221–226.

24. Ellis L, Nyborg H. Racial/ethnic variations in male testosterone levels: A probable contributor to group differences in health. *Steroids* 1992;57: 72–75.

25. Abdalla I, Ray P, Vijayakumar S. Race and serum prostate-specific antigen levels: Current status and future directions. *Semin Urol Oncol* 1998;16:207–213.

26. Powell IJ, Heibrun LK, Sakr W, et al. The predictive value of race as a clinical prognostic factor among patients with clinically localized prostate cancer: A multivariate analysis of positive surgical margins. *Urology* 1997;49:726–731.

27. Glover FE Jr, Coffey DS, Douglas LL, et al. The epidemiology of prostate cancer in Jamaica. *J Urol* 1998;159:1984–1986.

28. Gilliland FD, Key CR. Prostate cancer in American Indians, New Mexico, 1969 to 1994. *J Urol* 1998; 159:893–897.

29. Baquet CR, Horm JW, Gibbs T, et al. Socioeconomic factors and cancer incidence among blacks and whites. *J Natl Cancer Inst* 1991;83:551–557.

30. Polednak AP. Stage at diagnosis of prostate cancer in Connecticut by poverty and race. *Ethn Dis* 1997; 7:215–220.

31. Cooney KA. Hereditary prostate cancer in African-American families. *Semin Urol Oncol* 1998;16: 202–206.

32. Ghadirian P, Cadotte M, Lacroix A, Perret C. Family aggregation of cancer of the prostate in Quebec: The tip of the iceberg. *Prostate* 1991;19:43–52.

33. Spitz MR, Currier RD, Fueger JJ, et al. Familial patterns of prostate cancer: A case control analysis. *J Urol* 1991;146:1305–1307.

34. Carter BS, Carter HB, Isaacs JT. Epidemiologic evidence regarding predisposing factors to prostate cancer. *Prostate* 1990;16:187–197.

35. Carter BS, Beaty TH, Steinberg GD, et al. Segregation and linkage analyses of human prostate cancer [abstract]. *Am Assoc Cancer Res Proc* 1992; 33:240.

36. Carter BS, Beaty TH, Steinberg GD, et al. Mendelian inheritance of familial prostate cancer. *Proc Natl Acad Sci U S A* 1992;89:3367–3371.

37. Tulinius H, Egilsson V, Olafsdottir GH, et al. Risk of prostate, ovarian, and endometrial cancer among relatives of women with breast cancer. *BMJ* 1992; 305:855–857.

38. Gronberg H, Isaacs SD, Smith JR, et al. Characteristics of prostate cancer in families potentially linked to the hereditary prostate cancer 1 (HPC1) locus. *JAMA* 1997;278:1251–1255.

39. Gronberg H, Xu J, Smith JR, et al. Early age at diagnosis in families providing evidence of linkage to the hereditary prostate cancer locus (HPC1) on chromosome 1. *Cancer Res* 1997;57:4707–4709.

40. Cooney KA, McCarthy JD, Lange E, et al. Prostate cancer susceptibility locus on chromosome 1q: A confirmatory study. *J Natl Cancer Inst* 1997;89: 955–959.

41. McIndoe RA, Stanford JL, Gibbs M, et al. Linkage analysis of 49 high-risk families does not support a common familial prostate cancer-susceptibility at 1q24-25. *J Urol* 1998;160:265.

42. Jianfeng X, Meyers D, Freije D, et al. Evidence for a prostate cancer susceptibility locus on the X chromosome. *Nat Genet* 1998;20:175–179.

43. Schaid DJ, McDonnell SK, Blute ML, Thibodeau SN. Evidence for autosomal dominant inheritance of prostate cancer. *Am J Hum Genet* 1998;62:1425–1438.

44. Gronberg H, Damber L, Damber JE. Studies of genetic factors in prostate cancer in a twin population. *J Urol* 1994;152:1484–1489.

45. Haas GP, Sakr WA. Epidemiology of prostate cancer. *CA Cancer J Clin* 1997;47:273–287.

46. Hsing AW, McLaughlin JK, Schuman LM, et al. Diet, tobacco use, and fatal prostate cancer: Results from the Lutheran Brotherhood Cohort Study. *Cancer Res* 1990;50:6836–6840.

47. Fincham SM, Hill GB, Hanson J, Wijayasinghe C. Epidemiology of prostatic cancer: A case-control study. *Prostate* 1990;17:189–206.

48. Matzkin H, Soloway MS. Cigarette smoking: A review of possible associations with benign prostatic hyperplasia and prostate cancer. *Prostate* 1993; 22:277–290.

49. Lumey LH, Pittman B, Zang EA, Wynder EL. Cigarette smoking and prostate cancer: No relation with six measures of lifetime smoking habits in a large case-control study among U.S. whites. *Prostate* 1997;33:195–200.

50. Rohan TE, Hislop TG, Howe GR, et al. Cigarette smoking and risk of prostate cancer: A population-based case-control study in Ontario and British Columbia, Canada. *Euro J Cancer Prev* 1997;6:382–388.

51. Rodriguez C, Tatham LM, Thun MJ, et al. Smoking and fatal prostate cancer in a large cohort of adult men. *Am J Epidemiol* 1997;145:460–475.

52. Hayes RB, Pottern LM, Swanson GM, et al. Tobacco use and prostate cancer in blacks and whites in the United States. *Cancer Causes Control* 1994; 5:221–226.

53. Van der Gulden JW, Verbeek AL, Kolk JJ. Smoking and drinking habits in relation to prostate cancer. *Br J Urol* 1994;73:382–389.

54. De Stefani E, Fierro L, Barrios E, Ronco A. Tobacco, alcohol, diet and risk of prostate cancer. *Tumori* 1995;81:315–320.

55. Aronson KJ, Siemiatycki J, Dewar R, Gerin M. Occupational risk factors for prostate cancer: Results from a case-control study in Montreal, Quebec, Canada. *Am J Epidemiol* 1996;143:363–373.

56. Liff JM, Chow WH, Greenberg RS. Rural-urban differences in stage at diagnosis: Possible relationship to cancer screening. *Cancer* 1991;67:1454–1459.

57. Whorton MD, Amsel J, Mandel J. Cohort mortality study of prostate cancer among chemical workers. *Am J Ind Med* 1998;33:293–296.

58. Costantino JP, Redmond CK, Bearden A. Occupationally related cancer risk among coke oven workers: 30 years of follow-up. *J Occup Environ Med* 1995; 37:597–604.

59. Kamradt JM, Smith DC, Esper PS, Pienta KJ. The natural history of prostate cancer in Vietnam veterans exposed to Agent Orange [abstract 1199]. *Proc Am Soc Clin Onc* 1997;16:335a.

60. Keller-Byrne JE, Khuder SA, Schaub EA. Meta-analyses of prostate cancer and farming. *Am J Indust Med* 1997;31:580–586.

61. Keller JE, Howe HL. Case-controlled studies of cancer in Illinois farmers using data from the Illinois state cancer registry and the US census of agriculture. *Eur J of CA* 1994;30A(4):469–473.

62. Dich J, Wiklund K. Prostate cancer in pesticide applicators in Swedish agriculture. *Prostate* 1998; 34:100–112.

63. Van der Gulden JW, Vogelzang PF. Farmers at risk for prostate cancer. *Br J Urol* 1996;77:6–14.

64. Wilding G. Endocrine control of prostate cancer. *Cancer Surv* 1995;23:43–62.

65. Morgentaler A, Bruning CO III, DeWolf WC. Occult prostate cancer in men with low serum testosterone levels. *JAMA* 1996;276:1904–1906.

66. Andersson SO, Adami HO, Bergstrom R, Wide L. Serum pituitary and sex steroid hormone levels in the etiology of prostatic cancer—a population-based case-control study. *Br J Cancer* 1993;68:97–102.

67. Signorello JB, Tzonou A, Mantzoros CS, et al. Serum steroids in relation to prostate cancer risk in a case-control study. *Cancer Causes Control* 1997;8: 632–636.

68. Adlercreutz H, Markkanen H, Watanabe S. Plasma concentrations of phyto-oestrogens in Japanese men. *Lancet* 1993;342(8881):1209–1210.

69. Ebling DW, Ruffer J, Whittington R, et al. Development of prostate cancer after pituitary dysfunction: A report of 8 patients. *Urology* 1997;49:546–548.

70. Giovannucci E, Rimm EB, Stampfer MJ, et al. Diabetes mellitus and risk of prostate cancer. *Cancer Causes Control* 1998;9:3–9.

71. Strickler HK, Burk R, Shah K, et al. A multifaceted study of human papillomavirus and prostate carcinoma. *Cancer* 1998;82:1118–1125.

72. Cuzick J. Human papillomavirus infection of the prostate. *Cancer Surv* 1995;23:91–95.

73. Dillner J, Knekt P, Boman J, et al. Sero-epidemiological association between human-papillomavirus

infection and risk of prostate cancer. *Int J Cancer* 1998; 75:564–567.

74. Bowersox J. Experts confer on vasectomy and prostate cancer risk. *J Natl Cancer Inst* 1993;85:527–528.

75. Sandlow JI, Kreder KJ. A change in practice: Current urologic practice in response to reports concerning vasectomy and prostate cancer. *Fertil Steril* 1996;66:281–284.

76. Hsing AW, Wang RT, Gu FL, et al. Vasectomy and prostate cancer risk in China. *Cancer Epidemiol, Biomarkers Prev* 1994;3:285–288.

77. Platz EA, Yeole BB, Cho E, et al. Vasectomy and prostate cancer: A case-control study in India. *Int J Epidemiol* 1997;26:933–938.

78. Zhu K, Stanford JL, Daling JR, et al. Vasectomy and prostate cancer: A case-control study in a health maintenance organization. *Am J Epidemiol* 1996; 144:717–722.

79. Bernal-Delgado E, Latour-Perez J, Pradas-Arnal F, Gomez-Lopez LI. The association between vasectomy and prostate cancer: A systematic review of the literature. *Fertil Steril* 1998;70:191–200.

80. Demark-Wahnefried W, Conaway MR, Robertson CN, et al. Anthropometric risk factors for prostate cancer. *Nutr Cancer* 1997;28:302–307.

81. Andersson SO, Wolk A, Bergstrom R, et al. Body size and prostate cancer: A 20-year follow-up study among 135,006 Swedish construction workers. *J Natl Cancer Inst* 1997;89:385–389.

82. Cerhan JR, Torner JC, Lynch CF, et al. Association of smoking, body mass, and physical activity with risk of prostate cancer in the Iowa 65+ Rural Health Study (United States). *Cancer Causes Control* 1997;8:229–238.

83. Giovannucci E, Rimm EB, Stampfer MJ, et al. Height, body weight, and risk of prostate cancer. *Cancer Epidemiol, Biomarkers Prev* 1997;6:557–563.

84. Oliveria SA, Lee IM. Is exercise beneficial in the prevention of prostate cancer? *Sports Med* 1997;23: 271–278.

85. Brawley OW, Knopf K, Thompson I. The epidemiology of prostate cancer. Part II: The risk factors. *Semin Urol Oncol* 1998;16:193–201.

86. Fair WR, Fleshner NE, Heston W. Cancer of the prostate: A nutritional disease? *Urology* 1997;50: 840–848.

87. Whittemore AS, Kolonel LN, Wu AH, et al. Prostate cancer in relation to diet, physical activity, body size in blacks, whites, and Asians in the United States and Canada. *J Natl Cancer Inst* 1995;87: 652–661.

88. Le Marchand L, Kolonel LN, Wilkens LR, et al. Animal fat consumption and prostate cancer: A prospective study in Hawaii. *Epidemiology* 1994;5:271–273.

89. Slattery ML, Schumacher MC, West DW, et al. Food-consumption trends between adolescent and adult years and subsequent risk of prostate cancer. *Am J Clin Nutr* 1990;52:752–757.

90. West DW, Slattery ML, Robison LM, et al. Adult dietary intake and prostate cancer risk in Utah: A case-contol study with special emphasis on aggressive tumors. *Cancer Causes Control* 1991;2:84–94.

91. Rose DP. Dietary fatty acids and prevention of hormone-responsive cancer. *Proc Soc Exp Biol Med* 1997; 216:224–233.

92. Willett WC. Specific fatty acids and risks of breast and prostate cancer: Dietary intake. *Am J Clin Nutr* 1997;66(6 Suppl):1557S–1563S.

93. Zhou JR, Blackburn GL. Bridging animal and human studies: What are the missing segments in dietary fat and prostate cancer? *Am J Clin Nutr* 1997; 66(6 Suppl):1572S–1580S.

94. Godley PA, Campbell MK, Gallagher P, et al. Biomarkers of essential fatty acid consumption and risk of prostatic carcinoma. *Cancer Epidemiol, Biomarkers Prev* 1996;5:859–600.

95. Andersson SO, Wolk A, Bergstrom R, et al. Energy, nutrient intake and prostate cancer risk: A population-based case-control study in Sweden. *Int J Cancer* 1996;68:716–722.

96. Meyer F, Bairati I, Fradet Y, Moore L. Dietary energy and nutrients in relation to preclinical prostate cancer. *Nutr Cancer* 1997;29:120–126.

97. Giovannucci E. Epidemiologic characteristics of prostate cancer. *Cancer* 1995;87:1767–1776.

98. Clinton SK, Emenhiser C, Schwart SJ, et al. Cis-trans lycopene isomers, carotenoids and retinol in the human prostate. *Cancer Epidemiol, Biomarkers Prev* 1996;5:823–833.

99. Giovannucci E, Ascherio A, Rimm EB, et al. Intake of carotenoids and retinol in relation to risk of prostate cancer. *J Natl Cancer Inst* 1995;87:1767–1776.

100. Heinonen OP, Albanes D, Virtamo J, et al. Prostate cancer and supplementation with alpha-tocopherol and beta-carotene: Incidence and mortality in a controlled trial. *J Natl Cancer Inst* 1998;990: 440–446.

101. Feldman D, Skowronski RJ, Peehl DM. Vitamin D and prostate cancer. *Adv Exp Med Biol* 1995; 375:53–63.

102. Gann PH, Ma J, Hennekens CH, et al. Circulating vitamin D metabolites in relation to subsequent development of prostate cancer. *Cancer Epidemiol, Biomarkers Prev* 1996;5:121–126.

103. Giovannucci E, Rimm EB, Wolk A, et al. Calcium and fructose intake in relation to risk of prostate cancer. *Cancer Res* 1998;58:442–447.

104. Nomura AM, Stemmermann GN, Lee J, Craft NE. Serum micronutrients and prostate cancer in Japanese Americans in Hawaii. *Cancer Epidemiol, Biomarkers Prev* 1997;6:487–491.

105. Giles G, Ireland P. Diet, nutrition and prostate cancer. *Int J Cancer* 1997;10(Suppl):13–17.

106. Nomura AM, Kolonel LN. Prostate cancer: A current perspective. *Am J Epidemiol* 1991;13:200–227.

107. Ford LG, Brawley OW, Perlman JA, et al. The potential for hormonal prevention trials. *Cancer* 1994;74(9 Suppl):2726–2733.

108. Thompson IM, Coltman CA Jr, Crowley J. Chemoprevention of prostate cancer: The prostate cancer prevention trial. *Prostate* 1997;33:217–221.

109. Feigl P, Blumenstein B, Thompson I, et al. Design of the prostate cancer prevention trial (PCPT). *Control Clin Trials* 1995;16:150–163.

110. Kelloff GJ, Lubet RA, Lieberman R, et al. Aromatase inhibitors as potential cancer chemopreventives. *Cancer Epidemiol, Biomarkers Prev* 1998; 7(1):65–78.

111. Greenwald P. Cancer risk factors for selecting cohorts for large-scale chemoprevention trials. *J Cell Biochem* 1996;25S:29–36.

112. Pienta KJ, Esper PS, Zwas F, et al. Phase II chemoprevention trial of oral fenretinide in patients at risk for adenocarcinoma of the prostate. *Am J Clin Oncol* 1997;20(1):36–39.

113. Norrish AE, Jackson RT, McRae CU. Non-steroidal anti-inflammatory drugs and prostate cancer progression. *Int J Cancer* 1998;77:511–515.

114. Campbell SC. Advances in angiogenesis research: Relevance to urological oncology. *J Urol* 1997;158: 1663–1674.

115. Crawford ED, DeAntoni EP, Ross CA. The role of prostate-specific antigen in the chemoprevention of prostate cancer. *J Cell Biochem Suppl* 1996;25: 149–155.

116. Bostwick DG, Burke HB, Wheeler TM, et al. The most promising surrogate endpoint biomarkers for screening candidate chemopreventive compounds for prostatic adenocarcinoma in short-term phase II clinical trials. *J Cell Biochem* 1994; 19S:283–289.

117. Bostwick DG, Aquilina JW. Prostatic intraepithelial neoplasia (PIN) and other prostatic lesions as risk factors and surrogate endpoints for cancer chemoprevention trials. *J Cell Biochem* 1996;25S: 156–164.

118. Bostwick DG. Target populations and strategies for chemoprevention trials of prostate cancer. *J Cell Biochem* 1994;19S:191–196.

119. Mahon S. Cancer risk assessment: Conceptual considerations for clinical practice. *Oncol Nurs Forum* 1998;25:1535–1547.

120. Labrie F, Dupont A, Suburu R, et al. Serum prostate-specific antigen: A pre-screening test for prostate cancer. *J Urol* 1992;147:846–852.

121. Gerard MJ, Frank-Stromborg M. Screening for prostate cancer in asymptomatic men: Clinical, legal, and ethical implications. *Oncol Nurs Forum* 1998;25:1561–1569.

Chapter 2

SCREENING AND EARLY DETECTION

ANNE ROBIN WALDMAN

OVERVIEW

INTRODUCTION

CONTROVERSY OVER SCREENING

HIGH-RISK AND CONTRIBUTING FACTORS

Age

Family History

Race

Diet

Testosterone Levels

WHO SHOULD BE SCREENED?

American Cancer Society Screening Guidelines

FACTORS INFLUENCING SCREENING FOR CANCER

BARRIERS TO SCREENING

SCREENING TOOLS

Digital Rectal Examination

Prostate-Specific Antigen

Age- and Race-Related Prostate-Specific Antigen

Transrectal Ultrasonography

COST VERSUS BENEFIT OF EARLY DETECTION

DEVELOPMENT OF A SCREENING PROGRAM IN PHILADELPHIA

CONCLUSION

INTRODUCTION

Since the widespread adoption of serum prostate-specific antigen (PSA) as a screening test in the late 1980s, prostate cancer has become the most commonly diagnosed cancer in men in the United States. Because PSA and the digital rectal exam (DRE) are available for screening, it might be expected that prostate cancer screenings would be universally advocated. However, there is considerable disagreement. Some experts advocate screening for all men. Others believe that only those at high risk should be screened; some would not screen men with less than a potential 10-year life span or at high risk of dying from medical problems rather than from prostate cancer; and some recommend no screening at all.[1, 2]

CONTROVERSY OVER SCREENING

Because prostate cancer is the second leading cause of cancer death in men in the United States, the urology community has been investing a great deal of energy on how best to screen for this disease. Several studies[3–7] have shown that, since 1989 when PSA was initiated in screening for prostate cancer, early detection has actually increased the number of early-stage cancers diagnosed and that the majority of these cancers were potentially significant disease. Hoffman, Blume, and Gilliland[1] reported that the American Cancer Society (ACS), American Urological Association, American College of Radiology, and Prostate Education Council recommend screening for prostate cancer. However, until there is clear proof that early detection actually improves survival, the National Cancer Institute (NCI), U.S. Preventive Services Task Force, American College of Physicians, and Canadian Task Force on the Periodic Health Examination have not endorsed screening for prostate cancer.

The first study on early prostate cancer detection was published in abstract form in 1998. Labrie and colleagues[8] reported the results of their prospective, randomized study of 46,289 men. They compared two groups of men: One was screened using DRE and PSA in Year 1 and PSA only in subsequent years and the other was not screened. A benefit of early diagnosis and treatment of prostate cancer was a reduction in early death from the disease. By examining the annual death rates of all the men in the screened and unscreened groups, Labrie and others found a 2.7-fold advantage in favor of screening and early treatment. Thus, the researchers concluded that screening with PSA diagnosed clinically localized prostate cancer in close to 100% of cases, resulting in nearly eliminating the diagnosis of metastatic and noncurable cancers. Further studies substantiating these results are needed to secure the position of PSA as an effective screening tool.

HIGH-RISK AND CONTRIBUTING FACTORS

Three factors—age, race, and family history—are known to increase a man's risk for prostate cancer. Diet and testosterone levels have been associated with racial-ethnic differences.

AGE

Of men older than 50, more than 14% have been diagnosed with prostate cancer, and 95% of men who die after 90 have been found to have some area of disease in the prostate at autopsy. This has led some researchers to theorize that prostate cancer is a normal part of the aging process and that living to an older age puts men at higher risk for prostate cancer.[9]

FAMILY HISTORY

Familial carcinoma is the clustering of a disease within families. There is some evidence that prostate cancer may appear more commonly in families. Cannon and associates[10] evaluated 2,821 cases of prostate cancer among the Mormon population in Utah and found that prostate cancer had the fourth highest mean kinship after carcinoma of the lip, skin melanoma, and ovarian cancer. This represented a stronger link than that seen in two well-recognized familial cancers: colon and breast. They also found that relatives of men in whom prostate cancer developed before age 53 had a greater lifetime risk of developing the disease.

In another review of familial research, Gronberg and colleagues[11] found strong evidence that prostate cancer clusters in families. The closer a man is genetically to an affected relative and the greater the number of relatives affected in the family, the greater is his risk for prostatic carcinoma. Whittemore and coworkers[12] conducted a population-based case-control study of prostate cancer among African-Americans, Caucasians, and Asian-Americans in the United States and Canada. After matching age, region of residence, and ethnicity, 13% of the men with prostate cancer reported a father, brother, or son with prostate cancer compared with only 5% of the control group. In addition, they found that concentrations of sex hormone–binding globulin (SHBG) were slightly higher in the men with, compared with those without, a positive family history.

Hereditary cancer refers to familial carcinomas with a pattern of distribution consistent with mendelian inheritance of a susceptibility gene.[13] Family history has been associated with prostate cancer in approximately 25% of all men with the disease; however, only 9% are affected through a hereditary factor.[14] In an effort to learn more about hereditary prostate cancer, researchers at the Fred Hutchinson Cancer Research Center in Seattle are conducting the Prostate Cancer Genetics Research Study. They are enrolling families with three or more blood-related men with prostate cancer. Two of the men must be alive to complete a health questionnaire and submit blood samples for analysis in the hopes of identifying the gene responsible for the prostate cancer in the families.[15]

RACE

African-American men have a 30% higher incidence of prostate cancer—the highest incidence of prostate cancer in the world—and a 120% higher mortality rate than other ethnic groups.[16] Efforts to determine why these statistics prevail involve examining lifestyle differences, socioeconomic status (SES), and hormone levels. Polednak[17] examined whether racial differences in distribution of stage at diagnosis remained after controlling for an SES indicator as an ecologic variable. Using 8,155 Caucasian and 521 African-American patients reported to the Connecticut Tumor Registry and adjusting for the difference in numbers of cases diagnosed by race, age, and poverty rate census track, the proportion of prostate cancer cases diagnosed at distant sites was significantly higher in African-Americans, suggesting that biologic factors need to be explored for their potential role in this disease.

DIET

Asians, including Japanese, consume a mostly vegetarian diet. The vegetarian diet reduces serum testosterone levels. Asian males have the lowest incidence and mortality rates from prostate cancer.[18]

TESTOSTERONE LEVELS

High levels of testosterone are thought to be associated with an increased risk of prostate cancer in African-Americans. Serum testosterone levels are, on average, 15% higher in African-American males than in Caucasian males, and the incidence of prostate cancer is 30 to 37% higher for African-American men than for Caucasian men.[18] Wu and others[19] conducted a population-based case-control study of 1,127 African-American, Caucasian, Chinese-American, and Japanese-American men in which they examined the distribution of serum androgens, dihydrotestosterone (DHT), DHT-testosterone ratio, and SHBG. After adjusting for age, they found that the DHT-testosterone ratio corresponded to the respective incidence rates of prostate cancer; it was highest in African-Americans, intermediate in Caucasians, and lowest in Asian-Americans, thus offering some indirect evidence for ethnic differences.

WHO SHOULD BE SCREENED?

In an effort to determine who should be screened, in 1993, the NCI opened the Prostate, Lung, Colorectal, and Ovarian Cancer Screening Trial at 10 sites throughout the country. It is a 10-year randomized, controlled study in which 148,000 men and women between the ages of 60 and 74 are evaluated at periodic intervals. The goals of the study are to determine whether screening reduces site-specific mortality rates and to establish the sensitivity, specificity, and predictive value of these parameters as screening tools. The study calls for evaluating 37,000 men using DRE and PSA and matching them with 37,000 men who enter the health care system without periodic screening.[20]

AMERICAN CANCER SOCIETY SCREENING GUIDELINES

The ACS screening guidelines recommend that men discuss the significance of the screening findings with their physicians and then decide whether or not they wish to be screened. Screening should include an annual DRE and a test for the PSA level beginning at age 50 for men who are asymptomatic and who have at least a 10-year life expectancy. Men at high risk for prostate cancer should begin screening before age 50 (at approximately age 45). Two groups of men fall into this category: men of African-American descent and those with a strong family history of prostate cancer (i.e., two or more affected first-degree relatives). In addition, patients should be informed of the potential risks and benefits of intervention.[21] (See Table 2-1 for screening guidelines.)

TABLE 2-1. American Cancer Society Screening Guidelines*

Population	DRE	PSA
Asymptomatic men with no high-risk factors and at least a 10-year life expectancy	Annually after age 50	Annually after age 50
Men with high risk factors African-American Two or more first-degree relatives with prostate cancer	Annually before age 50 (at approximately age 45)	Annually before age 50 (at approximately age 45)

*Based on information from the American Cancer Society.
DRE, digital rectal examination; PSA, prostate-specific antigen.

FACTORS INFLUENCING SCREENING FOR CANCER

A significant factor promoting cancer screening is a recommendation by the patient's physician.[22] Several studies[23–25] identifying factors that influenced women in participating in cancer screenings have shown that appointment scheduling and reminding clients of the scheduled appointment result in a high compliance rate. In addition, McKee,[22] specifically studying prostate cancer screening, found that having a friend or family member diagnosed with prostate cancer positively influenced a man's decision to be screened. However, only 2% of the study sample were African-American. Weinrich and associates[26] found that African-American men were more likely to participate in prostate cancer screening programs if an ethnic role model shared his personal perspective on the importance of prostate screening and if individualized educational interventions are used.

BARRIERS TO SCREENING

A major barrier to screening and early detection efforts is the variety of cultural beliefs and practices of different ethnic or cultural groups. The differences consist of a variety of concepts of health, and these vary from group to group.[27] Because of African-Americans' high risk for prostate cancer, those health concepts specifically related to African-Americans are of great concern.

Barriers to screening for prostate cancer in African-American men include a fear of the DRE, fear of the diagnosis of cancer, fear of treatment resulting in loss of continence and potency, lack of insurance, and lack of access.[28]

Research suggests that, as a group, African-Americans are more frightened of cancer and may be deterred from any procedure involving examination of the rectum because of the mental images created by discussing the procedure. In four large research studies,[28] African-American enrollment ranged only from 2.2% to 5%. However, Gelfand and associates,[29] in their survey of 613 church-based African-American men, reported that those who had undergone a DRE found it was not as negative an experience as

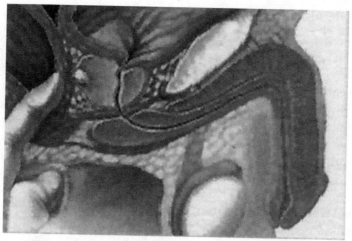

FIGURE 2-1. The digital rectal examination

expected. The effort of one institution—the North Philadelphia Cancer Awareness and Prevention (CAP) Program—to address these barriers—is described at the end of this chapter.

SCREENING TOOLS

DIGITAL RECTAL EXAMINATION

DRE of the prostate should be performed by a health care professional skilled in detecting abnormalities of the gland. The examination takes about 5 seconds and can be performed at least three different ways. The patient can (1) stand, flex his hips, and lean over an examination table with his upper body resting across the table; (2) lie on his side in a fetal position; or (3) kneel face-down on top of the examining table. The examiner inserts the index finger into the rectum and palpates the surface of the gland to assess for symmetry and texture (Figure 2-1). DRE is useful in detecting abnormalities in the posterior and lateral aspects of the gland. This also limits its sensitivity because up to 40% of tumors occur anterior to the midline and are undetectable by DRE.[30]

Another limitation is the difficulty in identifying small-volume tumors. It is generally agreed that detecting small-volume tumors and treating them aggressively improve survival rates compared with tumors found at later stages. When used alone, DRE has been shown to have missed approximately 40% of cancers detected during initial screenings[31]; however, the probability of the presence of clinically significant intracapsular prostate tumors as well as extracapsular disease increases when the DRE reveals abnormalities such as induration, marked asymmetry, and frank nodularity.[32]

PROSTATE-SPECIFIC ANTIGEN

Specific for prostate epithelial cells, PSA is a glycoprotein found in normal, benign hypertrophic and malignant cells. Any increase in the size of the gland will result in an increase in the PSA level. Thus, elevated levels may be seen in men with carcinoma as well as in those with benign prostatic hypertrophy. Procedures such as cystoscopy, prostate biopsy, and transurethral resection of the prostate (TURP) cause a rise in PSA that may last as long as 4 weeks, and, after biopsy or TURP, it is recommended that patients wait at least 6 weeks before having a PSA measurement.[33]

In the early years of PSA testing, there was concern that the DRE might affect the accuracy of the test. Crawford and coworkers[34] evaluated 2,754 men who presented to a prostate screening program to evaluate the effects of DRE on PSA levels. Each participant had a pre- and post-DRE PSA specimen taken. Men with values between 4 and 10 ng/mL had statistically insignificant changes in the serum PSA levels after DRE. The researchers concluded, therefore, that DRE caused no clinically important effects on serum PSA. Yuan and others[35] examined DRE, prostatic massage, and ultrasonography and found that all three had only minimal effect on PSA in most patients. They did find, however, that transrectal needle biopsy of the prostate caused an elevation of serum PSA in 92 of 100 men, with the increase lasting longer than the expected 2 to 3 days in more than 25% of the men. (See Table 2-2.)

In 1997, the U.S. Food and Drug Administration (FDA) approved the use of PSA combined with DRE as an aid in the detection of prostate cancer in men 50 years of age and older. The FDA currently approves six PSA assays for use in the United States (Table 2-3). Because results can vary slightly, men should have their PSA specimens processed by the same laboratory each year.[36]

In an effort to improve PSA sensitivity (a man having the disease will be correctly identified) and PSA specificity (a man having no disease will be correctly identified), other PSA tests have been identified and are being evaluated for use in patients. The tests being evaluated include age-related PSA values, PSA velocity or slope, PSA density, and the ratio of unbound or free PSA to total PSA. See Chapter 4 for details on the last three areas.

TABLE 2-2. Factors Affecting PSA*

Increase	Decrease
Acute prostatitis	Finasteride (Proscar)
Acute urinary retention	Bedrest
Benign prostatic hyperplasia (BPH)	
Ejaculation (up to 48 hours after)	
Prostate biopsy	
TRUS-guided biopsy	

*Based on information from Oesterling et al.,[33] Crawford et al.,[34] Yuan et al.,[35] and Oesterling and Moyad.[36]
PSA, prostate-specific antigen, TRUS, transrectal ultrasonography.

TABLE 2-3. PSA Tests Approved by the Food and Drug Administration

PSA Test	Manufacturer
Abbott IMX	Abbott Laboratories
Immunolite	Diagnostic Products Corporation
PSA I & II	Chiron Diagnostics
Tandem-E	Hybritech Inc.
Tandem-R	Hybritech Inc.
Toosh PSA	Toosh Medics Inc.

PSA, prostate-specific antigen.

Adapted from Oesterling JE, and Moyad MA. *The ABCs of Prostate Cancer: The Book That Could Save Your Life.* Lanham, MD: Madison Books, 1997. Used with permission of Madison Books.

TABLE 2-4. PSA Reference Ranges

Age Range (yr)	Asians	African-Americans	Caucasians
40–49	0–2.0	0–2.0	0–2.5
50–59	0–3.0	0–4.0	0–3.5
60–69	0–4.0	0–4.5	0–4.5
70–79	0–5.0	0–5.5	0–6.5

PSA, prostate-specific antigen.

Adapted from Oesterling JE, and Moyad MA. *The ABCs of Prostate Cancer: The Book That Could Save Your Life.* Lanham, MD: Madison Books, 1997. Used with permission of Madison Books.

❏ Age- and Race-Related Prostate-Specific Antigen

Because PSA has been used as an indicator of prostate growth, the normal reference range has been 0.0 to 4.0 ng/mL. This range was determined from the almost exclusively Caucasian northern European population residing in Olmstead County, Minnesota.[37] However, this range does not take into consideration age-dependent prostatic growth, variation in PSA production and secretion, and racial differences.

Age-specific reference ranges, when compared with the standard PSA reference ranges, seem to be a more sensitive marker in men younger than 60 and a more specific marker in men older than 60.[32] Increasing the sensitivity of the test in younger men has the potential for enabling the early detection of more curable, organ-confined tumors, and, increasing the specificity of the test in older men may avoid unnecessary biopsies.[38] However, Morgan and colleagues[39] found that the age-specific reference ranges developed for Caucasian men showed a poor sensitivity when applied to African-American men. Their study showed that African-American men had higher PSA values and that the values were more widely distributed, especially in older men.

Opinions vary as to these ranges. Oesterling[38] suggested the age-specific and race-specific ranges seen in Table 2-4, Morgan and colleagues[39] recommended those in Table 2-5, and Catalona and colleagues[40] prefer 4.0 ng/mL as the appropriate cutoff for all ages and races. As research continues on the clinical significance of age and race-

TABLE 2-5. Age-Specific Reference Ranges for the PSA Test According to Race

Age (yr)	Caucasians	African-Americans
40–49	0.0–2.5	0.0–2.0
50–59	0.0–3.5	0.0–4.0
60–69	0.0–3.5	0.0–4.5
70–79	0.0–3.5	0.0–5.5

PSA, prostate-specific antigen.

Adapted 1999 with permission from Morgan TO, Jacobsen SJ, McCarthy WF, et al. Age-specific reference ranges for serum prostate-specific antigen in black men. *N Engl J Med* 1996;335:304–310. Copyright © 1996 Massachusetts Medical Society. All rights reserved.

specific PSA reference ranges, using them may be useful in decreasing the number of false-positive test results when screening large groups.[41]

TRANSRECTAL ULTRASONOGRAPHY

Transrectal ultrasonography (TRUS) is primarily used to guide needle biopsies for staging of tumors, and it may also be used adjunctively in screening for prostate cancer when initial screening with PSA and DRE has resulted in abnormal findings in one or both of these parameters. TRUS facilitates accurate measurement of the size and shape of the gland, enabling estimation of volume to determine the density of the gland.[42] It is a costly procedure, averaging about $633[43] for a complete workup for suspicious results, and it is operator dependent. See Chapter 4 on diagnosis for more details of this procedure.

COST VERSUS BENEFIT OF EARLY DETECTION

Cost effectiveness of early detection programs are determined by incorporating the cost of the actual screening as well as the costs of any subsequent tests, treatment costs, and expected costs for treatment of complications. It is hoped that early detection and treatment will be effective, thus reducing the later costs that would be associated with treating the disease as it progresses. Coley and colleagues,[43] in evaluating the potential benefits, harms, and economic consequences of DRE and PSA for the early detection of prostate cancer, developed a cost-effectiveness model for a one-time DRE and PSA measurement to examine possible outcomes. They found that, given a combination of favorable assumptions and when compared with previously published estimates for other screening methods, using DRE and PSA might well be cost effective for men in their 50s and 60s.

DEVELOPMENT OF A SCREENING PROGRAM IN PHILADELPHIA

When a health care facility identifies a need for early detection screenings, their initial step should be the development of a needs assessment to identify health-specific problems and provide rationales for program goals, objectives, and activities.

In 1995, the Cancer Center at the Albert Einstein Medical Center, a community hospital located in the northern section of Philadelphia, performed a needs assessment of the surrounding community. The resident composition of this area included African-Americans, Asians, Hispanics, and Caucasians whose demographic information from the Pennsylvania Department of Health validated the need for earlier disease detection. On the basis of this information, the Albert Einstein Cancer Center, the local division of the ACS, and the LaSalle University Neighborhood Nursing Center received a grant from the Office of Minority Health funding the North Philadelphia CAP program.[44]

The goals of the CAP program were to (1) increase awareness within North Philadelphia minority populations regarding cancer prevention and early detection through outreach and educational programs; (2) increase participation of North Philadelphia minority populations in cancer screening programs; (3) provide appropriate follow-up and case management services for patients enrolled in the CAP to ensure delivery of appropriate medical care to participants with abnormalities; and (4) collect outcome data that will evaluate benefits and costs of the CAP interventions. To achieve these goals, the three agencies combined their joint resources to provide educational programs, screenings for breast, cervical, and prostate cancer, and follow-up.

The basic steps involved in developing the education and screening programs included identifying the client population, identifying the needs to be met, specifying the size and distribution of the client population, setting boundaries for the program services, clarifying the program and perspectives of the program, and identifying resources.

Once these were achieved, work began on implementing the program. Each of the agencies involved in the project identified their areas of expertise, staff responsibilities, and the support they could provide. The medical director of the cancer center was the project director, a public health nurse was the coordinator for the program, and master's degree–prepared nurses were assigned as case managers for each disease site. This professional staff assumed the responsibility for conducting training sessions and in-services on the mission, goals, and activities of the program and, in the process, developed slide and overhead presentations for the educational sessions associated with the screenings.

Registration forms and coordination and evaluation tools were developed as well as an inventory of equipment needs for the screenings. Provisions were made for ordering and storing supplies, for the delivery of heavy equipment to the screening site, and for processing of specimens. Portable boxes were purchased and labeled with supplies for each screening.

Community groups and agencies willing to hold a forum or a screening and an on-site leader were identified. The community leader was provided with a list of tasks and responsibilities as well as those for the CAP program personnel. Educational sessions preceding the screenings were scheduled based on the site availability, the time frame best for the target population, and the availability of the CAP program resources. With the date and site established, flyers were developed for release to local and regional newspapers and a local university cable television station as well as to the community leader for on-site outreach.

Monthly staff meetings, conducted by the project coordinator, were held to review upcoming activities, plan for staffing needs, and evaluate the completed programs, and a database was developed to record the results of the screenings.

Preparation time for the development of the CAP program was about 6 months, and it took about 1 year to eliminate some unforeseen pitfalls. Now, however, 3 years later, the CAP program has been refunded for another 3 years and is hoping to add colorectal and oral screenings to its repertoire.

CONCLUSION

Prostate cancer screening has the ability to detect cancer at an earlier stage. Patients at high risk should begin screening early compared with the majority of the population. Nurses can play an active role in educating men about the need for screening and as participants in screening programs in their community.

REFERENCES

1. Hoffman RM, Blume MD, Gilliland F. Prostate-specific antigen testing practices and outcomes. *J Gen Intern Med* 1998;13:106–110.
2. *U.S. Preventive Services Task Force: Guide to Clinical Preventive Services.* Baltimore, MD: Williams & Wilkins, 1996.
3. Lodding P, Aus G, Bergdahl R, et al. Characteristics of screening detected prostate cancer in men 50 to 66 years old with 3 to 4 ng/mL prostate specific antigen. *J Urol* 1998;159:899–903.
4. Mettlin CJ, Murphy GP, Babaian RJ, et al. Observations on the early detection of prostate cancer from the American Cancer Society National Prostate Cancer Detection Project. *Cancer* 1997;80: 1814–1817.
5. Newcomer LM, Stanford JL, Blunenstein BA, Brawer MK. Temporal trends in rates of prostate cancer: Declining incidence of advanced stage disease, 1774–1994. *J Urol* 1997;158:1427–1430.
6. Reissigl A, Horninger W, Fink K, et al. Prostate carcinoma screening in the county of Tyrol, Austria: Experience and results. *Cancer* 1997;80:1818–1829.
7. Smith DS, Humphrey PA, Catalona WJ. The early detection of prostate carcinoma with prostate specific antigen. *Cancer* 1997;80:1852–1856.
8. Labrie F, Dupont A, Candas B, et al. Decrease of prostate cancer death by screening: First data from the Quebec prospective and randomized study [abstract 4]. *Proc Am Soc Clin Oncol* 1998;17:2a.
9. Lind J. Nursing care of the client with cancer of the urinary system. In: Itano JK, Taoka KN (eds.) *Core Curriculum for Oncology Nursing,* 3rd ed. Philadelphia: WB Saunders,1998:421–447.
10. Cannon L, Bishop DT, Skolnick M, et al. Genetic epidemiology of prostate cancer in the Utah Mormon genealogy. *Cancer Surv* 1982;1:47–69.
11. Gronberg H, Damber L, Damber JE. Familial prostate cancer in Sweden. A nationwide register cohort study. *Cancer* 1996;77:138–143.
12. Whittemore AS, Wu AH, Kolonel LN, et al. Family history and prostate cancer risk in black, white, and Asian men in the United States and Canada. *Am J Epidemiol* 1995;121:732–740.
13. Walsh PC, Partin AW. Family history facilitates the early diagnosis of prostate carcinoma. *Cancer* 1997; 80:1871–1874.
14. Carter BS, Beaty TH, Steinberg GD, et al. Mendelian inheritance of familial prostate cancer. *Proc Natl Acad Sci U S A* 1992;89:3367–3371.
15. Fred Hutchinson Cancer Research Center. Prostate Cancer Genetics Research Study (PROGRESS). Seattle: Author, in press. (Available electronically at progress@fhcrc.org)
16. Wingo P, Bolden S, Tong T, et al. Cancer statistics for African-Americans. *CA Cancer J Clin* 1996;46: 113–117.
17. Polednak AP. Stage at diagnosis of prostate cancer in Connecticut by poverty and race. *Ethn Dis* 1997; 7:215–220.
18. Groenwald SL, Frogge MH, Goodman M, Yarbro CH (eds). *Comprehensive Cancer Nursing Review.* Sudbury, MA: Jones and Bartlett, 1998:552.
19. Wu AH, Whittemore AS, Kolonel LN. Serum androgens and sex hormone–binding globulins in relation to lifestyle factors in older African-Americans, white, and Asian men in the United States and Canada. *Cancer Epidemiol, Biomarkers Prev* 1995;4:735–741.

20. Kramer BS, Brown ML, Prorok PC, et al. Prostate cancer screening: What we know and what we need to know. *Ann Intern Med* 1993;119:914–923.
21. Von Eschenbach A, Ho R, Murphy GP, et al. American Cancer Society guidelines for the early detection of prostate cancer: Update. *Cancer* 1997;80: 1805–1897.
22. McKee JM. Cue to action in prostate cancer screening. *Oncol Nurs Forum* 1994;21:1171–1176.
23. Williams E, Vessey M. Randomized trial of two strategies offering women mobile screening for breast cancer. *BMJ* 1989;299:158–159.
24. Wilson A, Leemings A. Cervical cytology: A comparison of two call systems. *BMJ* 1987;295:181–182.
25. Wolosin R. Effect of appointment scheduling and reminder post cards on adherence to mammography recommendations. *J Fam Pract* 1990;30:542–547.
26. Weinrich SP, Boyd MD, Weinrich M, et al. Increasing prostate cancer screening in African American men with peer-educator and client-navigator interventions. *J Cancer Educ* 1998;13:213–219.
27. Kagawa-Singer M. Addressing issues for early detection and screening in ethnic populations. *Oncol Nurs Forum* 1997;24:1705–1714.
28. Powell IJ. Early detection issues of prostate cancer in African American men. *In Vivo* 1994;8:451–452.
29. Gelfand DE, Parzuchowski J, Cort M, Powell I. Digital rectal examinations and prostate cancer screening: Attitudes of African American men. *Oncol Nurs Forum* 1995;22:1253–1255.
30. Littrup PJ, Lee F, Mettlin C. Prostate cancer screening: Current trends and future implications. *CA Cancer J Clin* 1992;42:198–211.
31. Catalona WJ, Richie JP, Ahmann FR, et al. Comparison of digital rectal examinations and serum prostate specific antigen in the early detection of prostate cancer: Results of a multicentered clinical trial of 6,630 men. *J Urol* 1994;1551:1283–1290.
32. Coley CM, Barry MJ, Mulley AG. Screening for prostate cancer. *Ann Intern Med* 1997;126:480–484.
33. Oesterling JE, Rice DC, Glenski WJ, Bergstralh EJ. Effect of cystoscopy, prostate biopsy, and transurethral resection of prostate on serum prostate-specific antigen concentration. *Urology* 1993:42: 276–282.
34. Crawford ED, Schutz MJ, Clejan S, et al. The effect of digital rectal examination on prostate-specific antigen levels. *JAMA* 1992;267:2227–2228.
35. Yuan JJ, Copen DE, Petros JA, et al. Effects of rectal examination, prostatic massage, ultrasonography and needle biopsy on serum prostate specific antigen levels. *J Urol* 1992;147:810–814.
36. Oesterling JE, Moyad MA. *The ABCs of Prostate Cancer: The Book That Could Save Your Life.* Lanham, MD: Madison Books, 1997:40, 49.
37. Oesterling JE, Jacobsen SJ, Chute CG, et al. Serum prostate-specific antigen in a community-based population of healthy men: Establishment of age-specific reference ranges. *JAMA* 1993;270: 860–864.
38. Oesterling JE. Using prostate-specific antigen to eliminate unnecessary diagnostic tests: Significant world wide economic implications. *Urology* 1995;46 (3 Suppl A):26–33.
39. Morgan TO, Jacobsen SJ, McCarthy WF, et al. Age-specific reference ranges for serum prostate-specific antigen in black men. *N Engl J Med* 1996;335:304–310.
40. Catalona WJ, Smith DS, Ornstein DK, Prostate cancer detection in men with serum PSA concentations of 2.6 to 4.0 ng/mL and benign prostate examination: Enhancement of specificity with free PSA measurements. *JAMA* 1997;277:1452–1455.
41. DeAntoni EP. Age-specific reference ranges for PSA in the detection of prostate cancer. *Oncology* 1997; 11:475–485.
42. Olson MC, Posniak HV, Fisher SG, et al. Directed and random biopsies of the prostate: Indications based on combined results of transrectal sonography and prostate-specific antigen density determinations. *Am J Roentgenol* 1994;163:1407–1411.
43. Coley CM, Barry MJ, Fleming C, et al. Early detection of prostate cancer. Part II: Estimating the risks, benefits, and costs. *Ann Intern Med* 1997;126:468–479.
44. Tester WT, Starr S. *Replication manual of the North Philadelphia Cancer Awareness and Prevention Program.* Philadelphia: Unpublished work fully funded by the Office of Minority Health, submitted for publication to Department of Health and Human Services, 1998.

Chapter 3

CELLULAR CHARACTERISTICS, PATHOPHYSIOLOGY, AND DISEASE MANIFESTATIONS

JENNIFER CASH

OVERVIEW

INTRODUCTION

CARCINOGENESIS AND PATHOLOGY
  Prostatic Intraepithelial Neoplasia
  Pathophysiology of Prostate Cancer

GRADING AND PROGNOSTIC INDICATORS OF
  PROSTATE CANCER

FACTORS FOR TUMOR DEVELOPMENT,
  PROGRESSION, AND METASTASIS

  Genetic Changes
  Angiogenesis
  Location of Disease
  Progression of Disease
  Role of Androgens

CLINICAL MANIFESTATIONS

CONCLUSION

INTRODUCTION

An estimated 185,000 new cases of prostate cancer are diagnosed annually in the United States, and an estimated 39,000 men will die of the disease.[1] Prostate cancer is recognized as the most common malignancy affecting males and ranks second only to lung cancer in cancer-related deaths among males. Clearly, prostate cancer is an important disease process that deserves the attention of the clinician and researcher alike. Identification of disease is paramount for appropriate management; therefore, the purpose of this chapter is to discuss the incidence and significance of cellular changes, both premalignant and malignant, that occur in the prostate as well as other independent factors that may contribute to the development of a cancer. Clinical manifestations of disease and contemporary grading systems used to define the pathologic properties of a cancer also are discussed.

CARCINOGENESIS AND PATHOLOGY

Carcinogenesis is the process of cancer development. Prostate cancer occurs as a result of cumulative changes in a cell's genes that may cause uncontrolled cellular proliferation, metastatic spread, and altered differentiation.[2,3] The process of carcinogenesis involves three stages: initiation, promotion, and progression.[4,5] Initiation is characterized by cellular DNA damage caused by a carcinogen. As a result, the damaged DNA will either undergo repair or become permanently changed (mutated). Promotion also involves cellular damage by carcinogens, and cells are subsequently either reversibly or irreversibly damaged. Stimulation of cellular proliferation follows initiation and allows cancer cell transformation to occur.[5] Progression then leads to additional morphologic changes that more resemble malignant behavior. Additional changes involve invasion, angiogenesis, and growth factor stimulation.[5] Metastasis may then occur.

Oncogenes—genes that regulate cellular growth and repair and are the mutated genes responsible for transformation of a normal cell into a cancer cell—are affected by carcinogens.[4,5] When there is a disruption in the balance between the normal state of cell differentiation and cell death, genetic changes (mutations) can be observed in both premalignant and malignant states within a single prostate gland. Thus, each individual cancer arises from an accumulation of mutagenic changes within the cell that have transpired over time. Cells that are only partially transformed may result in a morphologically identifiable premalignant lesion. One of these lesions is prostate intraepithelial neoplasia (PIN), which is associated with progressive abnormalities between normal prostatic epithelium and cancer.

PROSTATIC INTRAEPITHELIAL NEOPLASIA

PIN has been considered to be a premalignant lesion as well as the main precursor of carcinoma of the prostate.[3,4,6–12] PIN mimics cellular changes of carcinoma, indicating impairment of cell differentiation and regulatory control. Atypical cellular proliferations have been described in the literature as early as the 1920s; however, the more contemporary and widely used term *prostatic intraepithelial neoplasia* was first described by L. E. McNeal in the 1960s and introduced as an actual term by Bostwick and Brawer in 1987.[8]

PIN encompasses morphologic changes of cellular proliferation that are usually associated with carcinoma (Table 3-1).[3,8,9] Based on a two-tier system developed by a workshop of the National Prostate Cancer Detection Project in 1989, PIN has been subdivided into low and high grades.[13,14] The greater the amount of dysplastic changes present in PIN, the greater is the risk of microinvasive cancer development.[4] To date, low-grade PIN has not been found to have a high correlation with clinical significance in the development of prostate cancer.[3,4,6,7,9,11,12] Conversely, high-grade PIN has been associated with the concomitant presence of carcinoma within the same specimen or in subsequent prostatic biopsies (needle biopsy, transurethral prostatic resection specimen, and whole prostate) (Table 3-2).[3,6,7,9,11,15,16] High-grade PIN is characterized by nuclear and nucleolar abnormalities, increased proliferative potential, and basal cell disruptions.[3,8,9,12]

TABLE 3-1. Prostatic Intraepithelial Neoplasia (PIN): Diagnostic Criteria

Feature	Low-grade PIN*	High-grade PIN†
Architecture	Epithelial cell crowding and stratification with irregular spacing	Similar to low-grade PIN; more crowding and stratification; four patterns; tufting, micropapillary, cribriform, and flat
Cytology		
Nuclei	Enlarged with marked size variation	Enlarged; some size and shape variation
Chromatin	Normal	Increased density and clumping
Nucleoli	Rarely prominent	Occasionally to frequently large and prominent, similar to invasive carcinoma; sometimes multiple
Basal cell layer	Intact	May show some disruption
Basement membrane	Intact	Intact

*Formerly PIN 1.   †Formerly PIN 2 and PIN 3.
From Bostwick DG. High-grade prostatic intraepithelial neoplasia: The most likely precursor of prostate cancer. *Cancer* 1995;75(Suppl):1823–1836. Copyright © 1995 American Cancer Society. Reprinted by permission of Wiley-Liss, Inc., a subsidiary of John Wiley & Sons, Inc.

TABLE 3-2. Prostatic Intraepithelial Neoplasia and Prostate Cancer: Incidence and Prevalence of PIN in Whole Prostates

Study	No Concomitant Prostatic Ca		Concomitant Prostatic Ca		PIN Grade	Mean Age (yrs.)
	No. Examined	No. PIN (%)	No. Examined	No. PIN (%)		
McNeal and[36] Bostwick	100*	43 (43)	100*	82 (82)	High and low	Not available
Oyasu et al[37]	37*	14 (38)	48†	51 (94)	High and low	70.0
Kovi et al[38]	176*†	81 (46)	253*†	150 (59)	Not available	54.5
Troncoso et al[39]	39†	28 (72)	61†	61 (100)	High and low	63.5
Sakr et al[40]	120*	51 (43)	32*	22 (69)	High and low	Less than 50
de la Torre et al[41]			54†	54 (100)	High and low	63.0
Qian and Bostwick[42]			195†	167 (86)	High	64.5

*Autopsy series.   †Prostatectomy series.   Ca, cancer.
From Häggman MJ, Macoska JA, Wojno KJ, Oesterling JE. The relationship between prostatic intraepithelial neoplasia and prostate cancer: Critical issues. *J Urol* 1997;158:14. Used with permission.

The clinical importance of recognizing high-grade PIN is based on its strong association with prostatic carcinoma. Predictive value of high-grade PIN has been evaluated through numerous comparative studies.[6, 8–12,16, 17] Davidson and colleagues[16] found subsequent prostate cancer on biopsy in 35 of 100 patients (35%) in a high-grade PIN-biopsy group and in only 15 of the 112 (13%) matched control group. Other studies reported subsequently diagnosed adenocarcinoma, in 35 to 100% of patients, identified through

TABLE 3-3. Cancer Detection on Subsequent Biopsies in Patients With Initial Isolated Prostatic Intraepithelial Neoplasia (PIN)

Study	Low-Grade PIN		High-Grade PIN	
	n	%	n	%
Brawer et al[43]	2/11	18.0	10/10	100.0
Ellis and Brawer[44]	—	—	5/5	100.0
Aboseif et al[45]	2/12	16.6	19/24	79.1
Weinstein and Epstein[46]	—	—	10/19	53.0
Keetch et al[47]	4/19	19.0	19/37	51.0
Davidson et al[48]	—	—	35/100	35.0
Markham[49]	3/23	13.0	13/32	40.0
Raviv et al[50, 51]	6/45	13.3	23/48	47.9

From Zlotta AR, Raviv G, Schulman CC. Clinical prognostic criteria for later diagnosis of prostate carcinoma iin patients with initial isolated prostatic intraepithelial neoplasia. *Eur Urol* 1996;30:250. Reproduced with permission of S. Karger AG, Basel.

needle core biopsy or aspiration biopsies from an immediate rebiopsy up to 8 years from initial diagnosis of high-grade PIN (Table 3-3).[8–12,16,17] Additionally, the likelihood of diagnosing cancer in patients with high-grade PIN was greater in those undergoing more than one follow-up biopsy (44%) as opposed to single biopsy (32%).[10–12,17]

The incidence and extent of PIN appear to increase with patient age, and PIN has been shown to predate the onset of carcinoma by up to 10 years.[3, 8, 10–12, 17] In addition, PIN was found to be more predictive of cancer in patients with a serum prostate-specific antigen (PSA) concentration greater than 4 ng/mL (normal 0.0–4.0 ng/mL) and in African-American men compared with Caucasian men.[8, 9, 12, 16]

Unfortunately, studies to date have not determined whether PIN remains stable, regresses, or progresses, although the implication is that it can progress.[12, 15, 16] Studies evaluating the use of androgen deprivation in the treatment of high-grade PIN demonstrate a decrease in the prevalence and extent of high-grade PIN in subsequent biopsies, which also suggests a possible role for chemoprevention.[9, 12, 16, 18, 19]

The diagnosis of PIN on prostate needle biopsy without associated prostatic adenocarcinoma raises difficult clinical issues. A major concern exists that prostate cancer is present but not detected in biopsy specimens with PIN as a result of sampling limitations. However, current evidence shows that high-grade PIN has a high correlation with foci of carcinoma and, therefore, may have merit to be used as an acceptable histologic marker for close patient follow-up and repeat biopsy for occult or latent prostate cancer. Because biopsy is the definitive method for detecting PIN and early cancer, recommended follow-up after initial diagnosis of high-grade PIN is suggested at 3- to 6-month intervals for 2 years and thereafter at 12-month intervals for life.[11, 12] Patient factors that may have an impact on aggressive follow-up biopsy are age and physical condition as well as the likelihood that the patient will undergo radical treatment for a subsequently diagnosed prostate cancer.

PATHOPHYSIOLOGY OF PROSTATE CANCER

Approximately 95% of all cancers that develop in the prostate are adenocarcinomas, which arise from one cell of origin, the embryonic urogenital sinus epithelium.[2, 3, 20] Within the classification of epithelial neoplasms are pure ductal and mucinous adenocarcinomas, small cell tumors, transitional cell carcinoma, and carcinoma in situ (includes intraepithelial neoplasia). Small cell tumors comprise only 1 to 2% of all prostatic cancers and tend to disseminate early in their course, similar to small cell counterparts in other primary sites.[3, 17, 20, 21] Transitional cell carcinomas (and squamous cell carcinoma, which is similar) often present with obstructive symptoms and also tend to metastasize early.[3, 20]

The second class of prostate neoplasms is carcinosarcoma, which is the coexistence of adenocarcinoma and sarcomas that have differentiated from malignant mesenchymal elements. Carcinosarcoma metastasizes early in its course and is usually resistant to systemic therapies.[3, 20]

The third class of prostate neoplasm includes nonepithelial neoplasms. These are composed of mesenchymal, both malignant and benign, and lymphoma.[3, 20] Malignant mesenchymal tumors comprise less than 0.3% of prostate cancers and have a poor prognosis because they are frequently diagnosed late in the course of the disease at an advanced stage.[3, 20] Lymphomas are rarely primary tumors of the prostate but are usually metastatic.[3, 20]

The final class of prostatic neoplasm includes germ cell tumors, which are very rare.[3] Secondary tumors, which germ cell tumors have sometimes been classified as, have also been reported in the literature and are defined as having prostatic involvement with tumor from contiguous, extensive locoregional disease or true metastatic disease.[20] Examples of secondary tumor sources include cancers of the bladder, urethra, colon, rectum, and anus; malignant lymphoma; bone or soft tissue sarcomas; alimentary tract carcinomas; and leukemia.[20]

GRADING AND PROGNOSTIC INDICATORS OF PROSTATE CANCER

Tumor grading, defined as the degree of cellular differentiation between cancerous cells and normal cells, is an effort to use histologic characteristics of a tumor to predict its biologic activity or aggressiveness.[20, 22] A variety of microscopic observations are made regarding configuration and arrangement of cells. Cellular characteristics are also observed, including distinctiveness of borders, nuclear distortion, nucleoli appearance, and significant behavioral patterns (i.e., invasion of lymphatic or vascular channels and tumor cell volume.)[20, 23]

The most widely accepted grading system for prostate cancer is the Gleason grading system. This system is based on the Veterans Administration Cooperative Urological Research Group Study of more than 4,000 patients between 1960 and 1975.[20, 22, 24] The Gleason classification system incorporates five histologic patterns based on the degree of cellular differentiation and assigns a value from 1 to 5: 1 represents well-differentiated cells and 5 represents poorly differentiated cells (Table 3-4). Gleason noted that approximately 50% of tumors found in the prostate will demonstrate more than one histologic pattern; therefore, the total histologic score is obtained by adding the scores of the two most dominant cell patterns, with a total possible score of 2 to 10.[2, 20, 22, 24]

Prognosis and treatment protocols are determined partially by the grade of a tumor. Tumor grade, which is based on cellular architecture, is a strong prognostic indicator. Other prognostic factors for therapeutic decision making include patient age and health, clinical stage, tumor location, tumor volume, and serum PSA level. Additionally, the likelihood of recurrence and survival are strongly correlated with cancer grade. The higher the Gleason score, 7 to 10, the higher is the risk of nodal metastatic disease and poor survival.[2, 20, 22, 24]

Tumor volume is also an important prognostic indicator for potential of extracapsular spread and is highly correlated with Gleason grade to predict progression of disease.[20, 22, 24] Low-grade tumors (Gleason Patterns 1 and 2) are rarely larger than 1cc, whereas high-grade tumors (Gleason Patterns 4 and 5) are almost always larger than 1cc.[20, 22, 24]

Other correlative factors with grade include PSA, pathologic stage, and tumor location. Cancer associated with an elevated serum PSA (greater than 10) is typically more likely to be of higher grade (Gleason score 7 or greater) because of the amount of tumor cells present, regardless of poorly differentiated cells expressing less PSA.[23, 24] As Gleason score increases (greater than 7), there is a strong correlation to increasing risk of capsular penetration, and if greater than 8, there is a greater risk of seminal vesicle invasion, lymph node metastasis, and bone metastasis.[20, 23, 24] Finally, cancers arising in the transition zone of the prostate appear to be of lower grade and less aggressive clinically than the more common cancers arising in the peripheral zone.[9, 20, 24]

Three other contemporary grading systems include the Mostofi, Gaeta, and Mayo Clinic systems; however, the Gleason system is the most widely used. There is an associated low but significant level of interobserver and intraobserver variability with the Gleason grading system. However, the consensus is that the Gleason grading system is important in predicting patient outcome and should be used in combination with other prognostic factors to allow more precise recommendations of treatment for patients.[2, 20, 24]

FACTORS FOR TUMOR DEVELOPMENT, PROGRESSION, AND METASTASIS

Characteristics of the natural history of carcinoma of the prostate have been researched for clinical importance. Specifically, several hereditary or genetic factors may play a role in the development of carcinoma: (1) The prevalence of carcinoma increases with each subsequent decade after age 40; (2) most carcinoma develops in the peripheral or outer prostate; (3) there are histologic and biochemical changes associated with most carcinomas; (4) histologic grade correlates with development of mass, invasion, and dissemination of carcinoma; (5) intra- and extragland local spread of carcinoma follows natural anatomic conduits; (6) the pelvic lymph nodes and bones of the axial skeleton are sites of initial dissemination; and (7) evidence of dependence on androgens for maintenance and

TABLE 3-4. Gleason Grading System for Prostatic Adenocarcinoma: Histologic Patterns

Pattern	Peripheral Borders of Tumor	Stromal Invasion	Appearance of Glands	Size of Glands	Architecture of Glands	Cytoplasm
1	Circumscribed, pushing, expansile	Minimal	Simple, round, monotonously replicated	Medium, regular	Closely packed, rounded masses	Similar to benign epithelium
2	Less circumscribed; early infiltration	Mild, with definite separation of glands by stroma	Simple, round, some variability in shape	Medium, less regular	Loosely packed, rounded masses	Similar to benign epithelium
3A	Infiltration	Marked	Angular, with variation in shape	Medium to large	Variably packed, irregular masses	More basophilic than Patterns 1 and 2
3B	Infiltration	Marked	Angular, with variation in shape	Small	Variably packed, irregular masses	More basophilic than Patterns 1 and 2
3C	Smoothed, rounded	Marked	Papillary and cribriform	Irregular	Round to elongate masses	More basophilic than Patterns 1 and 2
4A	Ragged infiltration	Marked	Microacinar, papillary, and cribriform	Irregular	Fused, with chains and cords	Dark
4B	Ragged infiltration	Marked	Microacinar, papillary, and cribriform	Irregular	Fused, with chains and cords	Clear (hypernephroid)
5A	Smoothed, rounded	Marked	Comedocarcinoma	Irregular	Round to elongate masses	Variable
5B	Ragged infiltration	Marked	Difficulty identifying gland lumina	Sheet of glands	Fused sheets and masses	Variable

Adapted from Bostwick DG. Grading prostate cancer. *Am J Clin Path* 1994;102:4(Suppl):540. Used with permission of the American Society of Clinical Pathologists.

stimulation of cells is also seen as substantial.[3, 4, 20] The remaining factors to be reviewed are genetic factors, angiogenesis, location of prostate tumors, patterns of spread of disease, and the role of androgens in relation to development of cancer.

GENETIC CHANGES

As outlined previously, genetic change that can induce neoplastic growth is usually the result of a combination of factors—genetic, hormonal, and environmental—that modulate the expression and function of specific genes. The loss of function of certain genes, antioncogenes (tumor-suppressing genes), that normally detoxify carcinogens, can predispose a man to cancer.[3, 20, 22] Protooncogenes provide the coding for producing cellular proteins in a normal genetic sequence. Oncogenes are the result of an alteration or mutation in the coding for protein development, which can lead to abnormal growth of cells and the development of a neoplasm.[3, 20, 22] The search for oncogenes related to prostate growth is ongoing, and to date no specific oncogenes are directly implicated in the initiation of prostate cancer. Current research on growth factor oncogenes such as *ras, myc,* and c-*erc B-2,* as well as *BCL2* and c-*kit,* are ongoing and indeterminate as to their possible role in the development of prostate cancer.[3, 22] Familial clustering of prostate cancer may be related to the heritable genetic risk factor along with the presence of environmental carcinogens that cause sufficient mutation of genes to cause carcinogenesis.[2, 3, 20, 22] Additionally, loss of expression of certain metastatic suppressor genes can promote metastasis of a cancer; the most studied to date is the p53 gene.[2, 3, 20] The p53 gene is thought to induce cell arrest in the G1 phase of the cell cycle and be responsible for the initiation of apoptosis (the active process of a cell's normal programmed cell death).[2, 3, 20, 25–27] In prostate cancer, the balance is lost between cell proliferation at an equal rate with programmed cell death, therefore producing continuous net growth of cells leading to cancer progression.[25, 26] Data also suggest DNA methylation, which plays an important role in the regulation of gene expression, when an imbalance may result in genetic instability, which can lead to tumor progression.[22]

ANGIOGENESIS

Angiogenesis, the ability of a tumor to induce its own blood supply, may play a role in the identification and extent of prostate cancer.[3, 20, 28, 29] Exponential growth of tumor cells requires the support of blood vessels to provide a vascular framework. This directed capillary network growth is important in understanding subsequent metastatic potential of a tumor. Microvessel density (a measure of tumor angiogenesis) is greatest in malignant tissue and has even been shown to have a significant difference between organ-confined and metastatic cancer.[2, 3, 20, 28, 29] Microvessel density appears to be an independent predictor of cancer progression, perhaps by facilitating microvascular invasion.[2, 3]

Folkman and associates[29] characterized two distinct stages as stepwise models of tumor progression: the prevascular and vascular phases. The prevascular phase is seen as an early development period with a limited number of tumor cells present and little to no tumor growth, whereas the vascular phase is marked by increased vascularity and increased tumor growth.[28, 29] It is speculated that stimulation of angiogenesis occurs as part of the transition of tumors to a malignant state because increased tumor cell population is preceded by increased capillaries supplying the tumor.[28–30] Subsequently, the progression to metastasis is also dependent on induction of a blood supply that may facilitate the process by engulfing tumor cells and instigating systemic spread.

LOCATION OF DISEASE

Two anatomic considerations of prostate carcinoma are regional distribution of the cancer and its multicentric origin.[3, 4, 20] Seventy to 75% of all prostate carcinomas are found in the peripheral zone of the prostate, which may affect the tumor's ability to invade surrounding tissue. Additionally, high-grade PIN is more consistent with higher grade (more aggressive) peripheral zone prostate cancer.[9, 20] With regard to the multicentric origin, there is an increased incidence of multiple separate tumor sites with differing size, cellular characteristics, and wide range of biologic malignancy. This is supported by observed changes in coexisting diagnosed PIN.[3, 11, 12, 20]

PROGRESSION OF DISEASE

Routes of growth and spread of carcinoma are important considerations in diagnosis and treatment. Prostate cancers tend to grow initially along normal intraprostatic and periprostatic tissue planes in the gland; however, it has been shown that higher grade tumors tend to invade other structures across natural planes.[31] Also transitional zone tumors infrequently spread to periprostatic tissue, unlike peripheral zone tumors. Sites of commonly recognized extraorgan spread are (1) local extension through the prostate capsule into the bladder base and seminal vesicles, (2) distant spread to the pelvic lymph nodes, and (3) bones of the axial skeleton.[3, 4, 31]

Extension into the urethra and rectum are uncommon. Breach of the prostate capsule may be due to defects occurring where adjoining organs meet the prostate, where neurovascular structures enter or exit the prostate, and the entry of ejaculatory ducts into the prostate.[3, 31] Higher risk of capsular penetration is associated with perineural invasion as well as cancers involving the apex or base.[3, 31]

Lymphatic spread most often occurs in the obturator lymph nodes followed by presacral, presciatic, hypogastric, common iliac, and inguinal lymph nodes.[3, 4, 31] Spread to periaortic, mediastinal, and supraclavicular lymph nodes are uncommon.[3, 4, 31]

Hematogenous spread of prostate cancer typically involves the lungs, liver, kidneys, and bone; metastasis to bone has been observed in up to 80% of patients who die from prostate cancer.[3, 4, 31] The spine is the most frequently involved, followed by the femur, pelvis, ribs, skull, and humerus.[3, 4, 31]

ROLE OF ANDROGENS

The prostate is dependent on androgens for maintaining normal structure and function. Testosterone, which originates from the testicles, converts into dihydrotestosterone (DHT) in prostate tissue and then binds to androgen receptors (AR) in prostate tissue cells.[27, 32] Dehydroepiandrosterone and androstenedione are circulating weak androgens produced by the adrenal glands that also have a role in the synthesis of DHT.[27, 32] The DHT-AR complex regulates the activity of the various androgen-responsive genes that are related to prostate growth and plays a crucial role in the growth regulatory processes of the prostate gland.[27, 32, 33]

Because epithelial cell differentiation in the prostate is driven by androgens and the majority of prostatic adenocarcinomas are initially androgen dependent, some speculate that androgens play a role in the development of prostate cancer.[27, 33, 34] Androgen-dependent cells are induced to die by programmed cell death regulated by the DHT-AR complex. The exact mechanism of signaling pathways in the prostate that maintain the growth regulatory balance promoted by DHT are not clearly understood.[33, 34] The clinical behavior of prostate cancers reflects their responsiveness to androgens by evidence of symptomatic relief experienced in up to 70 to 80% of patients treated with first-line endocrine therapy.[33, 34] These endocrine therapies are designed to prevent the activation of androgen-regulated genes.[33-35]

There are androgen-independent tumor cells that thrive and continue to grow in the absence of androgen influence. Three potential mechanisms may be responsible for androgen-independent clones: (1) alteration of the AR, causing the signal for cell death to be absent; (2) alteration of the responses of target genes that interact with the AR; and (3) alteration of the AR cellular content through mutation.[33-35] It is the progression of cancer cells to no longer undergo apoptosis (cell death) that leads to uncontrolled tumor growth and ineffectiveness of endocrine therapy.

CLINICAL MANIFESTATIONS

Prostate cancer is usually asymptomatic in its early stages. Presenting signs and symptoms vary in accordance with location of the cancer and extent of involvement.[1, 3, 4, 31] Because the majority of prostate cancers arise in the peripheral zone of the gland, there usually are no presenting symptoms. Those cancers that arise in the transitional zone or that enlarge and encroach on the urethra produce benign prostatic hyperplasia–type symptoms of urinary frequency, hesitancy, dysuria, and slow stream.[1, 3, 4, 31] If the obstruction worsens, symptoms can progress to nocturia, urgency, postvoid dribbling, hesitancy, intermittency, retention, and urgency incontinence.[3, 4, 31] Unfortunately, there is no one distinct voiding pattern that is diagnostic of prostate cancer. Infiltration of the seminal vesicles by tumor can result in hematospermia or decreased ejaculate volume if ejaculatory ducts are also involved.[3, 4, 31] Invasion of the neurovascular bundles can produce impotence.[3, 4, 31] Patients who present with bone metastasis frequently complain of bone pain, primarily in the lumbosacral spine.[3, 4, 31] Further metastatic manifestations of disease can include anemia, pancytopenia, weight loss, and perineal and leg pain.[3, 4, 31]

Physical findings needed as objective evidence to support a diagnosis of prostate cancer are obtained by a digital rectal exam (DRE).[3, 4, 31] The classic sign of the presence of carcinoma has been an abnormal exam reflecting indistinct, irregular margins; induration; or hard nodular areas. Alternate causes of a nodule or induration can include prostate calculus, prostatitis, focal infarction, or postbiopsy reaction.[3, 31] Clearly, a definitive diagnosis of carcinoma cannot be made on the basis of physical findings alone; subsequent objective workup and testing are needed to confirm the presence and extent of a prostate malignancy. Nonetheless, the DRE and patient symptomatology complaints are an integral part in determining the need for further testing and workup.

CONCLUSION

Effective management of prostate cancer is largely based on accurate detection and diagnosis. Knowledge of the natural history and cellular changes that occur within the prostate gland that can lead to carcinogenesis can enhance patient understanding of the disease process. Through proper grading techniques and determination of stage, appropriate treatment protocols are delineated. The identification of angiogenesis and the role of oncogenes and antioncogenes in the development of a cancer can lead to a better understanding of the progressive and biologic potential of the disease. A better understanding of prostate cancer pathogenesis will improve selection of contemporary treatment protocols, enhance patient management, and create a challenge for future research.

The nurse plays a role in facilitating the patient's understanding of the disease process, grading, potential for metastasis, and clinical manifestations. When signs and symptoms of disease are promptly recognized, management of the problem can be initiated, enhancing the patient's quality of life.

REFERENCES

1. American Cancer Society. *Cancer Facts & Figures.* Atlanta, GA: Author, 1998.

2. Bostwick DG. Evaluating prostate needle biopsy: Therapeutic and prognostic importance. *CA Cancer J Clin* 1997;47:297–319.

3. Oesterling J, Fuks Z, Lee CT, Scher HI. Cancer of the prostate. In: DeVita VT Jr, Hellman S, Rosenberg SA (eds). *Cancer: Principles & Practice of Oncology,* 5th ed. Philadelphia: Lippincott-Raven, 1997:1322–1345.

4. Held-Warmkessel J. Prostate Cancer. In: Groenwald SL, Frogge MH, Goodman M, Yarbro CH (eds). *Cancer Nursing Principles & Practice.* Sudbury, MA: Jones and Bartlett, 1997:1334–1354.

5. Volker DL. Carcinogenesis. In: Itano JK, Taoka KN (eds). *ONS Core Curriculum for Oncology Nursing,* 3rd ed. Philadelphia: WB Saunders, 1998:357–382.

6. Pacelli A, Bostwick DG. Clinical significance of high-grade prostatic intraepithelial neoplasia in transurethral resection specimens. *Urology* 1997;50: 355–359.

7. Wills ML, Hamper UM, Partin AW, Epstein JI. Incidence of high grade prostatic intraepithelial neoplasia in sextant needle biopsy specimens. *Urology* 1997;49(3):367–373.

8. Bostwick DG. High grade prostatic intraepithelial neoplasia: The most likely precursor of prostate cancer. *Cancer* 1995;75(Suppl):1823–1836.

9. Häggman MJ, Macoska JA, Wojno KJ, Oesterling JE. The relationship between prostatic intraepithelial neoplasia and prostate cancer: Critical issues. *J Urol* 1997;158:12–22.

10. Zlotta AR, Raviv G, Schulman CC. Clinical prognostic criteria for later diagnosis of prostate carcinoma in patients with initial isolated prostatic intraepithelial neoplasia. *Eur Urol* 1996;30:249–255.

11. Bostwick DG, Pacelli A, Lopez-Beltran A. Molecular biology of prostatic intraepithelial neoplasia. *Prostate* 1996;29:117–134.

12. Bostwick DG. Progression of prostatic intraepithelial neoplasia to early invasive adenocarcinoma. *Eur Urol* 1996;30:145–152.

13. Anonymous. Prostatic intraepithelial neoplasia: Significance and correlation with prostate-specific antigen and transrectal ultrasound. Proceedings of a workshop of the National Prostate Cancer Detection Project, March 13, 1989. Bethesda, MD. *Urology* 1989;34(Suppl):2.

14. Murphy GP, von Eschenbach AC, Bostwick, DG. International consultation on prostatic intraepithelial neoplasia and pathologic staging of prostatic carcinoma: Conference summary. *Cancer* 1996;78 324–325.

15. Bostwick DG, Qian I, Frankel K. The incidence of high grade prostatic intraepithelial neoplasia in needle biopsies. *J Urol* 1995;154:1791–1794.

16. Davidson D, Bostwick DG, Qian I, et al. Prostatic intraepithelial neoplasia is a risk factor for adenocarcinoma: Predictive accuracy in needle biopsies. *J Urol* 1996;154:1295–1299.

17. Berner A, Skjorten FJ, Fossa SD. Follow up of prostatic intraepithelial neoplasia. *Eur Urol* 1996;30: 256–260.

18. Ferguson J, Zincke H, Ellison E, et al. Decrease of prostatic intraepithelial neoplasia following androgen deprivation in patients with stage T_3 carcinoma treated by radical prostatectomy. *Urology* 1994;44: 91–95.

19. Wheeler TM. Influence of irradiation, and androgen ablation on prostatic intraepithelial neoplasia. *Eur Urol* 1996;30:261–264.

20. Kozlowski JM, Grayhack JT. Carcinoma of the prostate. In: Gillenwater JY, Grayhack JT, Howard SS, Duckett JW (eds). *Adult and Pediatric Urology,* 3rd ed. St. Louis, MO: CV Mosby, 1996: 1575–1713.

21. Aygun C. Small cell carcinoma of the prostate: A case report and review of the literature. *MD Med J* 1997;46:353–356.

22. Newman J. Epidemiology, diagnosis and treatment of prostate cancer. *Radiol Technol* 1996;68:39–68.

23. Stenman UH. Prostate specific antigen, clinical use and staging: An overview. *Br J Urol* 1997;79:53–60.

24. Bostwick DG. Grading prostate cancer. *Am J Clin Pathol* 1994;102:538–556.

25. Denmeade SR, Lin XS, Isaacs JT. Role of programmed (apoptotic) cell death during the progression and therapy for prostate cancer. *Prostate* 1996; 23:251–265.

26. Sakr WA, Grignon, DJ. Prostate cancer: Indicators of aggressiveness. *Eur Urol* 1997;32:15–23.

27. Boulikas T. Gene therapy of prostate cancer: p53, suicidal genes, and other targets. *Anticancer Res* 1997;17:1471–1506.

28. Siegal JA, Yu E, Brawer MK. Topography of neovascularity in human prostate carcinoma. *Cancer* 1995;75:2545–2551.

29. Folkman J, Watson K, Ingber D, Hanahan D. Introduction of angiogeneis during the transition from hyperplasia to neoplasia. *Nature* 1989;339: 58–61.

30. Ferrer FA, Miller LJ, Andrawis RI, et al. Angiogenesis and prostate cancer: In vivo and in vitro expression of angiogenesis factors by prostate cancer cells. *Urology* 1998;51:161–167.

31. McGinnis DE, Gomella LG. Tumors of the prostate. In: Babnson RR (ed). *Management of Urologic Disorders.* London: Wolfe, 1994:5.2–5.31.

32. Dorkin TJ, Neal DE. Basic science aspects of prostate cancer. *Semin Cancer Biol* 1997;8:21–27.

33. Griffiths K, Morton MS, Nicholson RI. Androgens, androgen receptors, antiandrogens and the treatment of prostate cancer. *Eur Urol* 1997;32:24–40.

34. Trapman J, Cleutjens KB, Kitty BJM. Androgen regulated gene expression in prostate cancer. *Semin Cancer Biol* 1997;8:29–36.

35. Habib FK, Grant ES. Molecular and cellular biology of the prostate: Is it clinically relevant? *Br J Urol* 1996;78:546–551.

36. McNeal JE, Bostwick DG. Intraductal dysplasia: A premalignant lesion of the prostate. *Human Pathol* 1986;17:64.

37. Oyasu R, Bahnson RR, Nowels K, Garnett JE. Cytological atypia in the prostate gland: Frequency, distribution and possible relevance to carcinoma. *Urology* 1986;136:959.

38. Kovi J, Mostofi FK, Heshmat MY, Enterline JP. Large acinar atypical hyperplasia and carcinoma of the prostate. *Cancer* 1988;61:555.

39. Troncosco P, Babaian RJ, Ro JY, Grignon DJ, Eschenbach AC, Ayala AG. Prostatic intraepithelial neoplasia and invasive prostatic adenocarcinoma in cysto-prostatectomy specimens. *Urology* 1989;34: 52.

40. Sakr WA, Haas GP, Cassin BF, Pontes JE, Crissman JD. The frequency of carcinoma and intraepithelial neoplasia of the prostate in young male patients. *J Urol* 1993;150:379.

41. de la Torre M, Haggman M, Brandstedt S, Busch C. Prostatic intraepithelial neoplasia (PIN) and

invasive carcinoma in total prostatectomy specimens: Distribution, volumes and DNA ploidy. *Brit J Urol* 1993;72:207.

42. Qian J, Bostwick DG. The extent and zonal location of prostatic intraepithelial neoplasia and atypical adenomatous hyperplasia: Relationship with carcinoma in radical prostatectomy specimens. *Path Res Pract* 1995;191:860.

43. Brawer MK, Bigler SA, Sohlberg OE, Nagle RB, Lange PH. Significance of prostatic intraepithelial neoplasia on prostate needle biopsy. *Urology* 1991; 38:103–107.

44. Ellis WJ, Brawer MK. Repeat prostate needle biopsy: Who needs it? *J Urol* 1995;153:1496–1498.

45. Aboseif S, Shinohara K, Weidner N, Narayan P, Carroll PR. The significance of prostatic intraepithelial neoplasia. *Br J Urol* 1995;76:355–359.

46. Weinstein MH, Epstein JI. Significance of high grade prostatic intraepithelial neoplasia on needle biopsy. *Human Pathol* 1993;24:624.

47. Keetch DW, Humphrey P, Stahl D, Smith DS, Catalona WJ. Morphometric analysis and clinical follow-up of isolated prostatic intraepithelial neoplasia in needle biopsy of the prostate. *J Urol* 1995:154:347–351.

48. Davidson D, Siroky M, Rudders R, Qian J, Oesterling J, Bostwick DG, Stilmant M. Prostatic intraepithelial neoplasia is a risk factor for adenocarcinoma: Predictive accuracy in needle biopsy of the prostate. *J Urol* 1995;154:1295–1299.

49. Markham CW. Prostatic intraepithelial neoplasia: Detection and correlation with invasive cancer in fine-needle biopsy. *Urology* 1989;35(Suppl):57–61.

50. Raviv G, Janssen TH, Zlotta AR, Descamps F, Verhest A, Schulman CC. Prostatic intraepithelial neoplasia: Influence of clinical and pathological data on the detection of invasive prostate cancer, in patients initially diagnosed on previous needle biopsy. *J Urol,* in press.

51. Raviv G, Zlotta AR, Janssen TH, Descamps F, Verhest A, Schulman CC. Does prostate-specific antigen and prostate-specific antigen density enhance the detection of prostate cancer in patients initially diagnosed to have prostatic intraepithelial neoplasia? *Cancer* 1996;77:2103–2108.

ASSESSMENT AND DIAGNOSIS

CINDY JO HORRELL

OVERVIEW

INTRODUCTION
CLINICAL PRESENTATION
HISTORY
PHYSICAL EXAMINATION
LABORATORY
  PSA Density
  Age-Specific PSA Reference Ranges
  Molecular Forms of PSA
    Free-PSA
    Reverse Transcriptase–Polymerase Chain
      Reaction Methodology

Prostate-Specific Membrane Antigen
E-cadherin
p27Kip 1
CD44
IMAGING
  Transrectal Ultrasonography
  Magnetic Resonance Imaging
  Computed Tomography
  Nuclear Scans
BIOPSY
CONCLUSION

INTRODUCTION

Cancer of the prostate is the most common noncutaneous malignancy in the United States. The American Cancer Society estimates 179,300 men will be diagnosed in 1999. The median age at diagnosis is 72 years. Many of those with prostate cancer, especially those in the early stage, will die of other illnesses without significantly experiencing the disability of the cancer. Survival of patients with prostate cancer depends on a number of factors, including tumor stage, grade, and serum prostate-specific antigen (PSA) level. Poorly differentiated tumors in particular are a high risk factor for early spread. This chapter discusses the clinical presentation, assessment, and diagnosis of the patient with prostate cancer.

CLINICAL PRESENTATION

Approximately 60% of patients have localized cancer when first diagnosed. Most of these patients will be asymptomatic or have only symptoms of lower urinary tract obstruction. Marked irritative symptoms in the absence of urinary tract infection should prompt a search for this malignancy.

The majority of these cancers (75%) will develop in the periphery of the prostate gland, where they will cause no symptoms. Local growth of the tumor causes obstructive voiding symptoms, including urinary hesitancy, diminished force of the urinary stream, intermittency, and postvoid dribbling (Figure 4-1). These may be misinterpreted as benign prostatic hyperplasia (BPH) (Table 4-1). As the detrusor muscle becomes less compliant, the bladder becomes unstable, causing urinary frequency, nocturia, and urgency incontinence. As the tumor extends, it can move outside the gland via the capsule or along the ejaculatory ducts to invade adjacent organs such as the seminal vesicles, bladder, rectum, and pelvic lymph nodes. The capsule is penetrated most often at the apex of the gland and least at the base. Seminal vesicle invasion, an independent predictor of disease progression, is associated with microscopic metastasis in lymph nodes.[1] Obstructed ejaculatory ducts can cause decreased volume of ejaculate. Impotence can occur as the tumor penetrates the prostatic capsule and invades the neurovascular bundles. Bone pain, frequently attributed to degenerative arthritis, especially in the axial and appendicular skeleton, may indicate metastatic disease. Characteristically osteoblastic, it

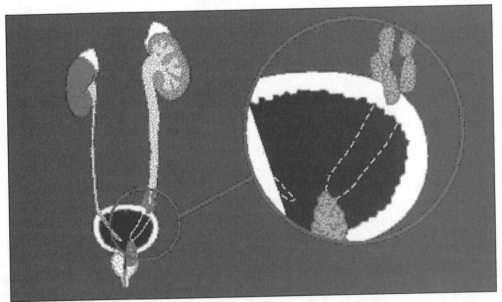

FIGURE 4-1. Obstruction of ureters resulting from prostate carcinoma
Reproduced with kind permission from Uronet [http://www.uronet.org].

TABLE 4-1. Comparison of Presenting Symptoms

Prostate Cancer	Benign Prostatic Hypertrophy
Decreased force of urinary stream; frequency, urgency, nocturia; residual urine	Same
Hermatospermia, decreased ejaculate volume	Not seen
Impotence	Uncommon
Lower extremity edema	Not seen
Bone pain	Not seen

is readily detected by bone scans. It is, therefore, mandatory to evaluate thoroughly patients with complaints of backache for impending spinal cord compression.

Lower extremity lymphedema suggests pelvic or inguinal adenopathy. Unusual presentations of prostate cancer include renal failure (as a result of bilateral ureteral obstruction), visceral metastasis, and pancytopenia (caused by bone marrow replacement). Patients with extensive bony metastasis can occasionally be minimally debilitated and have an excellent quality of life, although with disease progression the cancer cachexia syndrome is invariable.

HISTORY

There are three clearly established risk factors in the literature for prostate cancer: age, race, and family history. Every decade of aging nearly doubles the incidence of prostate cancer from 10% of men in their 50s to 70% of men in their 80s.

Conclusive evidence for a gene predisposing men to prostate cancer has been mapped to chromosome 1. The *HPC1* gene appears to cause about one in three of all inherited cases. This gene is especially common in African-American males, who are at a 30 to 50% higher risk than Caucasians for prostate cancer and have twice the mortality rate. Vasectomy is not a definite risk factor for the future development of prostate cancer, and individuals should be counseled accordingly.

Questions to be included in the history are found in Table 4-2. Medication history remains important because of the effects of certain drugs. Although these drugs have no effect on prostate cancer, identification of current medications can aid in the differential diagnosis. Anticholinergics (e.g., hyoscyamine sulfate [Levsin]), dicyclomine [Bentyl], meclizine [Antivert]) impair bladder contractility and alpha-sympathomimetics (e.g., over-the-counter cold and cough preparations containing pseudoephedrine) increase bladder outflow resistance.

PHYSICAL EXAMINATION

The gold standard for physical examination remains the digital rectal examination (DRE). When performed by a trained clinician, DRE allows for assessment of symmetry and texture of the prostate gland (Figure 4-2). The initial step is examination of the

TABLE 4-2. Patient History Questions

1. What is your age?
2. What is your race?
3. Is there any history in your family of prostate cancer?
4. What medications are you currently taking? (Include both prescription and over-the-counter medications.)
5. Have you ever had blood in your urine?
6. Have you ever had a urinary tract infection?
7. Do you have problems emptying your bladder completely? Have you ever had this problem?
8. Do you have diabetes?
9. Have you ever had problems passing your urine?
10. Have you ever had surgery on your urinary tract?

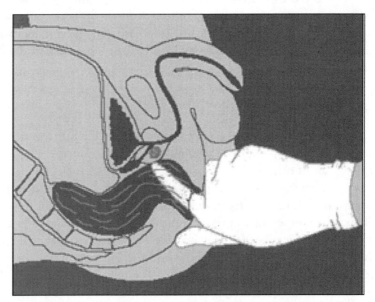

FIGURE 4-2. Cancer of the prostate may be detected on digital rectal exam as irregular, hard, or indurated areas with indistinct margins.
Reproduced with kind permission from Uronet [http://www.uronet.org].

external genitalia to exclude meatal stenosis or a palpable urethral mass. Next, the patient is examined from a posterior approach while he is supported in a bent-over or knee-chest position. The anal area is inspected. Using a well-lubricated gloved finger, the clinician assesses rectal sphincter tone on insertion. This provides evidence of the status of the somatic, sensory, and motor components of the sacral reflex arc. The rectum is thoroughly inspected, including the sacral hollow, to identify unsuspected rectal disease. The prostate gland, situated between the examining finger and the symphysis pubis, is palpated for size, consistency, and distinctness of margins. The gland is palpated for extension later-ally to the pelvic side wall, superiorly to seminal vesicles, and inferiorly at the apex to the pelvic floor diaphragm. Integrity of landmarks, including the median furrow and lateral sulci, is noted. The base of the seminal vesicle is examined for extension of induration.

Manifestation of an enlarged prostate includes increases in normal width (4.4 cm), length (3.4 cm), and thickness. Standardized nomenclature describing size has not been universally accepted. The common assessment includes estimation of dimensions. Classic signs of prostate cancer are irregular, stony, hard or indurated, and flat or nodular areas with indistinct margins. The presence of a noncancer cause for any palpable abnormality does not preclude carcinoma. Differential diagnoses include prostatitis, calculus, tuberculosis, focal infarction, postbiopsy tissue reaction, and BPH. Some patients with prostate cancer can present with a urinary tract infection that appears as prostatitis. Reexamination after a period of limited observation or active treatment should be done to confirm the abnormality. A disadvantage to the DRE is that only the posterior and lateral areas can be palpated, so precise tumor extent and volume cannot be assessed. Tumor size is an important prognostic indicator in prostate cancer. Minimum parameters used clinically to stage a patient with prostate cancer are the DRE in combination with serum PSA, biopsy, and Gleason scoring.

LABORATORY

The serum PSA is the single best test for early diagnosis of prostate cancer. In 1984, 6% of all prostate cancers were diagnosed by PSA elevations; in 1990, this rose to 68%.[2] A serine protease produced by normal, hyperplastic, and malignant cells of the prostate (Figure 4-3), PSA is involved in the liquefaction of the seminal coagulum, which is

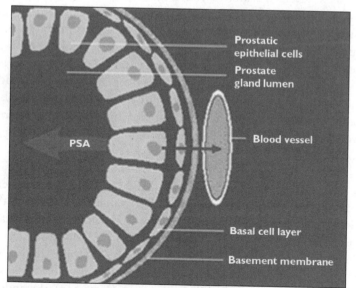

FIGURE 4-3. Prostate-specific antigen (PSA) is secreted exclusively by the prostatic epithelial cells.

Reproduced with kind permission from Uronet [http://www.uronet.org].

formed at ejaculation. The PSA is prostate specific, not cancer specific. The half-life in serum is approximately 3 days. Minute amounts, produced by the periurethral and anal glands, are not considered clinically significant.[3] Disrupting the normal prostatic architecture allows PSA to diffuse into the prostatic tissue, gaining access to the circulation. This can occur in the presence of prostate disease and with prostate manipulation (biopsy, DRE, massage). The change in PSA after DRE has been determined not to be clinically significant. The presence of prostate disease is the most important factor affecting PSA levels. Elevated levels in the blood are seen with BPH, prostatitis, acute urinary retention, cystoscopy, and transrectal ultrasonography (TRUS) of the prostate. PSA circulates in the blood in both bound and unbound forms. Most PSA is complexed to antiproteases. These protease inhibitors are present in large enough amounts to complex all enzymatically active PSA. Serum PSA concentrations of 4.0 ng/mL (monoclonal assay) are accepted as the upper limit of normal; however, more than 20% of men with prostate cancer have low levels.[4]

Treatment for BPH and prostate cancer can lower levels of PSA by decreasing the volume of prostatic tissue available to produce the protease. Finasteride is a 4-azasteroid inhibitor of one isoenzyme of 5α-reductase that converts testosterone to dihydrotestosterone (DHT). DHT stimulates growth in the transitional zone of the prostate, the site of initial BPH development. Finasteride, prescribed at a dosage of 5 mg/day for relief of symptomatic BPH, reduces the size of the gland, causing long-term symptomatic improvement.[5] After several months of treatment, PSA levels are decreased by approximately 50%. The drug is well absorbed after oral administration and undergoes extensive hepatic metabolism to essentially inactive metabolites that are eliminated through the bile and urine. Few adverse reactions are seen because the pharmacologic effects are specific to inhibition of the enzyme 5α-reductase, concentrated in the prostate gland, scalp, and genital skin. The most commonly reported adverse effects include loss of libido (3.3%) and sexual potency (2.8%), impotence (3.7%), breast tenderness, and enlargement.[6] Serum testosterone levels increase but do not exceed the upper limits of normal. One statistically significant drug interaction has been reported with the coadministration of finasteride and the α_1-adrenoceptor antagonist terazosin. Maximum plasma concentration and the area under the plasma concentration-time curve of finasteride, from 0 to 24 hours, were significantly higher. The clinical significance of this finding has not yet been determined.[7]

Studies were completed to describe the extent to which prostate cancer detection could be affected by treatment with finasteride. In 1997, the Finasteride PSA Study Group reported the effects of finasteride on PSA variability and found that the drug did not mask the detection of prostate cancer.[8] Two 1998 studies reported that, although total PSA serum levels decreased, the percent-free PSA (fPSA) did not change significantly ($P < .01$).[9, 10] In a randomized, double-blind, placebo-controlled trial, 3,040 men between the ages of 45 and 78 with no history of prostate cancer and a PSA less than 10 ng/mL were given either finasteride (N=1,524) or placebo (N=1,516). Prerandomization biopsy was negative for prostate cancer in 98% of men with a screening PSA of 4.0 ng/mL or more. End-of-study biopsy of the same patients verified negative pathology. Six hundred forty-four men (21%) underwent biopsy, and 201 (6.6%) underwent TRUS. Prostate cancer was diagnosed in 4.7% of men taking finasteride and in 34% of men taking placebo. Use of upper limit of normal for last PSA of 2.0 ng/mL for finasteride and 4.0 ng/mL for placebo yielded similar sensitivity (66% vs. 70%, P=.6) and higher specificity (82% vs. 74%, P < .0001). The researchers concluded that in men treated with finasteride, multiplying PSA by two and using normal ranges for untreated men preserves the usefulness of PSA for prostate cancer detection. PSA values must be interpreted in light of the presence of prostate disease, previous diagnostic procedures, and treatment directed at the prostate gland.

Combined with DRE, serum PSA detects histologically significant organ-confined disease. A major limitation of PSA levels is the considerable overlap between men with malignant disease and men with benign disease. This gray area includes measurements between 2 and 10 ng/mL. Methods to improve the ability of the PSA test to distinguish between men with BPH and those with cancer have led to the development of several PSA derivatives. These include PSA density, velocity, age-specific reference ranges, and others (fPSA, prostate-specific membrane antigen [PSMA], human glandular kallikrein [hK2]).

PSA DENSITY

PSA density is the ratio of serum PSA to the volume of the prostate gland estimated on TRUS. This technique of calculating approximate volume of the prostate is highly operator dependent. The justification for developing this measure is the assumption that prostate cancer tissue produces more PSA per gram of tissue than benign tissue of BPH. Therefore, levels greater than 0.15 suggest the presence of cancer. In a 1994 study, half of the tumors were missed using a PSA density cutoff of more than 0.15 for biopsy in men with PSA levels of 4 to 10 ng/mL and normal DRE.[11] The researchers concluded that men with PSA levels of 4.1 to 9.9 ng/mL should undergo biopsy based on serum PSA concentration rather than PSA density. Authors of a 1995 study concluded that PSA density compared with DRE was of limited additional value in correctly diagnosing prostate cancer in patients with intermediate PSA levels.[12]

AGE-SPECIFIC PSA REFERENCE RANGES

Age-specific measurements were developed to account for the normal enlargement of the benign prostate with age. BPH causes increased prostate volume. Therefore, elevated levels of PSA may be seen when, in fact, there is no malignancy. The value in this approach is the decrease in biopsies required in older men with PSA values greater than 4 ng/mL. Unfortunately, PSA age reference ranges have not been shown to be vastly superior to the usual PSA cut-off levels in diagnosing cancer.[13] The established reference ranges were based on studies of Caucasian males. A study to determine age-specific reference ranges in black men—who have a higher incidence of prostate cancer, are more likely to have advanced disease at diagnosis, and are more likely to die from the cancer—

was published in 1996.[14] PSA levels were measured in 3,475 men with no clinical evidence of prostate cancer (1,802 whites and 1,673 blacks) and 1,783 men with prostate cancer (1,372 whites and 411 blacks). The PSA concentrations were significantly higher in black men (geometric mean in controls, 1.48 ng/mL, and in patients, 7.46 vs. 1.33 ng/mL for white men; and in patients, 6.28). There was direct correlation of the values in the controls with age. Using traditional age-specific reference ranges with the test specificity at 95%, 41% of prostate cancers would have been missed. For 95% sensitivity among black men, the test's reference ranges would need to be modified. The authors concluded that maintaining the sensitivity at 95% as opposed to specificity was acceptable in identifying black men with prostate cancer. Similar racial differences in PSA levels have been described.[15]

MOLECULAR FORMS OF PSA

❑ Free-PSA

Studies have demonstrated that PSA exists in different molecular forms. The predominant forms are noncomplexed, or free form and a complexed form bound to α_1-antichymotrypsin (α_1-ACT), an endogenous protease inhibitor. Assays have been developed to distinguish the amount of PSA in the circulation that is unbound from the total amount present. This approach is based on the fact that BPH-produced PSA is predominately in the free form, whereas tumor-derived PSA is mainly complexed to ACT. Pannek and others[16] demonstrated the value of percent fPSA in staging clinically localized prostate cancer. A cut-off level of 12% fPSA provided a 72% positive predictive value and 52% negative predictive value for favorable diseases. With a cut-off value of 15% fPSA, 76% positive and 53% negative predictive values for organ-confined disease were seen. Catalona and colleagues[4] studied 914 men age 50 years or older with serum PSA levels of 2.6 to 4.0 ng/mL, a benign prostate examination, and no prior suspicious screening tests for prostate cancer. The purpose was to investigate the ability of percent fPSA to increase the sensitivity of total PSA. They discovered that the percent fPSA means for benign disease (20.2 ± 7.9%) and malignant cases (18.8 ± 6.9%) were not statistically significant (P=.10). The conclusion, based on 27% percent fPSA cutoff with 90% sensitivity and 18% specificity, was that percent fPSA could distinguish a group of benign diseases. The probability of cancer in the proposed normal group was not significantly different from that of the increased risk group (P=.16).

The objective of another study was to identify the lowest PSA level for which percent fPSA distributions differentiate between benign and malignant disease. The study also described at what percent fPSA level prostate cancer can be predicted.[17] Statistical analysis demonstrated that with a total PSA of 3.9 ng/mL, percent fPSA distributions for benign and malignant disease significantly differed and remained so when total PSA levels were 4.0 ng/mL. Men with malignant disease produced more complexed PSA as total PSA level increased. A strong negative correlation was established between total PSA and percent fPSA for malignant disease (P<.001). On the basis of the results of this study, the researchers suggested that the lower limit of percent fPSA reflex range should be 4.0 ng/mL.

Oesterling and colleagues[18] found that an increased ratio of protein-bound PSA to fPSA predicted cancer on biopsy independent of the total PSA level. The major proportion of serum PSA appears in complex with the protease inhibitor α_1-ACT. Brawer and associates[19] found measurement of complexed serum PSA yielded 95% sensitivity compared with fPSA–total PSA ratio. Studies are needed to confirm the findings, which could decrease false-positive PSA results as well as decrease the number of biopsies performed.

Preliminary data investigating whether the hK2 serum measurement improves the detection of prostate cancer in patient with total PSA levels of 4 to 0 ng/mL showed promise.[20] Of particular clinical interest was the finding that the hK2-fPSA ratio had a better specificity without loss of sensitivity for prostate cancer than total PSA or PSA-total ratio. Further studies are necessary to determine the significance of these findings, but hK2 in combination with fPSA may offer a new diagnostic study for the detection of prostate cancer.

❑ Reverse Transcriptase–Polymerase Chain Reaction Methodology

The development in molecular technology of a method termed *reverse transcriptase-polymerase chain reaction* (RT-PCR) allows identification of small amounts of prostate cells in tissues outside the prostate gland. The remarkable methodology identifies and amplifies the occurrence of specific DNA sequences in tissue. Using the enhanced RT-PCR assay, authors of a 1995 study demonstrated detection of as few as one PSA-synthesizing cell diluted into 10 million lymphocytes.[21] A positive PCR assay for PSA using peripheral blood suggests the presence of circulating prostate cells because the genetic message (messenger RNA) for PSA is prostate specific, not cancer specific. This diagnostic test has been used to detect prostate cells in the bone marrow, lymph nodes,[22] and peripheral blood specimens[23] of patients with metastatic prostate cancer. Ongoing multiinstitutional research continues in order to refine procedures and techniques to find reproducible sensitivity and reliability data that can be used as a basis for clinical decision making.

❑ Prostate-Specific Membrane Antigen

PSMA is an amino acid type II transmembrane glycoprotein highly specific for benign and malignant prostate epithelial cells. It is elevated in prostate cancers,[24] particularly in poorly differentiated,[25] metastatic, and hormone-refractory carcinomas.[26] Measured in serum using immunocompetitive and Western blot assays, its levels have been correlated with prediction of treatment failure and disease prognosis. A 1998 study published in *Cancer Research* showed the combined preoperative PSA-PSMA could predict extracapsular extension (P=.0001) and was superior to PSA, clinical stage, and Gleason score.[27] These data need to be verified because of the small numbers (N=11). PSMA is currently used as an immunoscintigraphic target using the antibody conjugate CYT-356 (ProstaScint, Cytogen, Princeton, NJ) to detect occult prostate cancer.

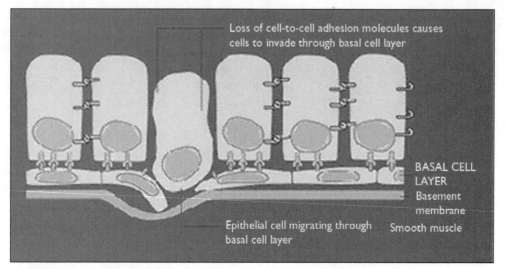

FIGURE 4-4. Deletion of E-cadherin causes loss of cell-to-cell adhesion molecules. Transformed epithelial cells can then migrate through the basal cell layer.
Reproduced with kind permission from Uronet [http://www.uronet.org].

❏ E-cadherin

Molecular tissue markers using histochemistry and cellular biological technologies are being developed. One molecular prognostic factor with potential is E-cadherin, a calcium-dependent cell surface glycoprotein found on epithelial cells that functions as an adhesion molecule. Loss of expression of this molecule enhances the invasiveness and motility of the epithelial cells (Figure 4-4). Correlation has been demonstrated between decreased E-cadherin expression and metastatic progression.[28] Two recent research studies[29, 30] concluded that, although there was a trend toward decreased expression of E-cadherin in metastatic prostate cancer, data did not support the marker as an independent prognostic indicator. This marker is being investigated in a prospective study for the Prostate Cancer Study Group.[31]

❏ p27Kip1

The protein p27Kip1 (also known as p27) is an inhibitor of the cell cycle with potential tumor suppressor function. Along with preoperative PSA, Gleason score, and pathologic stage, p27 immunohistochemistry was shown to be a strong independent predictor of disease-free survival.[32] The results of a study of 96 men with localized prostate cancer confirmed those findings.[33] Tumor samples were assayed for the presence of the p27 protein. Decreased p27 expression was significantly associated with an increased probability of recurrence ($P=.004$) and decreased survival ($P=.010$). The potential clinical and economic implications are significant in guiding the practitioner's choice of treatment. Current research is investigating whether levels of p27 expression play a role in tumor resistance to hormone therapy and chemotherapy.

❏ CD44

CD44, a metastasis-suppressor gene, was mapped to chromosome 11p13. Researchers using antibodies against CD44 analyzed a number of prostate cancer specimens.[34, 35] They concluded that CD44 expression was reduced in pelvic lymph nodes and in bone metastasis. The usefulness of this marker has not yet been established.

Several additional laboratory tests may aid in the differential diagnosis and formulation of the treatment plan. The complete blood count (CBC) with differential is done to assess the presence of anemia and infection. Urinalysis can analyze for glucose, protein, occult blood, and pH level. A requisition for a urine culture and sensitivity is sent, if indicated by elevated white blood cell count or presence of bacteria in the urinalysis. Creatinine and blood urea nitrogen (BUN) are analyzed to assess kidney function.

IMAGING

The major goal of imaging is to determine whether disease is confined to the prostate gland. Detection of metastasis in asymptomatic patients is dependent on the staging tests performed. Prognosis worsens when there is involvement of the pelvic lymph nodes. Lymphography, computed tomography (CT) scan, and magnetic resonance imaging (MRI) have been used to evaluate pelvic lymph nodes. Lymphography is of limited value because of inconsistent visualization of the hypogastric and obturator nodes. Common methods of imaging in the diagnosis of prostate cancer are described.

TRANSRECTAL ULTRASONOGRAPHY

TRUS uses a rectal ultrasound probe and ultrasonic energy. Currently, its main use is guiding needle biopsies. It cannot assess pelvic lymph node size. Volume of prostate tissue can be estimated from TRUS, but Brawer and others[36] found significant interobserver variability. In a National Institutes of Health–funded prospective multiinstitutional study, 386 patients underwent DRE and TRUS before radical prostatectomy.[37] The purpose was to determine the accuracy of these procedures in staging the local extent of biopsy-proven prostate cancer. After surgery, pathologic findings were correlated with preoperative TRUS and DRE. The calculated areas under the curve for transrectal ultrasound in predicting extracapsular tumor extension was 0.69 compared with 0.72 for DRE ($P=.64$) and for predicting seminal vesicle invasion, 0.74 and 0.69, respectively ($P=.36$). The researchers concluded that neither procedure proved superior to the other for staging local extent of prostate cancer. It is doubtful that procedures that depend on gross architectural changes will have high degrees of accuracy in detecting microscopic extension of tumor.

MAGNETIC RESONANCE IMAGING

MRI has undergone significant advances and has promise in the staging of prostate cancer. After pathologic confirmation of the cancer diagnosis, MRI is able to determine the extent by looking for capsular penetration, seminal vesicle and neurovascular bundle

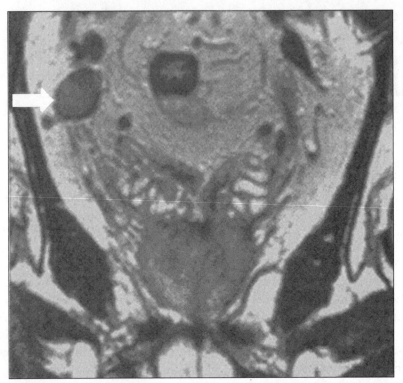

FIGURE 4-5. Magnetic resonance imaging reveals a large node (*arrow*) on the right
Reproduced with kind permission from Uronet [http://www.uronet.org].

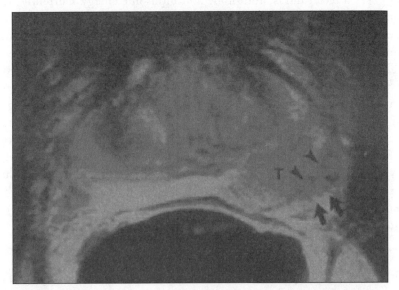

FIGURE 4-6. Endorectal magnetic resonance imaging with a posterolateral lesion involving the neurovascular bundle of that side
Reproduced with kind permission from Uronet [http://www.uronet.org].

invasion, regional lymph node metastasis, and bony metastasis (Figure 4-5). The endorectal MRI coil (Figure 4-6) for prostate imaging produces the highest sensitivity and specificity for identification of organ-confined and extracapsular disease.[38] The results were confirmed in a small study (N=70) using the endorectal coil MRI. The sensitivity and specificity in diagnosing capsular penetration were 77% and 81%, respectively. Seminal vesicle invasion was detected with 87% sensitivity and 96% specificity.[39] Addition of the pelvic-phased array (PPA) coils with the endopelvic coil array increased the signal anteriorly, providing high-quality images of the pelvis and lymph node sites.[40] Hricak and associates[41] demonstrated that the two coils were superior to PPA alone in detecting capsular penetration.

The significance of the radiologist's experience with interpretation of these particular MRIs cannot be overemphasized. Limitations to use of the MRI include expense, discomfort, and inability to obtain images and perform prostatic biopsy simultaneously.

COMPUTED TOMOGRAPHY

CT scan detects grossly enlarged lymph nodes but poorly defines the intraprostatic features. Factors that explain the failure of CT-documented disease may include low-volume disease, poor visualization of the prostate and surrounding structures, biopsy artifact, observer interpretation variability, and inability to distinguish between inflammation and neoplasm.[42] CT scans lack sensitivity and specificity in detecting extraprostatic extension.

Phase III clinical trials have shown promising results evaluating the use of radioimmunoscintigraphy in identifying sites of metastatic disease in lymph nodes.[43]

NUCLEAR SCANS

Some studies have shown that elevated PSA levels may predict positive bone scans.[44, 45] A bone scan is highly sensitive but relatively nonspecific. An equivocal positive finding needs to be correlated with plain radiographs. Lentle and colleagues[46] demonstrated that greater than 50% of bone density was replaced by tumor before routine radiographs identified bone metastasis. Radionuclide can localize in soft tissue areas, demonstrating calcification as well as infarction, inflammation, trauma, and tumor. In patients with PSA levels of 20 ng/mL and higher, a radionuclide bone scan is done to rule out metastases. A baseline chest radiograph is obtained to rule out lung metastases.

BIOPSY

Biopsy is required for definitive diagnosis and additional staging information. Traditional core biopsies have largely been replaced by sextant biopsies. In 1989, Hodge and coworkers[47] first described the concept of sextant biopsies for clinical staging. Using ultrasonography, six biopsies are taken transrectally in the parasagittal plane at the base, middle, and apex of the prostate gland plus directed biopsies of any hypoechoic defects (Figure 4-7). A disadvantage is the limited accuracy in detecting small-volume cancers (less than 5.1mL). Tissue is obtained using an 18-gauge needle aspiration (transrectally) or directly using ultrasound-guided approach.

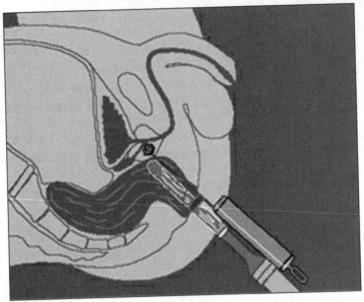

FIGURE 4-7. Transrectal ultrasound–guided biopsy of the prostate
Reproduced with kind permission from Uronet [http://www.uronet.org].

The transrectal approach is superior to transperineal or blind biopsy.[48] Eskew and colleagues[49] found detection rates improved using a five-region biopsy technique consisting of 13 or more biopsy cores per prostate. Compared with sextant (six-core) approach, 35% more cancers were identified. The 18-gauge needle is superior to the older 14-gauge needle. Rates of postbiopsy infections and hemorrhage with urinary clot retention have fallen to less than 1%. False-negative rates and quality of tissue specimen have improved.[48] As many as 18 biopsies can be obtained with relatively minor complications such as self-limiting hematuria, hematospermia, and low-grade fever.[49] These needles are also less likely to cause cancer seeding and implantation.[50] Prostate biopsy is performed on an outpatient basis. There is no special preparation by the patient. Nursing care involves assisting during the procedure and educating or instructing the patient and caregiver after the procedure. For TRUS-guided prostate biopsy, the patient lays on the table in the lithotomy position. Local anesthesia is given. An ultrasound probe is inserted into the rectum to guide the placement of the biopsy needle. The patient experiences a sensation of fullness or pressure. In the immediate postbiopsy period, fluids are encouraged, and the patient may be required to submit a urine specimen before discharge. This is an opportunity to examine the specimen for excessive hematuria. Table 4-3 summarizes patient postbiopsy discharge instructions.

In general, the degree of tumor differentiation and histology correlate directly with prognosis. There can be marked variability in the tumor from one area to another so many pathologists report the degrees of differentiation that are seen on the biopsy. The

TABLE 4-3. Postbiopsy Discharge Instructions

- Hematuria, with clots, is common for 24 hours.
- Bleeding and ecchymosis may occur at biopsy site.
- Avoid strenuous activity for 24 hours.
- Force fluids for 24 hours; avoid alcohol.
- Contact the physician if fever, chills, or dysuria occurs.
- Hermatospermia may occur up to 6 months after biopsy.

system used for histologic grading of the tumor is the Gleason system. In this system, prostate cancer cells are graded from 1 (well differentiated) to 5 (poorly differentiated) depending on the degree of anaplasia. Two numbers are assigned according to the two dominant grades observed. The sum of these two numbers equals the Gleason score. The higher the number, the more poorly differentiated is the tumor, and 95% of prostate cancers are adenocarcinomas.

Two commonly used systems for staging prostate cancer are the Jewett system (Stage A through D), which was introduced in 1975 and has since been modified, and the TNM system. The T stages are the same, with the TNM system using subcategories of the T to include those tumors found on screening. Several studies point to the importance of multimodality staging in the subset of patients with intermediate PSA levels (10–20 ng/mL) and Gleason scores of 5 to 7.[51–53]

CONCLUSION

Many questions still need to be answered regarding utilization of the PSA and the PSA derivatives. The role of MRI needs to be addressed. More sensitive and specific diagnostic and staging tools must be developed to decrease not only the morbidity and financial burden of prostate cancer but the psychological impact as well. Educating the patient about how the diagnostic tests are performed, the length of the procedure, and the sensations that may be experienced during the test will help reduce patient concerns and promote patient cooperation during the study. Afterward the patient needs to understand any pertinent self-care measures and when it is appropriate to contact his health care provider.

REFERENCES

1. Epstein JI, Carmichael M, Walsh PC. Adenocarcinoma of the prostate invading the seminal vesicle: Definition and relation of tumor volume, grade, and margins of resection to prognosis. *J Urol* 1993; 149:1040–1045.
2. Mettlin C, Jones G, Murphy G. Trends in prostate cancer care in the United States, 1974–1990: Observations from the Patient Care Evaluation Studies of the American College of Surgeons Commission on Cancer. *CA Cancer J Clin* 1993;43:83–91.
3. Lee W, Giantonio B, Hanks G. Prostate cancer. *Curr Probl Cancer* 1994;18:295–357.
4. Catalona WJ, Smith DS, Ornstein DK. Prostate cancer detection in men with serum PSA concentrations of 2.4 to 4.0 ng/mL and benign prostate examination. *JAMA* 1997;277:1452–1455.

5. Marberger MJ. Long-term effects of finasteride in patients with benign prostatic hypertrophy: A double blind, placebo-controlled, multicenter study. PROWESS Study Group. *Urology* 1998;51:677–686.

6. Hebel SL (ed.) *Drug Facts & Comparison.* 52nd ed. St. Louis, MO; Wolters Kluwer; 1998.

7. Vashi V, Chung M, Hilbert J, et al. Pharmacokinetic interaction between finasteride and terazosin, but not finasteride and doxazosin. *J Clin Pharmacol* 1998;38:1072–1076

8. Oesterling JE, Roy J, Agha A, et al. Biologic variability of prostate-specific antigen and its usefulness as a marker for prostate cancer: Effects of finasteride. The Finasteride PSA Study Group. *Urology* 1997;50:13–18.

9. Pannek J, Marks L, Pearson J, et al. Influence of finasteride on free and total serum prostate specific antigen levels in men with benign prostatic hyperplasia. *J Urol* 1998;159:449–453.

10. Andriole G, Guess H, Epstein J, et al. Treatment with finasteride preserves usefulness of prostate-specific antigen in the detection of prostate cancer: Results of a randomized, double-blind, placebo-controlled clinical trial. *Urology* 1998;52:195–201.

11. Catalona W, Ritchie J, deKernion J. Comparison of prostate specific antigen concentration versus prostate specific antigen density in the early detection of prostate cancer: Receiver operating characteristic curves. *J Urol* 1994;152:2031–2036.

12. Van Iersel MP, Witjes WP, de la Rosette JJ, et al. Prostate-specific antigen density: Correlation with histological diagnosis of prostate cancer, benign prostatic hypertrophy and prostatitis. *Br J Urol* 1995;76:47–53.

13. Catalona W, Hudson M, Scardino P. Selection of optimal prostate specific antigen cutoffs for early detection of prostate cancer: Receiver operating characteristic curves. *J Urol* 1994;152:2037–2042.

14. Morgan TO, Jacobsen SJ, McCarthy WF, et al. Age-specific reference ranges for prostate-specific antigen in black men. *N Engl J Med* 1996;335:304–310.

15. Smith DS, Bullock AD, Catalona WJ, Herschman JD. Racial differences in a prostate cancer screening study. *J Urol* 1996;156:1366–1369.

16. Pannek J, Rittenhouse H, Chan D, et al. The use of percent free prostate specific antigen for staging clinically localized prostate cancer. *J Urol* 1998;159:1238–1242.

17. Carlson GD, Calvanese CB, Childs SJ. The appropriate lower limit for the percent-free prostate-specific antigen reflex range. *Urology* 1998;52:450–454.

18. Oesterling JE, Jacobsen SJ, Klee GG, et al. Free, complexed and total serum prostate specific antigen: The establishment of appropriate reference ranges for their concentrations and ratios. *J Urol* 1995;154:1090–1095

19. Brawer M, Meyer G, Letran J, et al. Measurement of complexed PSA improves specificity for early detection of prostate cancer. *Urology* 1998;52:372–378.

20. Kwiatkowski MK, Recker F, Piironem T, et al. In prostatism patients the ratio of human glandular kallikrein to free PSA improves the discrimination between prostate cancer and benign hyperplasia within the diagnostic "gray zone" of total PSA 4 to 10 ng/mL. *Urology* 1998;52:360–364

21. Katz AE, de Vries GM, Begg MD, et al. Enhanced reverse-transcriptase polymerase chain reaction for prostate specific antigen as an indicator of true pathologic stage in patients with prostate cancer. *Cancer* 1995;75:1642–1648.

22. Vassella RL, Blouke KA, Stray JE, et al. The use of the polymerase chain reaction to detect metastatic prostate cancer in lymph nodes and bone marrow. *Proc Am Assoc Cancer Res* 1992;33:2376.

23. Moreno JG, Croce CM, Fischer R, et al. Detection of micrometastasis in patients with prostate cancer. *Cancer Res* 1994;54:6344

24. Bostwick DG, Pacelli A, Blute M, et al. Prostate specific membrane antigen expression in prostatic intraepithelial neoplasia and adenocarcinoma: A study of 184 cases. *Cancer* 1998;82:2256–2261.

25. Israeli RS, Powell CT, Lorr JG, et al. Expression of the prostate-specific membrane antigen. *Cancer Res* 1994;54:1807–1811.

26. Wright GL, Grob M, Haley C, et al. Upregulation of prostate-specific antigen after androgen deprivation therapy. *Urology* 1996;48:326–334.

27. Grasso Y, Gupta M, Levin H, et al. Combined nested RT-PCR assay for prostate-specific antigen and prostate-specific membrane antigen in prostate cancer patients: Correlation with pathologic stage. *Cancer Res* 1998;58:1456–1459.

28. Umbas R, Schalken JA, Aalders TW, et al. Expression of the cellular adhesion molecule E-cadherin is reduced or absent in high-grade prostate cancer. *Cancer Res* 1992;52:5104–5109.

29. Paul R, Ewing CM, Jarred DF, et al. The cadherin cell-cell adhesion pathway in prostate cancer progression. *Br J Urol* 1997;79(Suppl 1): 37–43.

30. Cheng L, Magabhushan M, Pretlow TP, et al. Expression of E-cadherin in primary and metastatic prostate cancer. *Am J Pathol* 1996;148: 1375–1380.

31. Ruijter E, van de Kaa C, Aalders T, et al. Heterogeneous expression of E-cadherin and p53 in prostate cancer: Clinical implications. BIOMED-II Markers for Prostate Cancer Study Group. *Mod Pathol* 1998;11:276–281.

32. Yang RM, Naitoh J, Murphy M, et al. Low p27 expression predicts poor disease-free survival in patients with prostate cancer. *J Urol* 1998;159:941–945.

33. Cote RF, Shi Y, Groshen S, et al. Association of p27Kip 1 levels with recurrence and survival in patients with stage C prostate carcinoma. *J Natl Cancer Inst* 1998;90:916–920.

34. Gao AC, Lou W, Dong JT, et al. CD44 is a metastasis suppressor gene for prostatic cancer located on human chromosome 11p13. *Cancer Res* 1997;57: 846–849.

35. DeMarzo AM, Bradshaw C, Sauvageot J, et al. CD44 and CD44v6 downregulation in clinical prostatic carcinoma: Relation to Gleason grade and cytoarchitecture. *Prostate* 1998;34:162–168.

36. Brawer M, Aramburu E, Chen G. The inability of prostate specific antigen index to enhance the predictive value of prostate specific antigen in the diagnosis of prostatic carcinoma. *J Urol* 1993;150:369–373.

37. Smith J, Scardino P, Resnick M, et al. Transrectal ultrasound versus digital rectal examination for the staging of carcinoma of the prostate: Results of a prospective multiinstitutional trial. *J Urol* 1997; 157:902–906.

38. Schiebler M, Schnall M, Pollack H. Current role of MRI imaging in the staging of adenocarcinoma of the prostate. *Radiology* 1993;189:339–352.

39. Masi A, Olmastroni M, Marin E, et al. Magnetic resonance with an endorectal coil and fast spin echo sequence in the staging of prostate carcinoma. The correlation with histopathological data. *Radiol Med* 1997;94:496–502.

40. Cheng D, Tempany C. MR imaging of the prostate and bladder. *Semin Ultrasound CT MRI* 1998;19: 67–89.

41. Hricak H, White S, Vigneron D, et al. Carcinoma of the prostate gland: MR imaging with pelvic phased array coils versus endorectal-pelvic phased array coils. *Radiology* 1994;193:703–709.

42. Manyak MJ. Clinical applications of radioimmunoscintigraphy with prostate-specific antibodies for prostate cancer. *Cancer Control* 1998;5:493–499.

43. Hinkle GH, Burgers JK, Neal CE, et al. Multi center radioimmunoscintigraphic evaluation of patients with prostate carcinoma using indium-111 capromab pendetide. *Cancer* 1998;83:739–747.

44. Oesterling J, Martin S, Bergstralh E. The use of PSA in staging patients newly diagnosed with prostate cancer. *JAMA* 1993;269:57–60.

45. Huncharek M, Muscat J. Serum PSA as a predictor of radiographic staging studies in newly diagnosed prostate cancer. *Cancer Invest* 1995;13:31–35.

46. Lentle BC, McGowan DG, Dierich H. Technetium-99m polyphosphate bone scanning in carcinoma of the prostate. *Br J Urol* 1994;46:543

47. Hodge K, McNeal J, Terris M, Stamey T. Random systematic versus directed ultrasound guided transrectal core biopsies of the prostate. *J Urol* 1989; 142:71.

48. Bostwick D. Evaluating prostate needle biopsy: Therapeutic and prognostic importance. *CA Cancer J Clin* 1997;47:297–319.

49. Eskew L, Bare R, McCullough D. Systemic 5 region prostate biopsy is superior to sextant method for diagnosing carcinoma of the prostate. *J Urol* 1997; 157:199–203.

50. Bostwick D, Vonk J, Picado A. Pathologic changes in the prostate following contemporary 18 gauge needle biopsy: No apparent risk of local cancer seeding. *J Urol Pathol* 1994;2:203–212.

51. Partin AW, Yoo J, Carter B, et al. The use of prostate-specific antigen, clinical stage and Gleason score to predict pathological stage in men with localized prostate cancer. *J Urol* 1993;150:110–114.

52. Partin AW, Kattan MW, Subong ENP, et al. Combination of prostate-specific antigen, clinical stage, and Gleason score to predict pathologic stage of localized prostate cancer. *JAMA* 1997;277:1445–1451.

53. D'Amico AV, Whittington R, Schnall M, et al. The impact of the inclusion of endorectal coil magnetic resonance imaging in a multivariate analysis to predict clinically unsuspected extraprostatic cancer. *Cancer* 1995;75:2368–2372.

Chapter 5

STAGING OF PROSTATE CANCER

MARY COLLINS

OVERVIEW

INTRODUCTION
CLASSIFICATION SYSTEMS
   Whitmore-Jewett System
   Tumor Node Metastasis Staging System
   1992 AJCC-UICC TNM System
   T1c Tumors
   Limitations of the 1992 AJCC-UICC TNM
     Classification System
   Benefits of the AJCC-UICC TNM System
CLINICAL STAGING
   Digital Rectal Examination
   Serum Tumor Markers
     Prostatic Acid Phosphatase

   Prostate-Specific Antigen
   Transrectal Ultrasonography
   Bone Scan
   Computed Tomography
   Magnetic Resonance Imaging
   Pelvic Lymphadenectomy
SIGNIFICANCE OF TUMOR STAGING
PATHOLOGIC STAGE
HISTOLOGIC GRADE
COMBINING CLINICAL FACTORS TO PREDICT
   PATHOLOGIC STAGE
CONCLUSIONS

INTRODUCTION

Staging or determining the extent of prostate cancer has two goals: (1) to define the extent of the disease; and (2) to guide appropriate therapy.[1] The volume of disease correlates directly with a prognosis in men who are newly diagnosed with prostate cancer. An accurate assessment of disease volume is critical when prostate cancer is initially diagnosed because there is no adjuvant therapy that affects survival if extracapsular disease is present. Pretreatment staging with a prostate-specific antigen (PSA), digital rectal examination (DRE), histologic grade, and imaging provides a way of differentiating among clinically localized, locally advanced, and metastatic disease in men with prostate cancer.

Understanding the general concepts of staging will assist healthcare workers in the care of patients with prostate cancer.

CLASSIFICATION SYSTEMS

WHITMORE-JEWETT SYSTEM

The most commonly used staging system for prostate cancer was developed by Whitmore in 1956.[2, 3] According to this system, the disease was divided into four categories: Stage A represents a tumor identified incidentally on transurethral resection of the prostate but not palpable; Stage B, palpable tumor confined to the prostate; Stage C, local extension beyond the prostate but without evidence of metastatic disease; and Stage D, metastatic disease.[4, 5]

In 1959, the American Joint Committee on Cancer (AJCC) Staging and End Results Reporting assigned a task force to stage urologic cancers.[5] As a result, Jewett revised the Whitmore system to include subclassifications. The Whitmore-Jewett staging system for clinically localized prostate cancer reflects the pathologic features of the tumor and provides significant prognostic information.[4, 5] Stage A disease is subclassified as focal or localized (A1) or diffuse or widespread (A2) and includes histologic differentiation of the tumor. Stage B is subclassified into tumor that involves either less than one lobe of the prostate (B1) or one lobe or more of the gland but without extracapsular involvement (B2). Stage C is subclassified into minimal extracapsular disease (C1) or extensive extracapsular disease resulting in bladder outlet or ureteral obstruction (C2).

The advantages of the Whitmore-Jewett system are that it is simple and widely recognized within the United States.[6] The disadvantage is that it is less accurate in reporting local or distant disease. For example, although only 25% of Stage B tumors will have lymph node metastases or Stage D1 disease, describing these as D1 does not specify the local extent of the tumor.

Another drawback to the Whitmore-Jewett system, or the American classification system as it is sometimes referred, is lack of uniformity in reporting results.[6] For example, some institutions may report a B1 tumor as smaller than 1.5 cm, whereas others may report it as less than 2.0 cm. Stage B may be separated into Stages B1 or B2, or some may report a Stage B tumor as B1, B2, and B3. There is no specific staging within the Whitmore-Jewett classification system for describing pathologic involvement of the capsule, no classification for metastatic sites, and no differentiation within the classification for local spread versus seminal vesicle involvement.

TUMOR NODE METASTASIS STAGING SYSTEM

In 1974, outside North America, a tumor, node, metastasis (TNM) classification system was introduced by the International Union Against Cancer (UICC).[7] Although this TNM system was accepted by AJCC Staging and End Results Reporting, the TNM system for prostate cancer never gained acceptance in North America. In 1988, the Organ

System Coordinating Center classification attempted to combine the TNM system and the North American system by adding A, B, C, and D after T to indicate the stage of the primary tumor and included the N and M as well.

Because of the initial confusion between UICC and AJCC, the continued conflicts with revisions of the system, and the complexity of this system in relation to the fairly simple Whitmore-Jewett system, the UICC-AJCC TNM system never gained acceptance in the United States, Japan, and Britain or with the European Organization for Research and Treatment of Cancer.[7]

1992 AJCC-UICC TNM SYSTEM

In 1992, after several revisions of the TNM system, AJCC and UICC proposed a TNM system for staging localized prostate cancer. The new system was developed with the following goals: (1) assist in the daily practice of urologic oncology; (2) retain basic principles of the Whitmore system; and (3) be flexible enough to include information derived from new technology[6] (see Table 5-1).

Stage A is now T1, which is the category for tumors not visible on imaging or palpable on DRE but discovered on tissue removed for bladder neck obstruction or after needle biopsy for elevated PSA.[8, 9] Stage A1 (T1a) disease is a well-differentiated tumor found in less than 5% of the resected tissue. Stage A2 (T1b) is less differentiated, more widespread disease involving greater than 5% of the resected tissue or disease with an elevated PSA (Stage T1c).

Stage T2 (B) disease is an organ-confined tumor with no definite evidence of local or distant spread found on DRE, imaging, or tumor markers.[8-10] Within Stage B1, there are two classifications that differentiate the amount of lobe involvement. T2a tumors occupy up to one half of one lobe or less, whereas T2b tumors involve more than one half of one lobe but not both lobes. A tumor that involves both lobes of the prostate without evidence of extension is considered stage T2c (B2).

Stage T3 (C) is further subdivided into T3a, T3b, and T3c (C1, C2, and C3, respectively).[9] This stage consists of tumors that have extended outside of the prostate, including the seminal vesicles, but without evidence of distant metastases. The incident of lymphatic metastases is approximately 50%, upstaging T3 (C) to D1 (positive pelvic nodes).[10]

Stage T1-4, N0-3, M0-1 (D) disease has been divided into several subsets.[9] Individuals with clinically localized prostate cancer who have positive pelvic lymph nodes removed at surgery or laparoscopic lymph node dissection are subclassified as N1-3 (D1). Stage N1 indicates disease in a single regional lymph node 2 cm or smaller; N2 indicates a regional node larger than 2 cm but smaller than 5 cm; N3 indicates a regional node larger than 5 cm. Patients with a persistently elevated serum acid phosphatase after surgery are designated as Stage D0 and have a particularly high risk of disseminated disease. A T4 category designates a tumor that is fixed or invades seminal vesicles other than adjacent structures and organs. Stage M1a-1c (D2) includes metastases to distant nodes, lungs, bones, and soft tissue.

TABLE 5-1. Comparison of TNM and Whitmore-Jewett Staging Systems

TNM	Description	Whitmore-Jewett	Description
TX	Primary tumor cannot be assessed	None*	None
T0	No evidence of primary tumor	None	None
T1	Clinically unapparent tumor—not palpable or visible by imaging	A	Same as TNM
T1a	Tumor found incidentally in tissue removed at TUR; 5% or less of tissue is cancerous	A1	Same as TNM
T1b	Tumor found incidentally at TUR; more than 5% of tissue is cancerous	A2	Same as TNM
T1c	Tumor identified by prostate needle biopsy because of PSA elevation	None	None
T2	Palpable tumor confined within the prostate	B	Same as TNM
T2a	Tumor involves half of a lobe or less	B1N	Tumor involves half of a lobe or less; surrounded by normal tissue
T2b	Tumor involves more than half a lobe but not both lobes	B1	Tumor involves less than one lobe
T2c	Tumor involves both lobes	B2	Tumor involves one entire lobe or more
T3	Palpable tumor extending through prostate capsule and/or involving seminal vesicle(s)	C1	Tumor <6 cm in diameter
T3a	Unilateral extracapsular extension	C1	Same as TNM
T3b	Bilateral extracapsular extension	C1	Same as TNM
T3c	Tumor invades seminal vesicle(s)	C1	Same as TNM
T4	Tumor is fixed or invades adjacent structures other than seminal vesicles	C2	Tumor > 6 cm in diameter
T4a	Tumor invades bladder neck and/or external sphincter and/or rectum	C2	Same as TNM
T4b	Tumor invades levator muscles and/or is fixed to pelvic wall	C2	Same as TNM
N	Involvement of regional lymph nodes	D1	Same as TNM
None	None	D0	Elevation of prostatic acid phosphatase only (enzymatic assay)
NX	Regional lymph nodes cannot be assessed	None	None
N0	No regional lymph node metastases	None	None
N1	Metastasis in a single regional lymph node, <2 cm in greatest dimension	D1	Same as TNM
N2	Metastasis in a single regional lymph node, > 2 cm but not > 5 cm in greatest dimension, or multiple regional lymph nodes, none > 5 cm in greatest dimension	D1	Same as TNM
N3	Metastasis in a regional lymph node > 5 cm in greatest dimension	D1	Same as TNM
M	Distant metastatic spread	D2	Same as TNM
MX	Presence of distant metastases cannot be assessed	None	None
M0	No distant metastases	None	None
M1	Distant metastases	D2	Same as TNM
M1a	Involvement of nonregional lymph nodes	D2	Same as TNM
M1b	Involvement of bones	D2	Same as TNM
M1c	Involvement of other distant sites	D2	Same as TNM
None	None	D3	Hormone refractory disease

None, no comparable category; TUR, transurethral resection; PSA, prostate-specific antigen.
Modified from Ballentine-Carter H, Carter AW. Prostate cancer staging. In: Walsh PC, Retik AB, Vaughn ED, Wein AJ (eds). *Campbell's Urology.* Philadelphia: WB Saunders, 1998. Reprinted with permission.

T1c TUMORS

Among the changes introduced by the 1992 AJCC-UICC TNM system was the classification of nonpalpable tumors discovered by an elevated PSA level and transrectal ultrasonography (TRUS) to a new category, T1c.[7] Staging of localized prostate cancer had traditionally been determined from results of the DRE or incidentally discovered on a transurethral resection of the prostate (TURP) procedure. Consequently, localized prostate cancer was divided into Stage A or B: palpable tumors confined to the prostate or nonpalpable tumors found on TURP. Between revisions of the 1987 and 1992 editions of the TNM system, TRUS and PSA were shown to be superior in predicting cancer than directed biopsies of visible or palpable nodules, which led to the new classification.

PSA has become the most useful tumor marker for screening men in whom prostate cancer will develop.[7] Therefore, on the basis of an abnormal PSA, men are having a biopsy in spite of a normal DRE or TRUS. The clinical significance of these T1c tumors seems to be similar to a T2 (palpable nodule) given similarities in findings from radical prostatectomy pathology specimens. Options for treatment of patients with a T2 nodule (surgery, observation with delayed treatment, and radiation therapy) are all presented to the patient with a T1c lesion because of the similarities in the natural history. Additional information such as grade and pathology of the biopsy are also critical variables.

LIMITATIONS OF THE 1992 AJCC-UICC TNM CLASSIFICATION SYSTEM

In spite of the advantages of the 1992 TNM system, areas of controversy remain.[6, 8] TRUS is the best imaging technique to identify a prostate nodule. However, because many urologists are doubtful that TRUS captures the extent of the disease, there is inconsistency in staging. If there is confidence that the TRUS identified a nodule in less than one half of the lobe, the stage would be T2a; if there is doubt that the TRUS identified the nodule, the tumor may be considered a T1c. This inconsistency can be very confusing but may not be clinically significant.[7] Data indicate that pathologic characteristics of T2a-T2b cancers are similar to T1c cancers and therefore, have the same prognosis.[7]

One of the drawbacks of any staging system is that new information dictates a change in the stage.[1] Stage migration suggests change from a lower stage to a higher stage based on more exact methods to define the extent of the disease. Advances in imaging studies, improvements in histopathologic tissue evaluation, and identification of micrometastases in pelvic lymph nodes all may indicate stage migration. For example, stage migration of patients from T2, N0, M0 to T3, N0, M0 or T2, N1, M0 may well influence the patient's survival rate on which the original stage classification was based.

Current staging is restricted by a significant amount of understaging, as much as 59%, as opposed to only 5% of overstaging demonstrated by results of pathologic specimens from resected prostate surgical specimens.[11] Accuracy of TRUS and DRE contribute to the upstaging of the tumor, as do limitations in subjectivity.

BENEFITS OF THE AJCC-UICC TNM SYSTEM

The AJCC-UICC TNM staging system retains the basis of the Whitmore system and offers a greater number of tumor categories than previous staging systems.[4] Although the AJCC-UICC TNM system defines the anatomic extent of the disease, that is not the only information that reflects prognoses. PSA, histologic grade, and DNA analysis are variables that, combined with the TNM system, can provide information to the physician and patient. With further improvements in diagnostic tools, there will probably be more changes and additions in the staging of prostate lesions, but presently it is the most accurate and practical system for clinicians as well as researchers.[4, 10]

CLINICAL STAGING

Primary tumor T stage is the clinical determination of the local extension of disease most commonly assessed by DRE, serum tumor markers, and histologic or cytologic confirmation of prostate cancer.[12, 13] Additional information from imaging and pelvic lymphadenectomy are also used for clinical staging. All information before initial definitive treatment may be included for clinical staging.

DIGITAL RECTAL EXAMINATION

DRE is the simplest method of evaluating the local extent of prostate cancer.[1] However, DRE lacks specificity (the ability of a test to detect that there is no disease) when determining organ-confined disease and sensitivity (the ability of a test to detect disease when it is present) for non-organ-confined disease when the predicted clinical stage is correlated with the pathologic findings.[13] Because DRE is so subjective, studies have found that even if one urologist performs the DRE as well as the radical prostatectomy and one individual pathologist reviews the specimens, the overall specificity for determining organ-confined disease by DRE was only 9%.[6, 13] Sensitivity was 98%, whereas overall accuracy was 57.7%. Conversely, DRE is a better predictor (80–93%) of non-organ-confined disease.[7, 13] For example, when a DRE categorizes the nodule as a stage T3A or greater, it is more than likely a non-organ-confined tumor. In spite of the limitations of DRE, clinical staging for prostate cancer begins with a carefully performed examination.

SERUM TUMOR MARKERS

❑ Prostatic Acid Phosphatase

Prostatic acid phosphatase (PAP) is secreted by the prostatic epithelial cells in men, but other isoenzymes are present in the liver, bone, muscle, and platelets.[6] PAP may be elevated in extracapsular disease but also in prostatitis and after prostate manipulations and DREs. PAP is also elevated in metastatic tumors to the bone and liver.

PAP correlates directly with the stage of prostate cancer.[6] PAP is rarely elevated in organ-confined disease but is elevated in approximately 67% of patients with extracapsular disease. A small contingent of patients present with clinically localized prostate cancer, normal bone scan, and even negative lymph node report but have an elevated PAP (D0) disease. This group of patients is at risk for progression within 18 months because their disease is already advanced at diagnosis but yet undetectable except by the elevated PAP.

❑ Prostate-Specific Antigen

PSA is an enzyme produced by the columnar epithelial cells of the prostate and peri-urethral glands.[14] Although PSA is organ specific, it is not cancer specific. In fact, benign hyperplastic tissue produces more PSA protein than malignant tissue produces. Serum PSA levels are normally less than 4 ng/mL, but disruption in the structure of the prostate as a result of trauma or disease allows PSA to escape into the bloodstream via the lymphatics or capillaries. PSA concentration only increases a small amount (0.3 ng/mL/g) in benign conditions compared with a larger increase with cancer (3.5 ng/mL/g) in malignant conditions.

Although advanced clinical and pathologic stage along with tumor volume tend to correlate with an increase in PSA value, PSA levels alone are not reliable to predict final pathologic stage.[14] PSA contributes approximately 0.3 ng/mL of benign prostatic hypertrophy (BPH) tissue, but the exact contribution that BPH tissue adds to total serum PSA is unknown. The pretreatment PSA is complicated by the volume of BPH tissue and the tumor grade, both of which influence PSA levels.[15, 16] This results in the overlap of serum PSA levels between stages, which prohibits prediction of the final pathologic stage.[1] As a general guideline, the majority of men with a PSA level lower than 4.0 ng/mL have organ-confined disease; greater than 50% of men with a PSA level higher than 10.0 ng/mL have capsular penetration; and the majority of men (75%) with a PSA greater than 50 ng/mL have positive lymph nodes.[15] Partin and colleagues[16] also reported that men with higher grade, higher volume prostate tumors produce less PSA per gram of tumor. More poorly differentiated tumors may not produce markers of more mature differentiation, like PSA.[16]

Establishing a threshold for PSA as a staging marker is not desirable because of the inaccuracy of negative values.[17] For example, if a PSA of 500 ng/mL was established as the level indicative of metastatic disease, there could be large numbers of men with metastatic disease with PSA below 500, thus, there would be little overall advantage from the established marker. Rather, the ability to predict a pathologic stage based on the PSA can be improved by combining PSA, tumor grade (from the biopsy specimen), and local clinical stage determined from the DRE.[14]

TRANSRECTAL ULTRASONOGRAPHY

Although there are multiple indications for TRUS of the prostate, the most common reason is for the evaluation of prostate cancer.[18] TRUS, in combination with prostatic needle biopsy, is usually recommended for an abnormal DRE or elevated PSA level. TRUS has the ability to provide imaging and simplifies biopsy of the prostate.

The ability of TRUS to provide helpful staging information is questionable.[18] One of the limitations of TRUS is the lack of sensitivity in distinguishing between benign and malignant tumors with any amount of certainty.[8] In addition, it is impossible to identify extracapsular microscopic foci of disease. There is also interobserver and intraobserver variability in categorizing a clinical stage.[9] Various staging studies have determined that there is generally more understaging than overstaging when ultrasonography results are compared with the radical prostatectomy specimens.[18] For example, in predicting localized disease, Rifkin and associates[19] reported the accuracy of TRUS in staging prostate cancer to be 58% (126 of 219 patients) with a sensitivity of 66% and specificity of 46%.[19]

BONE SCAN

Radionuclide bone scintigraphy for evaluating skeletal metastases continues to be part of the staging process for newly diagnosed prostate cancer.[20] To determine the correlation between PSA value and bone scan findings in newly diagnosed prostate cancer patients, Oesterling and others reviewed the medical records of more than 800 patients with newly diagnosed prostate cancer and PSA levels less than 20 ng/mL. Five hundred sixty-one patients had a PSA level of less than 10 ng/mL, and only 3 had an abnormal bone scan. Although there are instances of patients with a low PSA and an abnormal bone scan, the likelihood is less than 2%. Oesterling concluded that a bone scan in a newly diagnosed prostate cancer patient with a PSA less than 10 and no skeletal symptoms provides no additional information to what has been obtained from the serum PSA value.[21] Despite the results of Oesterling's study and documentation of cost savings (a total body bone scan costs $270–$1,153), proponents of bone scan indicate this allows a baseline for future evaluation.[13]

COMPUTED TOMOGRAPHY

Computed tomography (CT) is considered inferior to DRE and TRUS when evaluating the stage of prostate cancer.[13] Staging studies have failed to differentiate local from extracapsular disease because most local extension is microscopic.[8] Biopsy artifact is poorly demonstrated and can mislead interpretation of the extent of the local lesion. In patients with a PSA of 10 ng/mL or less, low volume of disease, and a good or moderately differentiated tumor, there is little need to use a CT scan in the initial staging workup. A CT scan may be valuable in prostate cancer if the PSA is greater than 25 ng/mL, a pathology report indicates a high-grade tumor, and there is a positive DRE. The addition of fine-needle aspiration (FNA) in patients with these characteristics or a lymph node larger than 6 mm seems to increase the sensitivity and decrease the false-positive rate.[21] For this group of patients, CT scan with FNA is warranted.

MAGNETIC RESONANCE IMAGING

Although magnetic resonance imaging (MRI) may contribute information about pelvic lymph nodes, it is not superior to CT, is more costly, and is inconvenient for the patient.[8] Overlap in appearance of benign and malignant processes contributes to a high degree of false-positive and false-negative results.[21] There is also considerable interobserver variability in reading MRI results of the prostate.

For patients at risk for extracapsular disease, an endorectal coil imaging study is fairly common and increases the accuracy of detecting lymph node metastases and seminal vesicle involvement.[8] Although MRI may have a slight advantage over CT in evaluating lymph nodes, the ability to combine CT with FNA outweighs the benefit.[21]

PELVIC LYMPHADENECTOMY

Histologic examination of the pelvic lymph nodes provides the most accurate staging information related to lymph node status.[2] Pelvic lymph node dissection has routinely been done at the time of radical prostatectomy but now can be achieved laparoscopically. The indication for pelvic lymph node dissection (PLND) is a strong suspicion for lymph node metastases based on (1) enlarged pelvic nodes on imaging; (2) a prebiopsy PSA level greater than 20 ng/mL; (3) poorly differentiated tumor on biopsy (Gleason score 8–10); or (4) palpable locally advanced tumor stages T3, T4.[22] PLND can be eliminated in patients with a PSA of 5 ng/mL or lower, Gleason score less than 5, or a combination of a PSA of 25 ng/mL, Gleason of 7, and a negative DRE.

SIGNIFICANCE OF TUMOR STAGING

Patients with low-volume tumors (Stage A1, T1a) have an exceptionally good long-term prognosis, but the prognosis is dimmer with each successive higher stage.[17] A critical prognostic factor is whether or not the tumor is confined to the prostate (Stage C). Disease-free survival rates for organ-confined disease are 90 to 94% at 5 years, 76% at 10 years, and 47% at 15 years, which are considerably higher than for tumors that extend beyond the prostate (59–77%, 54%, and 11%, respectively).[23] Extension into the seminal vesicles indicates a poor prognosis, and overall survival for patients with Stage C disease is less than for patients with Stage B disease. Approximately 62% of patients who are clinically staged A-B are pathologically Stage C or even Stage D.

Incidental histologic prostate cancers can be distinguished from clinically significant cancers by the volume, grade, and extent of the tumor when these features are analyzed at surgery.[23] It is more difficult to determine indolent cancers from clinical cancers by analyzing the clinical guidelines of stage, grade, and serum PSA levels. When early-stage prostate cancer is discovered, it is often difficult to determine those that should be treated conservatively from those that should be treated aggressively, because it can be argued that many men face a low probability of dying from their prostate cancer compared with other causes.

If the medical community is to detect and treat early-stage prostate cancer aggressively, strides must be made to identify correctly those tumors that are benign and can be observed versus those cancers that need to be treated.[23] The only factors that consistently show a correlation are serum PSA levels, Gleason grade, and clinical T classification. There is a critical need to identify and characterize prognostic factors that can be determined clinically before treatment that will predict with increased preciseness the rate of progression and response to therapy. This would be especially beneficial in deciding treatment options, particularly in older men.

PATHOLOGIC STAGE

There is no current pathologic staging system for prostate cancer.[2] Total prostatoseminal vesiculectomy, regional lymph node specimen, and histologic confirmation are required for pathologic T classification and provide the best accurate description of the extent of disease.[12, 13] If the tumor is not organ confined, the extent of surgical margins, seminal vesicles, pelvic lymph nodes, and periprostatic fibroadipose tissue are documented.

HISTOLOGIC GRADE

The purpose of the histologic grade is to assist in predicting pathologic grade and prognosis. The most widely used grading system for prostate cancer is the Gleason system.[2, 9, 13, 24] The Gleason system is based on a low-power microscopic description of the glandular pattern of the tumor. The primary and secondary patterns are identified and are graded from 1 (well differentiated) to 5 (least differentiated). The Gleason score is the sum of the primary (predominant) and secondary (second most prevalent) grades.

Gleason sums range from 2 ($1 + 1 = 2$), which represents tumors that are uniform in glandular shape, to 10 ($5 + 5 = 10$), which represents highly undifferentiated tumors. Gleason score and combined Gleason grade are synonymous for Gleason sum. Pathologists may assign only a Gleason pattern score rather than a total Gleason score in specimens with limited cancer on biopsy. Careful attention needs to be made when reviewing a pathology report that states Gleason Grade 4 (i.e., Gleason Pattern 4), which may be confused with Gleason score including a combined Gleason grade.

The histologic grade is an important prognostic factor in prostate cancer.[13] In early-stage prostate cancer, the grade and pathologic extent are closely linked. Badalament and associates[25] reported that a Gleason score of 7 or higher had a 58% accuracy rate when predicting the status of organ-confined disease using sextant biopsies in a study of 210 patients, of whom 167 (79.5%) had Gleason scores of 6 or 7. In their series of 703 patients (T1-T3), Partin and others[14] reported that 77% of the tumors were well differentiated (Gleason score 2–4) and were confined to the prostate, 61% were moderately differentiated (Gleason score 5–6), and 26% were poorly differentiated (Gleason score 7–10) (Table 5-2)

Ohori and colleagues[22] reviewed the records of 500 patients treated with radical prostatectomy to determine an algorithm for detecting high-grade cancer while still confined to the prostate. Only 34% of patients with a Gleason score of 7 had disease confined to the prostate. Patients with Gleason scores of 7 have somewhat of a lower risk of recurrence after a radical prostatectomy than those with a higher Gleason score and have a greater risk of recurrence than those with a Gleason score of 6 or less. Although the preoperative Gleason score correlates with final pathologic stage at either extreme of

TABLE 5-2. Histopathologic Grade

Grade (G)	Description
GX	Grade cannot be assessed
G1c	Well differentiated (slight anaplasia)
G2	Moderately differentiated (moderate anaplasia)
G3-4	Poorly differentiated or undifferentiated (marked anaplasia)

If grouping of Gleason scores is necessary for research purposes, the following grouping is suggested: Gleason score 2–4, well differentiated; 5–6, moderately differentiated; 7, moderately poorly differentiated; 8–10, poorly differentiated.

Adapted with permission of the American Joint Committee on Cancer (AJCC), Chicago, Illinois. The original source for this material is the *AJCC Cancer Staging Manual*, 5th edition (1997) published by Lippincott-Raven Publishers, Philadelphia, Pennsylvania.

the system (2–4 and 8–10), Gleason scores between 5 and 7 do not contribute to the prediction of the final pathologic stage. The Gleason score is an independent prognostic factor, as Partin and colleagues demonstrated, but only when it is used in combination with clinical stage and PSA does the Gleason score become significant in predicting pathologic stage.[4]

COMBINING CLINICAL FACTORS TO PREDICT PATHOLOGIC STAGE

Partin and colleagues[14] assessed clinical stage, Gleason score, and serum PSA of 703 men with clinically localized prostate cancer and compared the results with those obtained from prostatectomy. Results indicated that the combination of the three variables were good predictors of final pathologic stage. Probability tables and nomograms have been developed based on a logistic regression analysis for all three variables. This information is helpful in counseling patients with newly diagnosed prostate cancer about treatment options and the likelihood of a curative outcome.[2] For example, a man with a PSA of 3 ng/mL, a stage T2a tumor, and a Gleason score of 5 has an 81% chance of having organ-confined prostate cancer; whereas a man with a PSA of 15 ng/mL, a stage T1c tumor, and a Gleason score of 7 has only a 24% chance of having organ-confined disease (Tables 5-3 and 5-4).

CONCLUSIONS

Over the last several years, the 1992 TNM classification system has experienced increasing acceptance by the urology community. This system defines a greater number of tumor categories and is superior to the Whitmore-Jewett system.[4] The future of staging prostate cancer will rely on the AJCC-UICC TNM system but will need to incorporate other prognostic information to allow precise staging for individual patients.[8] One of the limitations of clinical staging is the lack of accuracy in predicting final pathologic stage. For example, there is need for a pathologic equivalent to the clinical staging of prostate cancer.[23]

In spite of continued efforts directed at research and therapeutic advances, little impact has been made in changing the mortality rate of prostate cancer.[2] Increased diag-

TABLE 5-3. Nomogram for Prediction of Final Pathologic Stage

Score	PSA 0.0–4.0 ng/mL						PSA 4.1–10 ng/mL						PSA 10.1–20 ng/mL						PSA > 20 ng/mL					
	T1a	T1b	T2a	T2b	T2c	T3a	T1a	T1b	T2a	T2b	T2c	T3a	T1a	T1b	T2a	T2b	T2c	T3a	T1a	T1b	T2a	T2b	T2c	T3a
Prediction of organ confined disease																								
2–4	100	85	88	76	82	—	100	78	83	67	71	—	100	—	61	52	—	—	—	—	20	7	—	—
5	100	78	81	67	73	—	100	70	73	56	64	43	100	49	58	43	37	26	—	—	32	—	3	—
6	100	68	72	54	60	42	100	53	62	44	48	33	—	36	44	28	37	19	—	—	14	11	4	5
7	—	54	61	41	46	—	100	39	51	32	37	26	—	24	36	19	24	14	—	—	18	4	5	3
8–10	—	—	48	31	—	—	—	32	39	22	25	12	—	11	29	14	15	9	—	—	3	1	2	2
Prediction of established capsular penetration																								
2–4	0	15	14	26	17	—	0	22	19	34	27	—	0	—	40	49	—	—	—	—	80	94	—	—
5	0	22	20	34	26	—	0	29	28	45	34	58	0	49	43	58	61	75	—	—	68	—	97	—
6	0	30	29	46	38	59	0	45	38	56	49	68	—	62	56	73	59	82	—	—	86	90	96	95
7	—	43	39	59	50	—	—	58	49	68	59	75	—	73	64	81	73	86	—	—	80	96	95	98
8–10	—	—	50	68	—	—	—	64	59	77	71	87	—	87	70	86	82	92	—	—	97	99	97	98

Numbers represent probability (%). Dash represents lack of sufficient data to calculate probability.   PSA, prostate-specific antigen.

From Partin A, Yoo J, Carter HB, et al. The use of PSA clinical stage and Gleason score to predict pathologic stage in men with localized prostate cancer. *Journal of Urology* 1993;150:110-114. Used with permission.

TABLE 5-4. Nomogram for Prediction of Final Pathologic Stage

Score	PSA 0.0–4.0 ng/mL						PSA 4.1–10 ng/mL						PSA 10.1–20 ng/mL						PSA > 20 ng/mL					
	T1a	T1b	T2a	T2b	T2c	T3a	T1a	T1b	T2a	T2b	T2c	T3a	T1a	T1b	T2a	T2b	T2c	T3a	T1a	T1b	T2a	T2b	T2c	T3a
Prediction of seminal vesicle involvement																								
2–4	0	1	1	2	2	—	0	2	1	3	3	3	—	7	5	8	12	11	—	—	12	30	—	—
5	0	3	2	4	4	—	0	4	3	6	6	5	—	15	11	19	17	18	—	—	11	—	29	31
6	0	6	5	9	9	8	0	9	6	11	12	11	—	28	19	33	33	31	—	—	35	40	53	55
7	—	12	9	17	17	—	0	18	12	22	23	18	—	55	29	50	53	49	—	—	31	73	63	55
8–10	—	—	17	29	—	—	—	29	22	38	40	40	—	—	—	—	—	—	—	—	81	93	73	65
Prediction of lymph nodal involvement																								
2–4	0	2	1	2	4	—	0	2	1	2	5	—	1	5	1	3	—	—	—	—	2	7	—	—
5	0	4	2	4	8	—	0	4	2	5	10	8	—	11	5	6	13	11	—	—	3	—	29	31
6	0	8	3	9	17	15	0	9	4	11	19	16	—	21	9	13	22	20	—	—	9	18	53	31
7	—	15	7	18	31	—	0	18	8	20	34	28	—	41	17	24	39	35	—	—	11	44	62	55
8–10	—	—	13	32	—	—	—	30	15	35	53	50	—	—	—	40	59	54	—	—	35	76	73	65

Numbers represent probability (%). Dash represents lack of sufficient data to calculate probability.   PSA, prostate-specific antigen.

From Partin A, Yoo J, Carter HB, et al. The use of PSA clinical stage and Gleason score to predict pathologic stage in men with localized prostate cancer. *Journal of Urology* 1993;150:110-114. Used with permission.

nostic and staging modalities are critical to assist in obtaining prognostic information and improving survival rates.

Nurses can be instrumental in helping patients and families understand the complexity of prostate cancer staging. Providing patient education and support can reduce the uncertainty while waiting for histologic and diagnostic imaging results. As patients attempt to sort out the information given them regarding diagnosis, staging modalities, and treatment options, nurses have the opportunity to help the patient process the information, answer questions in a knowledgeable and straightforward manner, and be a focal point during a confusing and overwhelming time.

REFERENCES

1. Montie J, Pienta K, Pontes JE. Staging systems and prognostic factors for prostate cancer. In: Vogelzang N, Scardino P, Shipley WL, Coffey DS (eds). *Comprehensive Textbook of Genitourinary Oncology.* Baltimore, MD: Williams & Wilkins, 1996:712–719.
2. Carter HB, Partin AW. Diagnosing and staging of prostate cancer. In: Walsh PC, Retik AB, Stamey TA, et al (eds). *Campbell's Urology,* 7th ed. Philadelphia: WB Saunders, 1998:2519–2530.
3. Levy D, Resnick M. Staging of prostate cancer. In: Raghavan D, Scher H, Leibel SA, Lange PH (eds). *Principle and Practices of Genitourinary Oncology.* Philadelphia: Lippincott-Raven, 1997:473–490.
4. Zagars GK, Geara FB, Pollack A, von Eschenbach AC. The T classification of clinically localized prostate cancer. *Cancer* 1994;73:1904–1912.
5. Jewett H. The present status of radical prostatectomy for stages A and B prostate cancer. *Urol Clin North Am* 1975;5:108–122.
6. Graham SD. Critical assessment of prostate cancer staging. *Cancer* 1992;70:269–274.
7. Ohori M, Wheeler T, Scardino P. The New American Joint Committee on Cancer and International Union Against Cancer TNM classification of prostate cancer. *Cancer* 1994;74:104–114.
8. Montie J. Staging of prostate cancer. *Cancer* 1995; 75:1814–1818.
9. Kozlowski J, Grayhack J. Carcinoma of the prostate. In Gillenwater J, Grayhack J, Howards, Duckett J (eds). *Adult Urology.* St. Louis, MO: CV Mosby, 1996:1575–1692.
10. McLeod DG. Prostate cancer: Past, present and future. In: Dawson N, Vogelzang N (eds). *Prostate Cancer.* New York: Wiley-Liss; 1994:1–18.
11. Bostwick D, Amin M. Male reproductive system: Prostate and seminal vesicle. In: Damjanov I, Linder J (eds). *Anderson's Pathology.* St. Louis, MO: CV Mosby, 1996:2197–2230.
12. Fleming J, Cooper J, Henson D, et al (eds). *Prostate: AJCC Cancer Staging Handbook,* 5th ed. Philadelphia: Lippincott-Raven, 1998:204–211.
13. O'Dowd G, Veltri R, Orozco R, et al. Update on the appropriate staging evaluation for newly diagnosed prostate cancer. *J Urol* 1997;158:687–698.
14. Partin A, Yoo J, Carter HB, et al. The use of PSA clinical stage and Gleason score to predict pathologic stage in men with localized prostate cancer. *J Urol* 1993;150:110–114.
15. Partin AW, Oesterling J. The clinical usefulness of PSA: Update 1994. *J Urol* 1994;152:1358–1368.
16. Partin AW, Carter HB, Chan DW, et al. Prostate specific antigen in the staging of localized prostate cancer: Influence of tumor differentiation, tumor volume and benign hyperplasia. *J Urol* 1990;143: 747–752.
17. Montie J, Meyers S. Defining the ideal tumor marker for prostate cancer. *Urol Clin North Am* 1997;24:247–259.
18. Brawer M, Chetner M. Ultrasonography of the prostate and biopsy. In: Walsh PC, Vaughn ED Jr, Wein A (eds). *Campbell's Urology,* 7th ed. Philadelphia: WB Saunders, 1998:2506–2517.
19. Rifkin MD, Zerhouni EA, Gatsonis CA, et al. Comparison of magnetic resonance imaging and ultrasonography in staging early prostate cancer. Results of a multiinstitutional cooperative trial. *N Engl J Med.* 1990;323:621.

20. Oesterling J, Martin S, Bergstralh E, Lowe F. The use of prostate-specific antigen in staging patients with newly diagnosed prostate cancer. *JAMA* 1993;269:57–60.

21. Rees M, Resnick M, Oesterling J. Use of prostate-specific antigen, Gleason score and digital rectal examination in staging patients with newly diagnosed prostate cancer. *Urol Clin North Am* 1997;24: 379–386.

22. Ohori M, Goad JR, Wheeler TM, et al. Can radical prostatectomy alter the progression of poorly differentiated prostate cancer? *J Urol* 1994;152:1843–1849.

23. Corless CL. Evaluating early-stage prostate cancer. *Hematol Oncol Clin North Am* 1996;10:565–579.

24. Epstein J. Pathology of adenocarcinoma of the prostate. In: Walsh PC, Retik AB, Vaughn ED, Wein A (eds). *Campbell's Urology,* 7th ed. Philadelphia: WB Saunders, 1998:2497–2505.

25. Badalament RA, Miller MC, Peller PA, et al. An algorithm for predicting nonorgan confined prostate cancer using the results obtained from sextant core biopsies with PSA level. *J Urol* 1996;156:1375–1380.

Chapter 6

TREATMENT DECISION MAKING

WILLIAM TESTER

MARIA DeVITO BROUCH

OVERVIEW

INTRODUCTION
PATIENT DATA COLLECTION
   Age
   Coexisting Medical Problems
   Prostate-Specific Antigen–Screened Patients
   Stage
   Tumor Factors
   Tumor Markers
TREATMENT OPTIONS
   Watchful Waiting
   Surgery
   Cryosurgery
   External Beam Radiation Therapy
   External Beam Radiation Therapy Plus
      Hormonal Therapy

   Interstitial Brachytherapy
   Systemic Radioisotopes
   Hormonal Therapy
   Chemotherapy
   Clinical Trials
COMMON COMPLICATIONS OF TREATMENT
   Surgical Complications
   Radiation Complications
   Hormonal Therapy Complications
   Chemotherapy Complications
TREATMENT SELECTION FOR THE
   INDIVIDUAL PATIENT
PSYCHOSOCIAL ISSUES
NURSING ISSUES AND CONCERNS

INTRODUCTION

For most men diagnosed with prostate cancer, more than one treatment option can be considered. The selection of treatment for an individual patient depends on the relative efficacy of various treatment choices and the likelihood of complications for that individual patient. In addition, a patient will express personal feelings about the degree of complications that are considered acceptable to him. Issues regarding, among others, anesthesia and surgical risks, impotency, incontinence, self-esteem, and bowel and bladder injury should be addressed before selecting the most appropriate treatment for a patient. Often consultation with physicians from more than one discipline is helpful. Depending on the patient's age, expected survival, coexisting medical problems, method of diagnosis, stage, tumor factors, expected side effects of treatment, and the patient's desires, a treatment decision can be made.

PATIENT DATA COLLECTION

AGE

Carcinoma of the prostate is predominantly a tumor affecting older men; the median age at diagnosis is 72 years. Older patients, especially those with localized tumors, may die of other illnesses without suffering significant disability from their cancer. Therefore, treatment decisions should be influenced by the patient's age and projected survival, independent of the cancer. Patients with limited life expectancy are generally not considered for radical treatments that can produce significant morbidity.

COEXISTING MEDICAL PROBLEMS

Curative treatment should be considered for men without significant comorbid medical illnesses because they are at greater risk of dying from prostate cancer than men with major comorbid medical illness. Because of increased morbidity and shorter expected survival benefit, radical prostatectomy is usually reserved for men who are younger than 70 and without significant medical illnesses.[1, 2] The incidence of coexisting medical problems increases with increasing age. A review of medical records of 584 men previously diagnosed with prostate cancer who died between 1980 and 1984 showed that only 54% of deaths were caused by prostate cancer. This retrospective review of medical records showed that the men who were more likely to die of prostate cancer were African-American, were younger than 65, had advanced-stage disease, or were treated with hormonal therapy. After adjusting for age, race, and stage, men with concurrent cardiovascular disease were more likely to die of other causes.[3]

Certain patients may be identified as poor surgical risks because of coexisting cardiac, pulmonary, renal, or cerebrovascular disease. These patients are generally better served by nonsurgical treatment, including watchful waiting, radiotherapy, hormonal therapy, or combined radiotherapy and hormonal therapy.

PROSTATE-SPECIFIC ANTIGEN–SCREENED PATIENTS

Controversy still exists regarding the value of prostate-specific antigen (PSA) screening and whether early treatment for patients with nonpalpable prostate cancers that are detected by PSA screening (Stage T1c) will produce improved long-term outcomes. Some studies suggested that PSA screening will diagnose more nonlethal tumors and that patients might be diagnosed and treated who were not destined to develop clinically significant cancers. A study from Sweden showed that long-term survival rates improved when PSA screening and ultrasonography for diagnosis of prostate cancer were introduced. An improvement in survival was observed even though watchful waiting and palliative hormonal treatment were the most common treatment strategies for localized prostate cancer during the study period.[4] Similarly, in the United States, with the increased use of PSA screening, prostate cancer patients are diagnosed with lower PSA levels, lower grade tumors, and lower stages.[5] Analysis of patients referred to Mayo Clinic for radical prostatectomy shows that after the introduction of PSA screening, patients are more likely to present with a lower stage and more favorable DNA ploidy.[6]

Whether improved outcomes will be related to treatment or to lead time and length biases remains under study. Only prospective, randomized trials will be able to determine whether PSA screening and earlier treatment will make a significant impact on survival. A National Cancer Institute (NCI) study* is presently under way to test the value of early detection on reducing mortality. This study will compare long-term outcomes between a population of men who undergo regular digital rectal exams and PSA screening with another population who receive usual medical care without formal screening. When completed, this study should clearly show the extent to which PSA screening and early treatment of prostate cancer will impact long-term outcomes.[7]

STAGE

Survival of the patient with prostatic carcinoma is related to the extent of tumor. When the cancer is confined to the prostate gland, median survival is greater than 5 years. Locally advanced cancer is not usually curable, and many patients will eventually die of their tumor, although median survival may be as long as 5 years. If prostate cancer has spread to distant organs, current therapy will not cure it. Median survival is usually 1 to 3 years, and the majority of such patients will die of prostate cancer. Even in this group of patients, however, some will have more indolent clinical courses lasting for many years.

Prognosis is worse in patients with pelvic lymph node involvement. Most patients should undergo lymph node dissection, either open or laparoscopic, before definitive treatment. Definitive therapy may be altered by the findings; patients with pathology-positive nodes are usually not considered good candidates for radical prostatectomy.[7] Also seminal vesicle biopsy may be useful in patients with palpable nodules who are being considered for radical prostatectomy. Seminal vesicle involvement is associated with a worse prognosis and is predictive of pelvic lymph node metastasis.[8]

In patients with clinically localized prostate cancer, Gleason score and serum prostatic acid phosphatase values predict the likelihood of capsular penetration, seminal vesicle invasion, and regional lymph node involvement.[9]

---

*Gohagan JK, Early Detection and Community Oncology Program, Division of Cancer Prevention, National Cancer Institute, National Institutes of Health: A 16-Year Randomized Screening Trial for Prostate, Lung, Colorectal, and Ovarian Cancer.

TUMOR FACTORS

The degrees of tumor differentiation and abnormality of histologic growth pattern directly correlate with likelihood of metastases and survival. The degree of differentiation can be expressed either with World Health Organization (WHO) or Gleason criteria. Tumor grade and Gleason score can be determined from surgical specimens or needle biopsy.[10, 11]

Tumor grade and other factors affecting the prognosis are useful in making therapeutic decisions. Poorly differentiated tumors are more likely to have already metastasized by the time of diagnosis and are associated with a poorer prognosis. Patients with stage T1 tumors and a favorable Gleason score can usually be offered watchful waiting, whereas those with the same stage but high-grade scores are more likely to develop symptomatic disease and deserve initial treatment. A retrospective study from Connecticut showed that men aged 65 to 75 years with low-grade tumors treated conservatively experienced no loss of life expectancy, whereas men with higher grade tumors experience a progressively increasing loss of life expectancy, depending on grade.[12]

For patients treated with radiotherapy, the combination of clinical tumor (T) stage, Gleason score, and pretreatment PSA level can be used to estimate more accurately the risk of relapse.[13] Most studies of flow cytometry have shown that nuclear DNA ploidy is an independent prognostic factor for disease progression and survival. Diploid tumors have a more favorable outcome than either tetraploid or aneuploid tumors.[14]

TUMOR MARKERS

Elevations of serum acid phosphatase are associated with poor prognosis in both localized and disseminated disease. However, PSA as a marker is associated with much greater sensitivity and specificity. It is of value in assessing prognosis as well as disease recurrence of patients treated with surgery, radiotherapy, or hormonal therapy.[15, 16]

TREATMENT OPTIONS

Treatment of patients with prostate cancer results in long disease-free survival for many patients with localized disease but is rarely curative in patients with advanced disease. Even when the cancer appears clinically localized to the prostate gland, metastases will develop in many after initial treatment. Patients with locally advanced or metastatic disease are usually treatable and derive significant palliation but are not curable.

WATCHFUL WAITING

Asymptomatic patients of advanced age or those with concomitant illness may warrant observation without immediate active treatment, especially those with low-grade and early-stage tumors. Patients can present with clinically silent tumors found at surgery for presumed benign disease. This incidental discovery of these occult cancers at prostatic surgery performed for other reasons accounts for the similar survival of men with Stage I prostate cancer compared with the normal male population, adjusted for age. Many of these cancers are well differentiated and only focally involve the gland (T1a, N0, M0), and the majority require no treatment other than careful follow-up. In a retrospective analysis, 828 men with clinically localized prostate cancer were managed by initial conservative therapy with subsequent hormone therapy given at the time of symptomatic disease progression. This study showed that the patients with Grade 1 or 2 tumors experienced a disease-specific survival of 87% at 10 years and that their overall survival closely approximated the expected survival among men of similar ages in the general population.[17]

A population-based study with 15 years of follow-up has shown excellent survival with watchful waiting in patients with well- or moderately well-differentiated tumors confined to the prostate.[18] A Connecticut Tumor Registry report[19] showed that men aged 55 to 74 at diagnosis faced a risk of dying from prostate cancer, depending on their Gleason score. Men with Gleason scores of 2 to 4 faced a 4 to 7% risk of dying, and men with scores of 5 faced a 6 to 11% risk of dying within 15 years. Another study of 94 patients with clinically localized prostate cancer managed by a watch-and-wait strategy gave very similar results at 4 to 9 years of follow-up.[20] Even in a selected series of 50 Stage C (T3) patients with well- and moderately well-differentiated tumors, the prostate cancer–specific survival rates at 5 and 9 years were 88% and 70%, respectively, when managed by a watch-and-wait strategy.[21]

Less differentiated cancers that involve more than a few chips of resected prostate tissue (T1b, N0, M0) are biologically more aggressive. Radical prostatectomy, external beam radiation therapy, interstitial implantation of radioisotopes, and watchful waiting yield apparently similar survival rates in uncontrolled selected series. The decision to treat should be made in the context of the patient's age, associated medical illnesses, and the patient's personal desires.[22]

The potential benefit of watchful waiting is that treatment-related morbidity will be avoided. The use of surgery or radiotherapy for patients with localized disease produces significant morbidity (see following discussion) and must be weighed against the curative potential and expected survival of the individual patient. The use of hormonal therapy will generally relieve cancer-related symptoms, such as bone pain. However, hormonal therapy can be withheld from the asymptomatic man with incurable, asymptomatic advanced disease.

SURGERY

Surgery is usually reserved for patients in good health who are younger than 70, who have no evidence of metastatic disease, and who elect surgical intervention.[2] Prostatectomy can be performed using either a perineal or a retropubic approach. Radical prostatectomy is not usually performed if frozen-section evaluation of pelvic nodes reveals metastases. Disease in these node-positive patients is generally considered not curable and can be treated with radiotherapy or hormonal therapy. The use of hormonal therapy before surgery has been evaluated at some medical centers, but it has not been shown to yield long-term survival advantage.[23, 24]

After radical prostatectomy, evaluation of the surgical specimen can divide patients into groups with organ-confined, specimen-confined, and margin-positive disease. When the tumor is organ confined, local or distant recurrence occurs rarely. The incidence of disease recurrence increases when the tumor is not specimen confined (extracapsular) or the margins are positive.[18, 21] Although there is no standard approach for patients with tumor outside the prostate, they often receive additional therapy, including postoperative radiation and hormonal treatment. It is presently unknown whether postoperative radiation or hormonal treatment will improve the long-term survival of patients with extracapsular and margin-positive disease.

CRYOSURGERY

Cryosurgery is a less proven surgical technique that destroys prostate cancer cells by freezing the prostate tissue with cryoprobes, usually directed by ultrasonography. It has been used as initial treatment or as treatment after radiation failures. Compared with prostatectomy and radiotherapy, the long-term outcomes are not as well known. The advantage of cryosurgery is that it can be performed as a 1-day procedure. Immediate surgical risks appear less than those of radical surgery. It can be performed under spinal anesthesia in patients with concurrent medical illnesses. However, serious complications that have been reported include bladder outlet injury, urinary incontinence, impotence, and rectal injury. Whether long-term results will prove that it produces less morbidity than radical prostatectomy or radiotherapy is unknown. This technique is still under development; its role as initial or second-line treatment remains under study.[25, 26]

EXTERNAL BEAM RADIATION THERAPY

Candidates for definitive radiation therapy must have a confirmed diagnosis of cancer that is clinically confined to the prostate or surrounding tissues (Stages I, II, and III). In general, patients selected for radiotherapy are older and have more coexisting medical problems than those selected for radical prostatectomy. Their staging is usually clinical (i.e., not determined at the time of planned prostatectomy). Patients chosen for definitive radiotherapy should have a negative bone scan, but when the PSA level is less than 10, it is extremely unlikely that the bone scan will reveal metastases.[27, 28] Lymph node dissection is usually not performed, but consideration should be given to staging with laparoscopic node sampling or computed tomographic scan–directed node biopsy before treating with definitive radiotherapy. Patients with more extensively staged tumors who are then treated with radiotherapy will have better results than those with clinically staged tumors because clinical staging often underestimates the true stage. If tumors are carefully staged, there is no difference in survival whether the patients receive radiotherapy to the prostate alone or to the prostate plus pelvic nodes.[29]

Long-term results with radiotherapy are dependent on stage. A retrospective review of 999 patients treated with external beam irradiation showed cause-specific survival rates to be significantly different at 10 years by T stage: T1 (79%), T2 (66%), T3 (55%), and T4 (22%).[30] In a series of 1,872 patients treated with external beam radiotherapy, interstitial radiotherapy, or radical prostatectomy, low-risk patients had similar treatment outcomes with all three treatment options. Intermediate- and high-risk patients had similar outcomes whether they were treated with either external beam radiotherapy or radical prostatectomy, as measured by freedom from PSA progression.[31] Patients considered poor medical candidates for radical prostatectomy can be treated with acceptably low complications if consideration is given to delivery technique. Some investigators claimed that conformal radiotherapy decreases acute radiation morbidity, especially bowel and bladder toxicity.[32, 33] In a series of 160 patients with nonpalpable tumors treated with conformal radiotherapy, the 5-year rate of biochemical control was 86%.[33]

EXTERNAL BEAM RADIATION THERAPY PLUS HORMONAL THERAPY

Hormonal therapy may be combined with radiation, especially for patients with locally advanced tumors. Several studies investigated whether hormonal treatment improves overall survival or just the time to disease progression. The Radiation Therapy Oncology Group (RTOG) performed a prospective, randomized trial in which patients with T3, N0, or any T, N1, M0 disease received external beam radiation therapy and then were randomized to receive goserelin or not. In patients assigned to receive goserelin, the drug was started during the last week of the radiation therapy course and was continued indefinitely or until signs of progression. The actuarial overall 5-year survival rate for the entire population of 945 analyzable patients was not statistically significantly different. However, the authors reported an improved actuarial 5-year local control rate (84% vs. 71%), improved freedom from distant metastasis (83% vs. 70%), and improved disease-free survival (60% vs. 44%), all in favor of goserelin.[34]

Additionally, the RTOG also conducted a study on node-negative patients: 456 men were evaluable and were randomly assigned to treatment with radiation alone or radiation plus androgen ablation. At 5 years, the overall survival of the two groups was identical, but local control (54% vs. 29%) and disease-free survival (36% vs. 15%) were improved with the addition of hormonal therapy.[35]

A similar trial was performed by a group of European investigators. Patients with T1, T2 (WHO Grade 3), N0-NX or T3, T4, N0 disease were randomized to receive either radiation or identical radiation and adjuvant goserelin (with cyproterone acetate for 1 month) starting with radiation and continuing for 3 years. The 401 patients available for analysis were monitored for a median of 45 months. The actuarial 5-year survival was 79% for the radiation plus hormonal therapy arm and 52% for the radiation alone arm. Similarly, the 5-year disease-free survival (85% vs. 48%) and local control (97% vs. 77%) were significantly improved with the addition of hormonal therapy.[36]

INTERSTITIAL BRACHYTHERAPY

Interstitial brachytherapy has been used at selected medical centers as treatment for patients with early-stage (T1 and T2) disease. The potential advantages of this treatment approach over radical prostatectomy are that it (1) is associated with less acute morbidity, (2) can be performed on an outpatient basis, and (3) can be performed on older patients with concurrent medical illnesses. The potential advantages of this treatment approach over standard external beam radiotherapy are that it appears to produce less long-term morbidity and less cystitis and proctitis and that it is completed in a much shorter period of time on an outpatient basis. Patients selected for interstitial brachytherapy are generally those with favorable characteristics, including low Gleason score, low PSA level, and organ-confined (Stage T1 and T2) tumors.[37, 38] Although this group of patients with early-stage small tumors appears to fare very well with this treatment, further study and longer follow-up are needed to define better the effects of modern interstitial brachytherapy on disease control and quality of life and to determine the contribution of favorable patient selection to outcomes.[39] Although long-term survival information is limited, this treatment has been shown to be effective in reducing PSA levels and producing negative biopsies.[37, 38] Some centers use the combination of interstitial brachytherapy followed by external beam radiation therapy. One series of 1,020 men so treated for T1 and T2 prostate cancer achieved 5- and 10-year survival rates of 79% and 72%, respectively, with this form of radiotherapy.[40]

This form of radiotherapy can presently be offered to men with other medical illnesses that preclude more standard treatments, such as radical prostatectomy or external beam radiation therapy. Alternatively, it may be offered to men who refuse standard treatments. Prospective, randomized trials are needed to determine the relative value of interstitial brachytherapy compared with more established treatment options. At present, it is not clear which radiotherapy technique (external beam radiation therapy, interstitial brachytherapy, or interstitial brachytherapy followed by external beam radiation therapy) will produce superior outcomes.[41]

SYSTEMIC RADIOISOTOPES

Patients with metastatic prostate cancer often have multiple areas of painful bone involvement. External beam radiation therapy for palliation of bone pain can be very helpful, but most patients will quickly develop other areas of painful metastatic disease. Systemic radioisotopes, such as strontium 89, have been shown to be effective in the palliative treatment of patients with osteoblastic metastases. When this isotope is given alone, it has been reported to decrease bone pain in 80% of patients treated.[42] For patients with multiple areas of bone involvement, it gave a similar response as hemibody radiation.[43] When used as an adjunct to external beam radiotherapy, strontium 89 was shown to slow disease progression and reduce analgesic requirements compared with external beam radiotherapy alone.[44]

HORMONAL THERAPY

The majority of patients with metastatic prostate cancer will respond to the initial hormonal therapy; median response duration is 18 months. Choices for initial palliative hormonal therapy include orchiectomy, luteinizing hormone-releasing hormone (LHRH) analogue alone, LHRH agonist with an antiandrogen, or estrogens. Estrogens are less often prescribed because of cardiovascular side effects. Total androgen blockade (TAB) can be achieved with LHRH agonist plus an antiandrogen or with orchiectomy plus an antiandrogen. TAB is theoretically better because it suppresses both gonadal and adrenal sources of androgen: however, its use remains controversial.[45] Current evidence suggests that the addition of an antiandrogen to orchiectomy does not improve survival but does increase the side effects of treatment.[46]

Most patients with metastatic disease do have significant symptoms and will derive meaningful palliation with initiation of hormonal therapy. For those patients with asymptomatic metastatic disease, some have questioned whether it is more appropriate to begin hormonal therapy when metastatic disease is diagnosed or to wait until the disease is symptomatic. The Medical Research Council Prostate Cancer Working Party Investigators Group addressed this issue in a prospective, randomized study. Their study compared immediate hormonal treatment (orchiectomy or LHRH) versus watchful waiting with hormonal therapy given at the time of disease progression. Patients included in the study were men with locally advanced or asymptomatic metastatic prostate cancer. An improved overall survival and prostate cancer–specific survival resulted with the use of immediate hormonal treatment. The incidence of pathologic fractures, spinal cord compression, and ureteric obstruction was also lower in the immediate treatment arm, supporting the role of immediate hormonal therapy.[47]

In patients who have symptomatic bone disease, several factors are associated with poor prognosis: poor performance status, elevated alkaline phosphatase, and short prior response to initial hormone therapy. Even among patients who relapse after response to initial hormonal therapy, some will retain a degree of hormone sensitivity. These patients can respond to a variety of second-line hormonal therapies.[48] Aminoglutethimide, hydrocortisone, flutamide withdrawal, progesterone, ketoconazole, and combinations of these therapies have produced PSA responses in 14 to 60% of patients treated and have also produced measurable clinical responses of 0 to 25%. The duration of these PSA responses has been in the range of 2 to 4 months.[49]

After disease progression on hormonal therapy, patients treated with LHRH agonists are usually maintained on LHRH, designed to maintain castrate levels of testosterone. However, it is not clear whether this policy is advantageous for the patient. One study from the Eastern Cooperative Oncology Group showed that a superior survival resulted when patients who failed their initial LHRH therapy were maintained on primary androgen deprivation.[50] However, another study from the Southwest Oncology Group did not show an advantage to continued androgen blockade after disease progression.[51]

CHEMOTHERAPY

Because hormonal therapy is less toxic and more effective than chemotherapy, it is always considered as the first-line option for patients with metastatic disease. Chemotherapy is generally considered for treatment of patients with metastatic prostate cancer when they have failed to respond to hormonal therapy and are believed to be unsuitable for additional hormonal treatment. In addition, ongoing clinical trials are now evaluating the role of chemotherapy combined with radiotherapy for patients with less advanced disease.

Phase II clinical studies report that several agents are capable of achieving short-term palliation of symptoms, decreasing bone pain, lowering PSA levels, and, in some studies, improving quality of life. Current chemotherapy agents do not prolong survival of patients refractory to hormonal therapy. Chemotherapy drugs that have shown clinical activity in the treatment of hormone refractory disease include mitoxantrone, paclitaxel, docetaxel, estramustine, suramin, oral etoposide, and various combinations of these agents.[52-55] No single chemotherapy agent or combination is considered standard at present. One prospective, randomized trial did show that pain was better controlled in hormone-resistant patients treated with mitoxantrone plus prednisone compared with those treated with prednisone alone. However, there were no statistically significant differences in overall survival or global quality of life between the two treatments.[54]

CLINICAL TRIALS

Clinical trials are available and appropriate for many patients with prostate cancer. Many trials are designed to improve on the efficacy of modern treatments, to evaluate the relative value of different treatment options, or to reduce the morbidity and improve the quality of life. An up-to-date listing of active clinical trials can be found in the Physicians Data Query service (PDQ) sponsored by the NCI. The following is an incomplete listing of ongoing current clinical trials taken from PDQ:

1. A 16-Year Randomized Screening Trial for Prostate, Lung, Colorectal, and Ovarian Cancer—PLCO Trial (National Institute of Health)
2. Phase I-II Dose Escalation Study of Three-Dimensional Conformal Radiotherapy for Stages I-III Adenocarcinoma of the Prostate (RTOG-9406)
3. Phase I-II Study of Weekly Intravenous Estramustine in Combination With Paclitaxel and Carboplatin in Patients With Advanced Prostate Cancer (Memorial Sloan Kettering Cancer Center-98032)
4. Phase III Randomized Study of Postoperative External Radiotherapy Versus No Immediate Further Treatment in Patients With pT3N0 Prostatic Adenocarcinoma (European Organization for Research and Treatment of Cancer-22911)
5. Phase III Randomized Study of Radiotherapy With Versus Without Neoadjuvant Flutamide/Goserelin in Good Prognosis, Locally Confined Adenocarcinoma of the Prostate (RTOG-9408)
6. Phase III Randomized Study of Prostatectomy Versus Expectant Observation With Palliative Therapy for Stage I-II Prostate Cancer (Veterans Administration-Cooperative Studies Program-407)
7. Phase II Study of Hyperthermia and Radiotherapy for Locally Advanced Adenocarcinoma of the Prostate (Dana Farber Cancer Institute-94153)
8. Phase II Randomized Study of Paclitaxel/Etoposide/Estramustine Versus Ketoconazole/Doxorubicin/Vinblastine/Estramustine for Androgen Independent Prostate Cancer (M. D. Anderson-DM-97022)

COMMON COMPLICATIONS OF TREATMENT

For all stages of prostate cancer, more than one treatment option can be considered. The selection of treatment depends on the relative efficacy of various treatment choices and the risks of significant complications. Most men will express strong feelings about the degree of complications that are considered acceptable. Issues regarding anesthesia and surgical risks, impotency, incontinence, self-esteem, and bowel and bladder injury should be addressed before selecting the most appropriate treatment for a patient. Often consultation with physicians from more than one discipline is helpful.

SURGICAL COMPLICATIONS

Complications of radical prostatectomy can include urinary incontinence, urethral stricture, impotence, and the morbidity associated with general anesthesia and surgery. A review of 10,600 men undergoing radical prostatectomy found a 30-day mortality rate of 2% and a cardiovascular morbidity rate of 8%. Morbidity and mortality increased with age and were appreciably greater in those patients older than 75.[56] In one large case study of men undergoing the nerve-sparing technique of radical prostatectomy, only about 6% of men required the use of pads for urinary incontinence, but some additional men reported occasional urinary dribbling. About 40 to 65% of men who were sexually potent before surgery retained potency adequate for vaginal penetration and sexual intercourse. Preservation of potency with this technique is dependent on tumor stage and patient age, but the operation probably induces at least a partial deficit in nearly all patients.[57]

A national survey of Medicare patients who underwent radical prostatectomy in 1988–1990 reported more morbidity than most single-institution reports.[58] In the Medicare survey, more than 30% of men reported the need for pads or clamps to control wetness, and 63% of all patients reported some problem with wetness. About 60% reported having no erections since surgery. Other series of men treated with radical prostatectomy by experienced surgeons showed similarly high rates of impotence as in the national Medicare survey.[59, 60]

RADIATION COMPLICATIONS

Definitive external beam radiation therapy can result in acute cystitis, proctitis, and occasionally enteritis. These are generally reversible but may be chronic and rarely require surgical intervention. Potency, in the short term, is generally preserved but may diminish over time. A cross-sectional survey of prostate cancer patients treated in a managed-care setting by radical prostatectomy, radiation, or watchful waiting showed substantial sexual and urinary dysfunction in the radiation therapy group.[61]

Morbidity is reduced with the use of sophisticated radiation techniques, such as the use of linear accelerators, and careful simulation and treatment planning. The treatment field should not include the dissected pelvic nodes. Prior transurethral resection of the prostate (TURP) increases the risk of stricture above that seen with radiation alone; if radiation is delayed 4 to 6 weeks after the TURP, the risk of stricture can be minimized.[62] A survey of Medicare recipients who received radiation therapy as primary treatment showed substantial differences in morbidity between surgery and radiation.[63] The men who underwent radiation were less likely to report the need for pads or clamps to control urinary wetness (7% vs. > 30%). More patients treated with radiation reported the ability to have an erection sufficient for intercourse in the month before the survey (men younger than 70 years, 33% who received radiation vs. 11% who underwent surgery alone; men 70 years or older, 27% who received radiation vs. 12% who underwent surgery alone). However, men receiving radiation were more likely to report problems with bowel function, especially frequent bowel movements (10% vs. 3%).

HORMONAL THERAPY COMPLICATIONS

Several different hormonal approaches can benefit men with advanced stage prostate cancer. These treatments are designed to be palliative but also can have significant side effects. In the treatment of patients with advanced disease, these treatments will often improve bone pain, appetite, and overall sense of well-being. Various hormonal options include bilateral orchiectomy, estrogen, LHRH agonists, antiandrogens, ketoconazole, and aminoglutethimide.

Benefits of bilateral orchiectomy include ease of the procedure, compliance, immediacy in lowering testosterone levels, and low cost. Disadvantages include psychological effects, loss of libido, impotence, hot flashes, and osteoporosis.[64] In the past, many have advocated the use of TAB, the combined use of orchiectomy or LHRH agonist with an antiandrogen. However, a large prospective clinical trial suggested that there is no advantage to the addition of an antiandrogen to orchiectomy. In addition, patients who took flutamide experienced more side effects with a negative impact on quality of life.[46]

Estrogens, in the form of diethylstilbestrol (3 mg/day), will achieve castrate levels of testosterone. Similar to orchiectomy, estrogens may cause loss of libido and impotence. Gynecomastia may be prevented by low-dose radiation to the breasts. However, estrogen is seldom used today because of the risk of serious side effects, including myocardial infarction, cerebrovascular accident, and pulmonary embolism.

LHRH agonists such as leuprolide, goserelin, and buserelin will lower testosterone to castrate levels. Similar to orchiectomy and estrogens, LHRH agonists cause impotence, hot flashes, and loss of libido. Tumor flare reactions may occur transiently but can be prevented by antiandrogens or by short-term estrogens at low dose for several weeks. The antiandrogen flutamide may cause diarrhea, breast tenderness, and nausea. There have been case reports of fatal and nonfatal liver toxicity.[65] Bicalutamide may cause nausea, breast tenderness, hot flashes, loss of libido, and impotence.[66]

The steroidal antiandrogen megestrol acetate suppresses androgen production incompletely and is generally not used as initial therapy. Long-term use of ketoconazole can result in impotence, pruritus, nail changes, and adrenal insufficiency. Aminoglutethimide commonly causes sedation and skin rash. Additional studies are required to evaluate further the effects of these hormone therapies on global quality of life.[67]

CHEMOTHERAPY COMPLICATIONS

Side effects of chemotherapy are dependent on the choice of agent or agents used, the schedule of drug administration, and the medical condition of the patient. Men with symptomatic hormone-refractory disease who have a good performance status (generally Eastern Cooperative Oncology Group 0-1) and adequate organ function can be offered a trial of chemotherapy using mitoxantrone, paclitaxel, docetaxel, estramustine, vinblastine, suramin, etoposide, or combinations of these agents. Commonly encountered side effects include fatigue, anemia, leukopenia, thrombocytopenia, alopecia, nausea, and phlebitis. Other side effects specific for each chemotherapy agent are possible.[52–55]

TREATMENT SELECTION FOR THE INDIVIDUAL PATIENT

For each patient, several treatment options are available. In decision making, the relative benefits and risks must be weighed. Depending on the patient's age, expected survival, concurrent medical illnesses, stage, tumor factors, expected side effects of treatment, and the patient's desires, a treatment decision can be made. In this section, treatment guidelines according to stage of disease are reviewed.

- Stage I

  T1a, N0, M0, G1 (WHO grade)
  1. Careful observation without further immediate treatment in most patients.
  2. Definitive treatment can be considered for young patients without significant medical illness, although treatment at this stage is not likely to impact long-term survival.

- Stage II

  T1a, N0, M0, G2, 3-4 (WHO grade)
  T1b, N0, M0, any G
  T1c, N0, M0, any G
  T1, N0, M0, any G
  T2, N0, M0, any G
  1. Radical prostatectomy.
  2. External beam irradiation.
  3. Interstitial implantation of radioisotopes.
  4. Watchful waiting. This is especially appropriate for patients with low-grade tumors, advanced age, or coexisting medical problems.
  5. Cryosurgery is under clinical evaluation; its impact on long-term survival and its long-term complications are unknown.

- Stage III

  T3, N0, M0, any WHO grade
  1. External beam irradiation. Hormonal therapy may be considered in addition to external beam irradiation. Prospective trials have shown improvement in disease-free survival with the addition of hormonal therapy to radiotherapy (see prior discussion).

2. Hormonal manipulations (orchiectomy or LHRH agonist).
3. Radical prostatectomy (rare patients). Consideration may be given to postoperative radiotherapy for patients found to have positive margins or a detectable level of PSA after surgery, although its impact on long-term survival is unknown.
4. Watchful waiting for asymptomatic patients with coexisting medical problems.

- Stage IV
T4, N0, M0, any WHO grade
Any T, N1, M0
Any T, any N, M1
1. Hormonal therapy.
   Orchiectomy alone.
   LHRH agonist alone or with an antiandrogen.
   Estrogens (less favored because of cardiovascular side effects).
2. External beam irradiation to the prostate and involved nodes for highly selected Stage M0 patients.
3. Palliative radiation therapy to sites of painful bone metastases.
4. Systemic radioisotopes for patients with generalized bone pain.
5. Watchful waiting for selected asymptomatic patients.
6. Chemotherapy for hormone-refractory patients.

PSYCHOSOCIAL ISSUES

The impact of a diagnosis of prostate cancer is profound. For many individuals, a diagnosis of cancer is closely connected with fears of death, disability, pain, and suffering and imparts an abrupt sense of uncertainty regarding the future quality and quantity of one's life. Initial emotional responses of anger, sadness, grief, and loss are common. Anxiety and disbelief ranging to shock can overwhelm and significantly impair the patient's and family's comprehension of initial information provided regarding diagnosis and treatment alternatives. Psychological distress related to a perceived sense of powerlessness and loss of control over the situation is not uncommon, and spiritual distress may be encountered as the patient attempts to assign personal meaning or significance to the diagnosis and its impending impact on his life.[68, 69]

As stated earlier, the majority of prostate cancer patients are men older than 65. Although it is frequently assumed that a diagnosis of cancer is not as traumatic an event for an elderly person compared with his younger counterpart, the elderly patient is vulnerable to the same array of distress reactions commonly seen in younger patients.[70] The diagnosis of cancer has the potential to compound inherent developmental challenges related to aging already faced by the majority of this population, including loss of role identity and loss of income through retirement, diminishing social support networks, and loss of spouse or loved ones, declines in physiologic and psychological performance, and increasing incidence of comorbid conditions such as arthritis, diabetes, heart disease, and hypertension. As O'Connor and Blesch[71] stated, "many elderly cancer patients do not cope just with cancer, but with other diseases as well" (p 181). In fact, the presence of other comorbid conditions at diagnosis is associated with an increased risk for poorer psychological outcome.[72] Generally, older individuals have more limited resources overall to use in managing a cancer diagnosis and its treatment, which holds the potential for further deprivation of physical health, autonomy, and self-esteem.[73]

A diagnosis of cancer often poses an immediate threat to body image.[74] The impact of a diagnosis of prostate cancer poses an additional threat to the patient's perceptions of masculinity, physical self, and identity and should not be minimized. Treatment-related complications such as urinary incontinence and bowel dysfunction can represent a source of embarrassment and can prompt withdrawal from participation in social activities. Sexual impairment, including erectile dysfunction secondary to radical prostatectomy or radiation therapy and loss of libido and feminization resulting from hormonal manipulation, can present tremendous adjustment issues for the patient and his partner. As Ofman[75] stated, "disruption in functioning or changes of appearance trigger reactions in some patients far greater than the medical team expects" (p 125). Singer and colleagues,[84] in their 1991 study of 50 men with localized prostate cancer, found that some men, particularly those with lower levels of education, were willing to trade off improved survival in an effort to preserve their level of sexual functioning, even if it was impaired at the outset and they only hoped for an improvement in functioning. Additionally, constitutional symptoms such as pain, fatigue, and nausea can significantly hamper feelings of masculinity, sexual desire, and overall well-being. Issues surrounding potential impairment of sexual function are frequently compounded in elderly patients, who are likely already experiencing age-related impairment of function and are often subject to societal misconceptions that sexual interest and activity are no longer of issue to them.[73]

Finally, one cannot address the psychosocial impacts of a diagnosis of cancer without discussing its impact on the family. The patient's experience with cancer has been described as an assault on the entire family.[76] It is now known that spouses experience significant levels of emotional distress, similar to those of patients themselves, and are often manifested as appetite-sleep disturbances, anxiety, and depression. The initial period surrounding diagnosis has been shown to be a time of particularly acute distress.[76] Complicating matters further, male patients typically fare better using denial as a defense mechanism, whereas the female partners may suffer increased distress if their style of coping is geared toward open communication of thoughts and emotions.[79] Additionally, as families struggle to adjust to the diagnosis and its implications for their loved one, members often experience heightened anxiety and interpersonal tension.[78] Amid all this emotional turmoil and psychological distress, the daily maintenance activities of the family must continue.

NURSING ISSUES AND CONCERNS

The nurse can be instrumental in facilitating patient and family adjustment to the diagnosis and participation in treatment decision making after a diagnosis of prostate cancer. Patient and family anxiety will be high, a factor that can often inhibit adequate comprehension of initial information provided regarding diagnosis and treatment alternatives as well as communication with health care providers. Nurses can play a key role in reducing anxieties through the provision of concrete information and nonjudgmental listening and support of the patient and family.

Because the ideal medical management of early-stage prostate cancer remains controversial, patients and their families have no clear-cut answers regarding treatment decisions.[79] The uncertainty of a diagnosis of cancer is compounded by the dilemma of not having a definite path for how "best" to proceed. When newly diagnosed prostate cancer patients were surveyed to ascertain the types of information they were seeking, three preferred themes emerged: (1) likelihood of cure; (2) stage and extent of disease; and (3) treatment alternatives available.[80] Among other beneficial outcomes, the provision of information to cancer patients has been demonstrated to improve the patient's sense of personal control, increase participation in treatment decision making, decrease levels of anxiety and distress, and facilitate communication of illness-related information to family members.[68]

Nurses working with newly diagnosed prostate cancer patients need to ascertain the extent of the patient's and family's understanding of information provided by physicians, clarify any misconceptions, and reinforce explanations as needed. Optional interventions nurses can use to enhance patient and family assimilation of information include one-on-one education, provision of written literature, identification of questions and concerns to be directed to the physician, and suggestions to audiotape initial consultations regarding diagnosis and treatment options. Nurses need to recognize that patients often obtain misinformation from friends and family members and lay literature and often underuse resources from the American Cancer Society and other agencies as potential sources of information.[79]

It is important to identify patient preferences and values when considering treatment alternatives. Clear, honest explanation of associated treatment complications such as erectile dysfunction and urinary incontinence and their overall incidence needs to be provided as well as whether potential benefit (i.e., improved survival) is likely to be gained. This is particularly true for patients with clinically localized, well-differentiated disease and for patients of advanced age or with significant comorbid illness. It should be noted as well that a course of watchful waiting is not without its potential for psychological distress; patients and family members may experience heightened uncertainty because nothing tangible is being done to treat the disease. Nurses need to serve as patient advocates in helping the patient and family make an informed decision regarding treatment and help the patient and family establish realistic expectations of treatment and goals for rehabilitation, whether the desired outcome is disease cure, control, or palliation. It is important also for nurses to respect and support the patient's decisions regarding treatment.

Nurses should seek to perform a comprehensive psychosocial assessment of the patient and family to assess adequacy of formal and informal support systems, potential for complying with therapy, existing financial resources, and prior coping style.[71, 77] Also important is a discussion of the patient's and partner's sexual concerns and potential side effects of treatment, which should be initiated when a decision is made regarding treatment.[75] Enhanced sexual functioning and improved overall adjustment have been demonstrated when sexual information and counseling were made available to patients.[81] Nurses can create an environment conducive to discussion of sexual concerns, suggest practical interventions to use for managing sexual side effects (such as timing sexual activity when fatigue is least problematic), and refer patients and partners to a trained sex therapist or counselor.[75, 82]

Referral to patient or family support groups can be quite beneficial. The important benefits of support during illness (as well as the potential negative impacts of its absence) have been well characterized.[83] Types of support groups vary, ranging from quite informal peer discussion groups, outings, and recreational activities to more formalized information sessions covering issues such as treatment side effects and their management. Support groups may be particularly useful in the elderly patient population, whose own peer and social support networks have often diminished.

In summary, nurses play a pivotal role in facilitating patient and family adjustment to a diagnosis of prostate cancer as well as in helping the patient and family decide on a course of treatment that is best for that individual within the context of his own unique circumstances. At a time of great uncertainty and upheaval, nurses may serve as a supportive, reassuring presence, guiding the patient and family through the initial difficult phases of diagnosis and treatment decision making.

REFERENCES

1. Corral DA, Bahnson RR. Survival of men with clinically localized prostate cancer detected in the eighth decade of life. *J Urol* 1994;152:1326–1329.
2. Zincke H, Bergstralh EJ, Blute ML, et al. Radical prostatectomy for clinically localized prostate cancer: Long-term results of 1,143 patients from a single institution. *J Clin Oncol* 1994;12:2254–2263.
3. Satariano WA, Ragland KE, Van Den Eeden SK. Cause of death in men diagnosed with prostate carcinoma. *Cancer* 1998;83:1180–1188.
4. Helgesen F, Holmberg L, Johansson JE, et al. Trends in prostate cancer survival in Sweden, 1960 through 1988: Evidence of increasing diagnosis of nonlethal tumors. *J Natl Cancer Instit* 1996;88:1216-1221.
5. Vijayakumar S, Vaida F, Weichselbaum R, Hellman S. Race and the Will Rogers phenomenon in prostate cancer. *Cancer J Sci Am* 1998;4:27–34.
6. Amling CL, Blute ML, Lerner S, et al. Influence of prostate-specific antigen testing on the spectrum of patients with prostate cancer undergoing radical prostatectomy at a large referral practice. *Mayo Clin Proc* 1998;73:401–406.
7. Schuessler WW, Pharand D, Vancaillie TG. Laparoscopic standard pelvic node dissection for carcinoma of the prostate: Is it accurate? *J Urol* 1993; 150:898–901.
8. Stone NN, Stock RG, Unger P. Indications for seminal vesicle biopsy and laparoscopic pelvic lymph

node dissection in men with localized carcinoma of the prostate. *J Urol* 1995;154:1392–1396.

9. Oesterling JE, Brendler CB, Epstein JI, et al. Correlation of clinical stage, serum prostatic acid phosphatase and preoperative Gleason grade with final pathological stage in 275 patients with clinically localized adenocarcinoma of the prostate. *J Urol* 1987;138:92–98.

10. Gleason DF. Histologic grading and clinical staging of prostatic carcinoma. In: Tannenbaum M. (ed). *Urologic Pathology: The Prostate.* Philadelphia: Lea & Febiger, 1977:171–197.

11. Algaba F, Epstein JI, Aldape HC, et al. Assessment of prostate carcinoma in core needle biopsy: Definition of minimal criteria for the diagnosis of cancer in biopsy material. *Cancer* 1996;78: 376–381.

12. Albertsen PC, Fryback DG, Storer BE, et al. Long-term survival among men with conservatively treated localized prostate cancer. *JAMA* 1995;274: 626-631.

13. Partin AW, Steinberg GD, Pitcock RV, et al. Use of nuclear morphometry, Gleason histologic scoring, clinical stage, and age to predict disease-free survival among patients with prostate cancer. *Cancer* 1992;70:161–168.

14. Lieber MM. Pathological stage C (pT3) prostate cancer treated by radical prostatectomy: Clinical implications of DNA ploidy analysis. *Semin Urol* 1990;8:219–224.

15. Takayama TK, Vessella RL, Lange PH. Newer applications of serum prostate-specific antigen in the management of prostate cancer. *Semin Oncol* 1994;21:542–553.

16. American Society for Therapeutic Radiology and Oncology Consensus Panel: Consensus statement: Guidelines for PSA following radiation therapy. *Int J Radiat Oncol Bio Phys* 1997;37:1035–1041.

17. Chodak GW, Thisted RA, Gerber GS, et al. Results of conservative management of clinically localized prostate cancer. *N Engl J Med* 1994;330:242–248.

18. Johansson JE, Holmberg L, Johansson S, et al. Fifteen-year survival in prostate cancer: A prospective, population-based study in Sweden. *JAMA* 1997;277: 467–471.

19. Albertsen PC, Hanley JA, Gleason DF, et al. Competing risk analysis of men aged 55 to 74 at diagnosis managed conservatively for clinically localized prostate cancer. *JAMA* 1998;280:975–980.

20. Waaler G, Stenwig AE. Prognosis of localised prostatic cancer managed by "watch and wait" policy. *Br J Urol* 1993;72:214–219.

21. Adolfsson J, Ronstrom L, Lowhagen T, et al. Deferred treatment of clinically localized low grade prostate cancer: The experience from a prospective series at the Karolinska hospital. *J Urol* 1994;152: 1757–1760.

22. Graversen PH, Nielsen KT, Gasser TC, et al. Radical prostatectomy versus expectant primary treatment in stages I and II prostatic cancer: A fifteen-year follow-up. *Urology* 1990;36:493–498.

23. Witjes WP, Schulman CC, Debruyne FM. Preliminary results of a prospective randomized study comparing radical prostatectomy versus radical prostatectomy associated with neoadjuvant hormonal combination therapy in T2-3 N0 M0 prostatic carcinoma. *Urology* 1997;49(Suppl 3A): 65–69.

24. Fair WR, Cookson MS, Stroumbakis N, et al. The indications, rationale, and results of neoadjuvant androgen deprivation in the treatment of prostatic cancer: Memorial Sloan-Kettering Cancer Center results. *Urology* 1997;49(Suppl 3A):46–55.

25. Bales GT, Williams MJ, Sinner M, et al. Short-term outcomes after cryosurgical ablation of the prostate in men with recurrent prostate carcinoma following radiation therapy. *Urology* 1995;46:676–680.

26. Shinohara K, Connolly JA, Presti JC, et al. Cryosurgical treatment of localized prostate cancer (stages T1 to T4): Preliminary results. *J Urol* 1996; 156:115–121.

27. Oesterling JE, Martin SK, Bergstralh EJ, et al. The use of prostate-specific antigen in staging patients with newly diagnosed prostate cancer. *JAMA* 1993;269(1):57–60.

28. Huncharek M, Muscat J. Serum prostate-specific antigen as a predictor of radiographic staging studies in newly diagnosed prostate cancer. *Cancer Invest* 1995;13:31–35.

29. Asbell SO, Martz KL, Shin KH, et al. Impact of surgical staging in evaluating the radiotherapeutic outcome in RTOG #77-08, a phase III study for T1bN0M0 and T2N0M0 prostate carcinoma. *Int J Radiat Oncol Biol Phys* 1998;40:769–782.

30. Duncan W, Warde P, Catton CN, et al. Carcinoma of the prostate: Results of radical radiotherapy (1970–1985). *Int J Radiat Oncol Biol Phys* 1993;26: 203–210.

31. D'Amico AV, Whittington R, Malkowicz B, et al. Biochemical outcome after radical prostatectomy, external beam radiation therapy, or interstitial radiation therapy for clinically localized prostate cancer. *JAMA* 1998;280:969–974.

32. Soffen EM, Hanks GE, Hunt MA, et al. Conformal static field radiation therapy treatment of early prostate cancer versus non-conformal techniques: A reduction in acute morbidity. *Int J Radiat Oncol Biol Phys* 1992;24:485–488.

33. Horwitz EM, Hanlon AL, Pinover WH, et al. The treatment of nonpalpable PSA-detected adenocarcinoma of the prostate with 3-dimensional conformal radiation therapy. *Int J Radiat Oncol Biol Phys* 1998;41:519–523.

34. Pilepich MV, Caplan R, Byhardt RW, et al. Phase III trial of androgen suppression using goserelin in unfavorable-prognosis carcinoma of the prostate treated with definitive radiotherapy: Report of Radiation Therapy Oncology Group protocol 85-31. *J Clin Oncol* 1997;15:1013–1021.

35. Pilepich MV, Krall JM, Al-Sarraf M, et al. Androgen deprivation with radiation therapy compared with radiation therapy alone for locally advanced prostatic carcinoma: A randomized comparative trial of the Radiation Therapy Oncology Group. *Urology* 1995;45:616–623.

36. Bolla M, Gonzalez D, Warde P, et al. Improved survival in patients with locally advanced prostate cancer treated with radiotherapy and goserelin. *N Engl J Med* 1997;337:295–300.

37. Ragde H, Blasko JC, Grimm PD, et al. Interstitial iodine-125 radiation without adjuvant therapy in the treatment of clinically localized prostate carcinoma. *Cancer* 1997;80:442–453.

38. Sharkey J, Chovnick SD, Behar RJ, et al. Outpatient ultrasound-guided palladium 103 brachytherapy for localized adenocarcinoma of the prostate: A preliminary report of 434 patients. *Urology* 1998;51:796–803.

39. D'Amico AV, Coleman CN. Role of interstitial radiotherapy in the management of clinically organ-confined prostate cancer: The jury is still out. *J Clin Oncol* 1996;14:304–315.

40. Critz FA, Levinson AK, Williams WH, et al. Simultaneous radiotherapy for prostate cancer: I-125 prostate implant followed by external beam radiotherapy. *Cancer J Sci Am* 1998;4:359–363.

41. Vicini FA, Horwitz EM, Kini VR, et al. Radiotherapy options for localized prostate cancer based on pretreatment serum prostate-specific antigen levels and biochemical control: A comprehensive review of the literature. *Int J Radiat Oncol Biol Phys* 1998;40:1101–1110.

42. Robinson RG. Strontium-89: Precursor targeted therapy for pain relief of blastic metastatic disease. *Cancer* 1993;72(Suppl):3433–3435.

43. Bolger JJ, Dearnaley DP, Kirk D, et al. Strontium-89 (Metastron) versus external beam radiotherapy in patients with painful bone metastases secondary to prostatic cancer: Preliminary report of a multicenter trial. *Semin Oncol* 1993;20(Suppl 2):32–33.

44. Porter AT, McEwan AJ, Powe JE, et al. Results of a randomized phase-III trial to evaluate the efficacy of strontium-89 adjuvant to local field external beam irradiation in the management of endocrine resistant metastatic prostate cancer. *Int J Radiat Oncol Biol Phys* 1993;25:805–813.

45. Cabet JF, Tosteson TD, Dong EW, et al. Maximum androgen blockade in advanced prostate cancer: A meta-analysis of published randomized controlled trials using nonsteroidal antiandrogens. *Urology* 1997;49:71–78.

46. Eisenberger MA, Blumenstein BA, Crawford ED, et al. Bilateral orchiectomy with or without flutamide for metastatic prostate cancer. *N Engl J Med* 1998;339:1036–1042.

47. Medical Research Council Prostate Cancer Working Party Investigators Group. Immediate versus deferred treatment for advanced prostatic cancer: Initial results of the Medical Research Council Trial. *Br J Urol* 1997;79:235–246.

48. Small EJ, Vogelzang NJ. Second-line hormonal therapy for advanced prostate cancer: A shifting paradigm. *J Clin Oncol* 1997;15:382–388.

49. Kelly WK, Scher HI, Mazumdar M, et al. Prostate-specific antigen as a measure of disease outcome in metastatic hormone-refractory prostate cancer. *J Clin Oncol* 1993;11:607–615.

50. Taylor CD, Elson P, Trump DL. Importance of continued testicular suppression in hormone-refractory prostate cancer. *J Clin Oncol* 1993;11:2167–2172.

51. Hussain M, Wolf M, Marshall E, et al. Effects of continued androgen-deprivation therapy and other prognostic factors on response and survival in phase II chemotherapy trials for hormone-refractory

prostate cancer: A Southwest Oncology Group report. *J Clin Oncol* 1994;12:1868–1875.

52. Pienta KJ, Redman B, Hussain M, et al. Phase II evaluation of oral estramustine and oral etoposide in hormone-refractory adenocarcinoma of the prostate. *J Clin Oncol* 1994;12:2005–2012.

53. Hudes GR, Greenberg R, Krigel RL, et al. Phase II study of estramustine and vinblastine, two microtubule inhibitors, in hormone-refractory prostate cancer. *J Clin Oncol* 1992;10:1754–1761.

54. Tannock IF, Osoba D, Stockler MR, et al. Chemotherapy with mitoxantrone plus prednisone or prednisone alone for symptomatic hormone-resistant prostate cancer: A Canadian randomized trial with palliative end points. *J Clin Oncol* 1996;14:1756–1764.

55. Myers C, Cooper M, Stein C, et al. Suramin: A novel growth factor antagonist with activity in hormone-refractory metastatic prostate cancer. *J Clin Oncol* 1992;10:881–889.

56. Lu-Yao GL, McLerran D, Wasson J, et al. An assessment of radical prostatectomy: Time trends, geographic variation, and outcomes. *JAMA* 1993;269:2633–2636.

57. Catalona WJ, Basler JW. Return of erections and urinary continence following nerve sparing radical retropubic prostatectomy. *J Urol* 1993;150:905–907.

58. Fowler FJ, Barry MJ, Lu-Yao G, et al. Patient-reported complications and follow-up treatment after radical prostatectomy—the National Medicare experience: 1988–1990 (updated June 1993). *Urology* 1993;42:622–629.

59. Jonler M, Messing EM, Rhodes PR, et al. Sequelae of radical prostatectomy. *Br J Urol* 1994;74:352–358.

60. Geary ES, Dendinger TE, Freiha FS, et al. Nerve sparing radical prostatectomy: A different view. *J Urol* 1995;154:145–149.

61. Litwin MS, Hays RD, Fink A, et al. Quality-of-life outcomes in men treated for localized prostate cancer. *JAMA* 1995;273:129–135.

62. Greskovich FJ, Zagars GK, Sherman NE, et al. Complications following external beam radiation therapy for prostate cancer: An analysis of patients treated with and without staging pelvic lymphadenectomy. *J Urol* 1991;146:798–802.

63. Fowler FJ, Barry MJ, Lu-Yao G, et al. Outcomes of external-beam radiation therapy for prostate cancer: A study of Medicare beneficiaries in three Surveillance, Epidemiology, and End Results areas. *J Clin Oncol* 1996;14:2258–2265.

64. Daniell HW. Osteoporosis after orchiectomy for prostate cancer. *J Urol* 1997;157:439–444.

65. Wysowski DK, Freiman JP, Tourtelot JB, et al. Fatal and nonfatal hepatotoxicity associated with flutamide. *Ann Intern Med* 1993;118:860–864.

66. Soloway MS, Schellhammer PF, Smith JA, et al. Bicalutamide in the treatment of advanced prostatic carcinoma: A phase II multicenter trial. *Urology* 1996;47(Suppl 1A):33–37.

67. Kirschenbaum A. Management of hormonal treatment effects. *Cancer* 1995;75(Suppl):1983–1986.

68. Davison BJ, Degner LF. Empowerment of men newly diagnosed with prostate cancer. *Cancer Nurs* 1997;20:187–196.

69. McCray ND. Psychosocial and quality-of-life issues. In: Otto SE (ed). *Oncology Nursing*, 2nd ed. St. Louis, MO: CV Mosby, 1997:817–834.

70. Engelking C. Comfort issues in geriatric oncology. *Semin Oncol Nurs* 1988;4:198–207.

71. O'Connor L, Blesch KS. Life cycle issues affecting cancer rehabilitation. *Semin Oncol Nurs* 1992;8:174–185.

72. Barsevick AM, Much J, Sweeney C. Psychosocial responses to cancer. In: Groenwald MH, Frogge M, Goodman M, Yarbro CH (eds). *Cancer Nursing: Principles and Practice*, 4th ed. Sudbury, MA: Jones and Bartlett, 1997:1393–1410.

73. Shell JA, Smith CK. Sexuality and the older person with cancer. *Oncol Nurs Forum* 1994;21:553–558.

74. Burt K. The effects of cancer on body image and sexuality. *Nurs Times* 1995;91:36–37.

75. Ofman U. Preservation of function in genitourinary cancers: Psychosexual and psychosocial issues. *Cancer Invest* 1995;13:125–131.

76. Northouse LL, Peters-Golden H. Cancer and the family: Strategies to assist spouses. *Semin Oncol Nurs* 1993;9:74–82.

77. Ofman U. Psychosocial and sexual implications of genitourinary cancers. *Semin Oncol Nurs* 1993;9:286–292.

78. Lewis FM. Psychosocial transitions and the family's work in adjusting to cancer. *Semin Oncol Nurs* 1993;9:127–129.

79. O'Rourke ME, Germino BB. Prostate cancer treatment decisions: A focus group exploration. *Oncol Nurs Forum* 1998;25:97–104.

80. Davison BJ, Degner LF, Morgan TR. Information and decision-making preferences of men with prostate cancer. *Oncol Nurs Forum* 1995;22:1401–1408.

81. Anderson B. Sexual functioning morbidity among cancer survivors. *Cancer* 1985;55:1835–1842.

82. Fisher SG. The psychosexual effects of cancer and cancer treatment. *Oncol Nurs Forum* 1983;10:63–67.

83. Peters-Golden H. Breast cancer: Varied perceptions of social support in the illness experience. *Soc Sci Med* 1982;16:463–491.

84. Singer PA, Tasch ES, Stocking C, et al. Sex or survival: Trade-offs between quality and quantity of life. *J Clin Oncol* 1991;9:328–334.

Chapter 7

EXPECTANT MANAGEMENT: THE ART AND SCIENCE OF WATCHFUL WAITING

MAUREEN E. O'ROURKE

ANDREW S. GRIFFIN

OVERVIEW

INTRODUCTION

RATIONALE FOR EXPECTANT MANAGEMENT

RATIONALE AGAINST EXPECTANT MANAGEMENT

THERAPEUTIC GOAL OF EXPECTANT MANAGEMENT

PATIENT ELIGIBILITY CRITERIA

PATIENT AND PARTNER VIEWS OF THE EXPECTANT MANAGEMENT OPTION

PROTOCOL FOR EXPECTANT MANAGEMENT

WHEN SHOULD TREATMENT BE PURSUED?

NURSING MANAGEMENT OF PATIENTS CHOOSING THE EXPECTANT MANAGEMENT OPTION

PSYCHOEDUCATIONAL INTERVENTIONS TO MINIMIZE UNCERTAINTY

CONCLUSION

INTRODUCTION

Prostate cancer continues to be the most common malignancy among men in the United States, accounting for an estimated 37,000 deaths annually.[1] This disease has been shrouded by a cloak of controversy and uncertainty, extending from initial decisions regarding the value and efficacy of screening and early detection to uncertainty regarding treatment choices and the management of treatment-related side effects and recurrent disease. The rising incidence of prostate cancer over the last decade has been paralleled by dramatic increases in media coverage. This coverage has included the personal testimony of male celebrities such as Intel chief executive officer Andy Groves, Persian Gulf war hero General Norman Schwarzkopf, and presidential candidate Bob Dole regarding their aggressive approaches to treatment and cure and frank discussion of previously taboo issues such as impotence and incontinence.[2, 3] Equal press, however, has not been given to the treatment option of watchful waiting, or expectant management. The American public would be hard-pressed to identify a single public figure who has spoken about his own personal experience with prostate cancer who has chosen this option.

Within the confines of Western medicine, three basic options are offered for the treatment of early-stage prostate cancer: radical prostatectomy, radiation therapy (either external beam or brachytherapy), and expectant management. The latter (also known as watchful waiting, observation, and surveillance therapy) has been defined as initial surveillance followed by active treatment if and when tumor progression causes bothersome symptoms.[4] Although the time to progression varies greatly depending on myriad factors, including histologic grade of the tumor, average time to initiation of such treatment is up to 10 years.[5] A common misconception is that patients are ignored while being monitored by surveillance only, when in fact they are monitored at regular intervals primarily through digital rectal examination (DRE) and prostate-specific antigen (PSA) testing.[6]

Important factors for patients and physicians in selecting among the available options are consideration of potential treatment side effects (e.g., incontinence, impotence, bowel dysfunction), estimation of life expectancy, and threat of increased morbidity and accelerated mortality associated with foregoing active treatment. Equally important considerations are the personal, marital, and cultural implications of each treatment option.

The focus of this chapter is a review of the option of expectant management, examining the scientific rationale for recommending this strategy in the case of early-stage prostate cancer, the therapeutic goals, and the criteria for patient eligibility. Additionally, the medical and nursing management of patients selecting this option is discussed with emphasis on the psychosocial support of patients and their families.

RATIONALE FOR EXPECTANT MANAGEMENT

The scientific rationale for offering expectant management as an option for early-stage prostate cancer has its basis in empiric observation: The incidence rates for prostate cancer far exceed the death rates, leading to the conclusion that more men are dying *with* the disease than *of* the disease.[7] The lifetime risk of an American male developing prostate cancer is 10%, whereas the risk of an American male dying of the disease is only 3%.[8] Proponents of this strategy cite the slow-growing nature of prostate tumors as further justification for the avoidance of aggressive therapy with its resultant side effects. Yet this strategy may not be applicable to African-American males. Incidence rates for males in the United States for 1995 to 1999 indicate that 150.3 Caucasian males per 100,000 and 224.3 African-American males per 100,000 are affected. Additionally, differential survival statistics among these two racial groups suggest that African-American males fare significantly worse than Caucasian males. Between 1989 and 1994, 5-year survival for Caucasian males was 95%; however, for African-American males during that same period, it was only 81% (significant at $P < .05$).[1]

The discovery of PSA and the widespread adoption of this screening test has made it possible (and indeed probable) to detect tumors before they are palpable on DRE, and perhaps, as some speculate, to detect tumors that are clinically insignificant.[6] Cancers detected through PSA-based screening programs are more likely to be organ confined and thus potentially amenable to early intervention.[7] However, these same tumors may not, over the patient's lifetime, cause any significant morbidity. The phenomenal increase in the number of diagnosed cases of prostate cancer since the introduction of PSA testing has not been universally hailed as advantageous, and critics contend that it has led to improvement of neither quantity of life nor quality of life (QOL).[9, 10]

Research has provided mounting evidence that surgery or radiation may not improve overall survival,[9] and, increasingly, concerns have been raised in the literature regarding QOL among previously asymptomatic men who developed distressing side effects after treatment. Guidelines published by the American College of Physicians (ACP)[11] cite a 3-year gain in life span for men diagnosed with prostate cancer who are treated aggressively with radical prostatectomy or radiation therapy, only a 1.5-year gain for men in their 60s, and a mere 0.4-year gain for men in their 70s.

Expectant management has been favored as a treatment option in the European community for more than 30 years. However, interest in this treatment option has increased in the United States only over the past 4 to 5 years after the publication of several reports indicating comparable survival at 10 and 15 years for men treated with this approach versus curative intent therapies.[12–14] Johansson and colleagues'[12] frequently quoted study consisted of retrospective observation of 233 patients (mean age, 72 years) with early-stage prostate cancer who received no treatment until symptomatic progression occurred. At this point the men received hormonal therapy. After a mean of 15 years follow-up, disease-specific survival rates were calculated to be 81%, a rate comparable to that of men who had undergone medical or surgical treatment. The investigators concluded that expectant management is a reasonable alternative for men with localized prostate cancer.[12] Because of the lack of prospective, randomized trials, justification for recommending this conservative option is based largely on retrospective data.

Goodman and colleagues[15] retrospectively reviewed 69 cases of men in whom prostate cancer was diagnosed incidentally at subtotal prostatectomy. The men received no further treatment despite the malignant diagnosis. Only six deaths were attributable to tumor progression. When progression was noted, men received hormonal therapy. Men younger than 70 with diffuse, high-grade (T1b) disease were at greater risk for symptomatic progression, most notably skeletal metastasis (60%) within 3 years. Other studies cited in the oncology and urologic literature indicate similar findings.

Adolfsson[4] reviewed various survival endpoints from 12 research publications, including overall survival, progression-free survival, and disease-specific survival. He concluded that overall survival at 10 years among prostate cancer patients choosing the expectant management option ranged from 34 to 72%. Progression-free survival, if based on bone scans as the measure of metastatic disease, ranged from 43 to 77% at 10 years. Finally, he reported disease-specific survival, which represents the chance of being alive at a specific point in time if not having died from some other disease, and noted that this measure is dependent on accurate establishment of cause of death. Although Adolfsson suggested that this is a less robust survival endpoint than overall survival, he reported disease-specific survival rates among the series reviewed to range from 74 to 87% at 10 years. Criticisms of the data emerging from these retrospective studies include patient selection bias concerns, including the observation that men in the conservatively managed group often were older, had smaller tumors, and had slower disease progression; thus, it is understandable that such men are dying of other causes.[16,17]

The U.S. Preventive Health Services, the Canadian Task Force on Periodic Health Examination, and the ACP have recommended against routine PSA screening for prostate cancer.[11, 18] Such recommendations stem in part from concerns over the lack of randomized clinical trials demonstrating the efficacy of treatment in reducing morbidity and mortality compared with expectant management alone. A single randomized trial comparing radical prostatectomy with expectant management failed to demonstrate significant differences in survival rates over 15 years; however, this study has been severely criticized for its design flaws.[19] In light of this lack of scientific evidence, the National Cancer Institute and the Veterans Affairs Cooperative Studies Group has undertaken a large-scale, randomized trial comparing radical prostatectomy with palliative expectant management for the treatment of clinically localized prostate cancer (Prostate Intervention Versus Observation Trial [PIVOT]). Additional studies are currently under way in Europe.

PIVOT, launched in 1995, was expected to enroll 2,000 patients over a 3-year period and will monitor these men over 12 years (for a total of 15 observable years). Eligibility requirements include age (patient of 75 years or younger with an estimated 10-year life expectancy) clinically localized prostate cancer of T1a,b,c/T2a,b,c and NX and M0 status (see Chapter 5 for explanation of prostate cancer staging), and diagnosis with prostate cancer in the preceding 6 months.[20] The trial is active and ongoing but has had difficulties with recruitment. In 1997 after a little more than 2 years of recruitment, PIVOT had enrolled slightly more than 400 men.[21] The slow rate of patient accrual has required a decrease in the sample size from 2,000 to 1,050 as well as extension of the recruitment period from 3 to 7 years.[22] Until data collection and analysis-interpretation are complete, healthcare providers and patients must continue to deliberate the value of expectant management as a treatment option based on a combination of factors, one of which is not solid scientific evidence.

RATIONALE AGAINST EXPECTANT MANAGEMENT

Just as early intervention strategies (radical prostatectomy, radiation) involve potential risks, so does expectant management. Scientific evidence supports the premise that radical prostatectomy and radiation therapy offer the possibility of complete tumor eradication and cure. Additionally, active treatment may reduce patient anxiety and uncertainty. Treatment with either radiation or surgery may also reduce the risk of metastasis and the need for subsequent interventions for disease.[23]

Early enthusiasm for the expectant management approach in patients with localized prostate cancer has been tempered by reports indicating that the full impact of intervention versus no intervention may not be detectable until 10 to 15 years.[24] Aus and colleagues[14] found that, among men with nonmetastatic disease at diagnosis who survived for more than 10 years, 63% eventually died from prostate cancer. Studies have demonstrated that younger men with T2 disease undergoing conservative management have a high risk of developing incurable disease and dying from prostate cancer itself.[14, 25] McLaren and associates[26] monitored 113 previously untreated men (mean age, 75 years) diagnosed with prostate cancer. Forty percent of the T1 patients and 51% of the T2 patients had clinical progression within 2 years; 60% had clinical progression by 3 years.

In perhaps the most comprehensive review of the arguments against expectant management of prostate cancer, Hugosson, Aus, and Norlen[27] posed three fundamental questions: Is prostate cancer a major health problem? Is current prostate cancer mortality acceptable? Is it worthwhile to decrease prostate cancer mortality? The magnitude of prostate cancer as a public health problem is obvious. In 1999 alone, 179,300 new cases are expected to be diagnosed in the United States, with 37,000 deaths anticipated.[1] Hugosson and colleagues[27] presented data suggesting that the relative costs of prostate cancer care should not be solely attributed to curative intent treatment (e.g., prostatectomy, radiation). Rather, consideration must be given to the cost of prolonged and intense morbidity associated with untreated disease, specifically the sequelae of metastasis: pain management, obstruction, palliative radiation, and upper urinary tract diversions. They cautioned that the dominant costs associated with prostate cancer care are those involving hospital care, often required for men in the final year of life. These same authors maintained that conservatively treated prostate cancer patients who do not die from the disease actually die from comorbidities already present, which do not allow them sufficient time to develop prostate cancer progression. They concluded that surveillance is a poor option because of the high financial and personal costs associated with pain, suffering, and death from progressive disease.

THERAPEUTIC GOAL OF EXPECTANT MANAGEMENT

The therapeutic goal of expectant management is to spare early-stage prostate cancer patients unnecessary treatment-related toxicity and to maintain reasonable QOL without compromising overall survival. Implicit in this therapeutic goal is maintaining the patient's sense of well-being, even in the face of considerable uncertainty.

Unfortunately, there is a lack of research to document the assumption that expectant management offers better QOL than other active treatment options. The majority of the medical literature published in the last 5 years examined QOL issues related to men receiving some form of active treatment for prostate cancer, either early stage or advanced. A single study was found that examined QOL in early-stage prostate cancer that included an observation or expectant management group.[28] In this study, Litwin and colleagues examined health-related QOL and disease-specific QOL among men treated for localized prostate cancer with radical prostatectomy (N=98), radiation therapy (N=56), and expectant management (N=60). Treatment groups were compared with each other and a group of age-matched controls. Findings revealed that surgical patients scored significantly worse than both the expectant management and the comparison groups in the area of sexual functioning. Additionally, the surgical patients scored significantly worse than the radiation, expectant management, and comparison groups in the area of urinary functioning. Radiation patients experienced more bowel dysfunction than the other three groups. With respect to overall health-related QOL, there was only one significant difference between groups. The expectant management (observation) group reported more role limitations because of emotional problems than patients in either treatment group or the comparison group. These data suggest that, although the physiologic aspects of QOL may be better for observation-only patients, the emotional aspects of selecting this option require further investigation. The data also suggest that disease-specific QOL measures may be more sensitive indicators of QOL disruptions than more global instruments.

The nursing literature offers no further insight into evaluating the QOL of men choosing the expectant management option. A single study was located examining QOL among men treated with radiation versus prostatectomy.[29] The findings were consistent with prior studies in that men choosing surgery experienced significantly worse urinary and sexual functioning but better bowel functioning than their radiation therapy counterparts. The sample did not include men choosing the expectant management option, however.

Although expectant management has been a treatment standard in European countries for years, evaluation of this option has been largely confined to survival statistics as opposed to patients' own subjective ratings of their QOL. Until prostate cancer treatment QOL investigations include all three standard treatment options (surgery, radiation, expectant management), healthcare providers have few data to support claims that patients choosing this latter option experience better QOL. Both psychological and physiologic sequelae may include, but are not limited to, uncertainty and urologic symptoms such as urinary obstruction and frequency. How these affect QOL remains to be determined.

PATIENT ELIGIBILITY CRITERIA

It has become increasingly apparent that prostate cancer exists as two distinct entities: (1) tumors that are clinically insignificant and pose little threat to men's lives and overall well-being, and (2) clinically significant tumors that pose significant threats to men's lives in terms of both morbidity and mortality. The distinguishing features characterizing tumors as clinically significant versus clinically insignificant include large tumor volume, elevated PSA, rapidly rising PSA, and high Gleason score.[30](See Chapter 3 for explanation of Gleason scoring.) Although there is no general consensus as to which patients are the most appropriate candidates for the expectant management approach, it has been considered a plausible option for men with a life expectancy of 10 to 15 years or less because of illness or advanced age, asymptomatic men with tumors too advanced to cure, and men with favorable pathologic findings, defined as Gleason scores of less than 7, low PSA density (0.10–0.15), and cancer involving less than three core biopsy specimens or less than 50% of any core.[31] Additional considerations that have been cited in the literature include a PSA level of less than 10 ng/mL and the absence of palpable disease on DRE.[32] Guidelines published by the American Urological Association[33] only specify that those patients who are most likely to benefit from surveillance are those with a shorter life expectancy or a low tumor grade. Published criteria for patient selection have failed to identify one other critical variable in the prostate cancer treatment decision: the patient's and partner's attitude toward this option and their overall tolerance of uncertainty.

PATIENT AND PARTNER VIEWS OF THE EXPECTANT MANAGEMENT OPTION

Little research has been conducted to ascertain the attitudes of men and their spouses or partners toward the expectant management watch and wait option. Healthcare professionals have minimal data as to the process by which prostate cancer patients themselves, or couples, arrive at a treatment decision. Such data are critical in light of the continued controversy surrounding prostate cancer treatment and the scientific ambiguity regarding which treatment, if any, is superior. Several studies suggested that the expectant management, or watch-and-wait, option is viewed negatively, at least within American culture,[34, 35] and some speculation has been made as to the basis of this negative viewpoint.

Using hypothetical case scenarios, Mazur and Merz[34] surveyed 148 male patients (aged 30–85) recruited through a Veterans Affairs Medical Clinic regarding their willingness to choose surgery versus expectant management as therapy for localized prostate cancer. None of the participants actually had prostate cancer but were presented with hypothetical scenarios, which varied treatment options and their expected survival benefits along with defined sets of complications. Forty-three percent of men preferred surgery over expectant management, even in the case of no expected survival benefit and high associated morbidities. However, this study suffers from some inherent biases. The age range of participants was broad, and it is likely that younger men viewed potential side effects such as impotence and incontinence differently than older participants. The expectant management scenario was biased in its presentation as an option that would only delay inevitable intervention, presupposing that symptoms would appear requiring yet another patient decision. Despite these concerns, the study does provide evidence that patients may have a strong bias toward surgery as the optimal treatment for prostate cancer.

O'Rourke[35] examined the decision-making process in prostate cancer treatment selection over an 18-month period, interviewing patients and their spouses individually and conjointly. She noted that couples swiftly rejected the expectant management, or watch-and-wait, option, which they consistently referred to as "doing nothing." This option was scrutinized through comparisons with other cancer patients (not necessarily prostate cancer patients) they had known who took this path and died painful deaths and comparisons with positive role models who were fighters and never gave up (General Schwartzkopf). This option did not hold up when patients and spouses confronted their worst fears: that, left untreated, the cancer would spread and cause a slow, painful death. Participants in this study spoke of the waiting they had already done, over months or years of monitoring rising PSA levels, and pursuing a diagnosis through numerous biopsies. Both the men and their wives identified "doing nothing" as an option presented to them for consideration by the urologist and in these precise terms. Patients and spouses identified the potential for cure and a minimized risk of recurrence associated with active treatment as the main reasons for opting against the watch-and-wait option. Women were more likely to favor active treatment for prostate cancer at almost any cost, based on their expressed desire to prolong their husband's lives, whereas men gave more consideration to potential treatment-related complications.[36, 37]

Other data have suggested that patients tend to overestimate their survival probabilities, and these estimates influence cancer treatment preferences, leading to a pursuit of more aggressive options.[38] Mazur and Merz[39] demonstrated that older patients were consistently willing to trade off adverse urologic side effects for a better chance of 5-year survival in the case of prostate cancer. This is of particular concern because healthcare providers are presently unable to predict prostate cancer patient survival accurately, despite the publication of complex decision algorithms intended to guide such counseling. Difficulties interpreting survival projections may influence patients' treatment choices in another fashion. Men and their partners may overestimate their survival potential and thus choose to delay treatment, believing that a more effective treatment is yet to be developed. They may opt to watch and wait to buy themselves time and avoid potential side effects associated with the current treatment options.

The sociocultural influences on patients' and couples' view of the expectant management option cannot be overlooked. For older couples facing prostate cancer treatment decisions, such factors as their tendency to defer treatment decisions to perceived omniscient physicians must be considered. Younger patients may be more influenced by access to high-tech modes of information access such as the Internet. In O'Rourke's study,[35] couples were profoundly influenced by past family experiences with cancer and cancer treatment. Finally, celebrity role models may influence attitudes toward prostate cancer treatment options, including expectant management. This effect was noted to be a powerful one in the case of Nancy Reagan's choice of mastectomy versus breast conservation surgery and radiation therapy, particularly among persons who were demographically similar and those of low income and educational status.[40]

PROTOCOL FOR EXPECTANT MANAGEMENT

No published clinical guidelines exist establishing a firm standard of care for expectant management of prostate cancer. Physicians are guided by their best clinical judgment and by collegial consensus. The protocol used in PIVOT is as follows: Patients are seen every

3 months for the first year and then every 6 months thereafter. Each visit includes the assessment of urologic symptoms and QOL, both disease specific and global measures. Physical examination and DRE are performed and PSA levels assessed at each follow-up visit. All patients have an annual bone scan.[23]

Some sources[41] operationalize "carefully observed and monitored at regular intervals" (p 935) to be every 3 months, without any further specification of what tests should be performed at these intervals. No published guidelines exist regarding when patients should undergo a repeat biopsy. The cost effectiveness of annual bone scans has been questioned.

Although practices are highly variable, one approach for men with less than 10 to 15 years of life expectancy and normal age-specific PSA values recommends that a DRE be performed and PSA evaluated every 3 months for 1 year and then every 6 to 12 months thereafter. Patients should be instructed to have their PSA levels drawn before their follow-up visit with the urologist so that interpretation of the results can be accomplished and questions and concerns addressed at the appointment. If these men have an abnormal DRE or increased PSA values, restaging is performed, including bone scan and transrectal ultrasonography (TRUS)–guided biopsies of the prostate. Treatment considerations then would be based on clinical stage, patient age, comorbidities, and personal preferences. Other approaches include PSA, DRE, and TRUS monitoring every 4 to 6 months.

The continued lack of understanding of the biology and natural course of untreated prostate cancer hampers the establishment of formal guidelines. Pending further research, clinicians are guided more by local standards of care than evidence-based medicine, and significant geographic variation in follow-up should be anticipated.

WHEN SHOULD TREATMENT BE PURSUED?

It is generally accepted that active treatment with hormonal manipulation should be pursued when patients who have chosen the expectant management option experience bothersome symptoms.[4] Delaying the initiation of hormonal therapy is based on the observation that the efficacy of hormonal manipulation is limited to 2 to 3 years.[42] For those patients who are not candidates for radical therapy (surgery or radiation), and who psychologically are intolerant of a no-treatment option, early hormonal manipulation may be preferable. This has been cited as a common approach in Latin American countries.[42]

A number of studies have attempted to use PSA as a biologic marker of prostate cancer disease activity. Carter and colleagues[43] demonstrated that the rate of PSA increase in men with prostate cancer is significantly greater (0.75 ng/mL/yr) than in men with benign prostatic hypertrophy only. However, once the diagnosis is established, determining what change in PSA is significant enough to warrant restaging is controversial. PSA doubling time also correlates with clinical disease progression, time to treatment for disease progression, and stage progression[43] and has not yet been demonstrated to be a more powerful indicator of disease activity than the Gleason score, tumor grade, or tumor stage.

NURSING MANAGEMENT OF PATIENTS CHOOSING THE EXPECTANT MANAGEMENT OPTION

Nurses can perform a vital role in educating men and their partners regarding the necessity of vigilant follow-up and in their comprehensive assessment of both overall QOL and disease-specific QOL. Consistent utilization of patient-focused QOL measures at each follow-up interval is essential. Patients and partners should be instructed to call and report any changes in symptoms and to inform their caregivers regarding the extent to which such symptoms interfere with lifestyle.

Herr[44] reviewed a number of QOL studies on prostate cancer, highlighting instruments that have been used with this population. Several prostate cancer–specific QOL instruments with established validity and reliability are available, including University of California at Los Angeles Prostate Cancer Index,[28] Prostate Cancer Treatment Outcome Questionnaire (PCT-Q),[45] Prostate Symptom Score,[46] and Functional Assessment of Cancer Therapy-Prostate.[47] Clinicians should be cautioned that such instruments were originally designed and intended for use in the research rather than the clinical setting and may require some adaptation. Other adaptations may be necessary because the focus of these instruments has been on measuring QOL as a function of treatment-related side effects versus QOL associated with no active treatment. Finally, nurses must consider the validity of QOL instruments when used with culturally diverse populations. Warnecke and colleagues[48] reviewed one QOL instrument (Ferrans and Powers' Quality of Life Index[49]) and noted that several changes were necessary related to interpretation of the questions. Some concepts were not linguistically transferable, response scales required alteration, and readability levels needed to be lowered to accommodate African-American and Mexican-American populations. The authors provided guidance on possible areas for revision enhancing cultural sensitivity.

PSYCHOEDUCATIONAL INTERVENTIONS TO MINIMIZE UNCERTAINTY

One of the most distressing concerns expressed by patients and their partners regarding selection of the expectant management option is living with continual uncertainty.[35] Although uncertainty has not been systematically examined in the prostate cancer population, Mishel and others described uncertainty in several cancer populations and suggested that uncertainty is associated with depression, diminished hope and optimism, and adjustment problems for patients and their family members.[50–52].

Treatment options may be viewed by patients and their families as being associated with varying degrees of certainty or uncertainty. These perceptions may affect treatment choices. Couples in O'Rourke's study[35] perceived surgical removal as curative, leaving no trace of the dreaded malignancy behind. Radiation therapy was viewed as less than curative, leaving a lingering doubt of recurrence, and expectant management was viewed as "doing nothing," forestalling the inevitable need for treatment and ultimately leading to a premature and painful death. In the case of both radiation and expectant management, couples spoke of their difficulties dealing with "not knowing" and of "always wondering" when the malignancy would cause problems and abruptly change their lives. They alluded to the uncertainty associated with these options, and this was a deterrent factor in their treatment choice. Their inclination was to "get it [treatment] over with" and not prolong their anxiety. Given these data, it seems that, in order for the expectant management or watchful waiting treatment option to be acceptable and tolerable over the long run, strategies must be used by individuals and their partners to minimize the negative aspects of uncertainty.

Research in this area has been sparse, given that interest in the expectant management treatment option has only recently taken hold within the United States, and QOL research in prostate cancer is also a recent development. Only one published study to date has specifically examined uncertainty management strategies used by men electing expectant management as a treatment option for prostate cancer.[52] In the nursing literature, Bailey and Mishel[53] and O'Rourke[35] reported that men and their spouses used a number of cognitive schemas to reframe uncertainty. One such strategy was reframing. Treatment was reframed as negative, associated with severe and debilitating side effects. Expectant management, or watchful waiting, was viewed as positive, the optimal choice.

O'Rourke[35] noted that, in making their treatment decision, men often compared themselves with others who were worse off than themselves, and such comparisons allowed them to view their situation more positively. The use of social comparisons or upward social affiliations has been found to be a successful method of maintaining hope and inspiration.[54]

Other strategies used by men included attempts to minimize the cancer threat by focusing on the small size of the tumor, low Gleason scores, and their own low PSA values compared with other men they knew with prostate cancer.[35, 53] Outright dismissal of the cancer threat was also attempted and entailed both not talking about the cancer and attempting to put it out of one's mind.[53]

Bailey and Mishel[53] did note that some men who had opted for expectant management self-medicated with shark cartilage and antioxidants in an effort to fight disease and build up their own immune systems, perhaps alleviating some of the anxiety associated with taking no active treatment for their disease.[35] O'Rourke[35] also reported that several men in her sample (one of whom chose expectant management) used saw palmetto berry extract and a variety of vitamins, minerals, and dietary supplements, including bee pollen and black walnut shell oil, as supplementary treatments.

The use of prayer has also been suggested to be a powerful strategy for dealing with uncertainty. Interest in this phenomenon has sparked considerable research, especially in the area of coping with cancer.[55-57]

Participation in support groups has long been advocated as an effective means of coping with the cancer diagnosis and the sequelae of treatment. This form of social support may not be appropriate, however, for those individuals who use dismissal as their dominant coping strategy. A number of local and nationally affiliated support groups specific to prostate cancer are available, including the US TOO support group and the Man-to-Man program. Nurses should assess both patient's and partner's needs before initiating referrals. Some support groups are structured to include both the men and their partners simultaneously, whereas others are structured to allow for parallel meetings, with men and their partners meeting separately. The unique needs of gay partners must also be considered because partner groups have been traditionally structured as support and educational groups for wives or female partners.

A variety of Internet web sites are available directed at both patients and their partners. Nurses should advise patients and their partners that medical information available at such sites may not be scientifically accurate. The best approach in terms of dealing with alternate treatment modalities and anecdotal information obtained through the Internet or other nontraditional sources is to maintain an open dialogue with patients and their partners and address their underlying concerns.

Cultural and ethnic differences in the uncertainty experiences of men and their families have only recently been explored. Germino and associates[58] reported that, among African-American men with prostate cancer, higher levels of uncertainty were related to a poorer social environment. High levels of uncertainty did not affect adult role functioning among African-American men to the extent that it did among Caucasian men. Emerging research suggests that the centrality of spirituality in QOL is important to African-Americans, particularly the aged. Further attention to both cultural and ethnic differences in the management of uncertainty is warranted. In the interim, nurses must be aware of the possibility of such differences and incorporate such sensitivity into QOL assessments.

The needs of patients and their partners are not always synchronous. Nurses and physicians must be prepared to deal with their concerns individually. Strategies that may be highly effective in managing uncertainty and anxiety for one partner may be poorly received by the other. Although patients and their partners have a shared history, they are also profoundly influenced by their own individual histories and coping styles. The public coping persona and the private coping persona may be quite different. Healthcare providers must take time to address both couple concerns and the concerns of patients and their partners as individuals.

Finally, nurses must address the possibility that the follow-up process itself may trigger increased anxiety and uncertainty. The lack of standardized guidelines for appropriate follow-up may lead to concern about variations among physicians. Additionally, the frequency of the follow-up may exacerbate stress. Recognition of factors potentiating uncertainty and anxiety, allowing for discussion about concerns, and encouragement of uncertainty management strategies tailored to individual patients' and spouses' needs are the critical elements of nursing care for those patients electing to pursue the expectant management option.

CONCLUSION

Johansson and colleagues' hypothesis[12] that expectant management is a viable treatment option for men with early-stage prostate cancer has been tested and seems correct for men with a low risk of biologic disease progression. On the basis of current data, the population of patients most appropriate for expectant management includes those with clinically confined disease; low Gleason scores, PSA values, and PSA densities; and a life expectancy of 10 to 15 years or less.[30–32]

The decision to elect this option is fraught with uncertainty. Follow-up recommendations and clear guidelines as to when treatment should be initiated are vague, with high geographic variability. Nurses and physicians must work with both patients and their partners to develop and maintain strategies to cope with multiple sources of uncertainty if the viability of this option is to extend beyond on-paper survival benefits to true-life benefits in terms of enhanced QOL.

REFERENCES

1. Landis SH, Murray T, Bolden S, Wingo PA. Cancer statistics, 1999. *CA Cancer J Clin* 1999;49:8–31.
2. Jaroff L. The man's cancer. *Time* 1996, April 1:58–63.
3. Grove A. Taking on prostate cancer. *Fortune* 1996, May 13:54–72.
4. Adolfsson J. Deferred treatment for clinically localized prostate cancer. *Eur J Surg Oncol* 1995;21:333–340.
5. Madsen PO, Graversen P, Gasser TC, et al. Treatment of localized prostate cancer. Radical prostatectomy versus placebo: A 15 year follow-up. *Scand J Urol Nephrol Suppl* 1988;100:95–100.
6. Palmer JS, Chodak G. Defining the role of surveillance in the management of localized prostate cancer. *Urol Clin North Am* 1996;23:551–556.
7. Mettlin CJ, Murphy GP. Why is the prostate cancer death rate declining in the United States? *Cancer* 1998;82:249–251.
8. Steinberg GD, Bales GT, Bredler CB. An analysis of watchful waiting for clinically localized prostate cancer. *J Urol* 1998;159:1431–1436.
9. Wilt TJ. Prostate cancer screening: Practice what the evidence preaches. *Am J Med* 1998;104:602–604.
10. Collins MM, Ransohoff DF, Barry MJ. Early detection of prostate cancer. Serendipity strikes again. *JAMA* 1997;278:1516–1519.
11. American College of Physicians. Clinical Guideline: Part III. Screening for prostate cancer. *Ann Intern Med* 1997;126:480–484.
12. Johansson JE, Holmberg L, Johansson S, et al. Fifteen year survival in prostate cancer: Results and identification of high-risk patient population. *JAMA* 1997;277:467–471.
13. Adolfsson J, Carstensen J, Lowhagen T. Deferred treatment in clinically localised prostate carcinoma. *Br J Urol* 1992;69:183–187.
14. Aus G, Hugosson J, Norlen L. Long-term survival and mortality in prostate cancer treated with noncurative intent. *J Urol* 1995;154:460–465.
15. Goodman CM, Busttil A, Chisholm GD. Age, size, and grade of tumor predict prognosis in incidentally diagnosed carcinoma of the prostate. *Br J Urol* 1988;62:576–580.
16. Albertsen PC, Fryback DG, Storer BE, et al. Long-term survival among men with conservatively treated localized prostate cancer. *JAMA* 1995;274:626–631.
17. Chodak GW. The role of watchful waiting in the management of localized prostate cancer. *J Urol* 1994;152:1766–1768.
18. United States Preventive Health Services Task Force. *Guide to Clinical Preventive Services.* 2nd ed. Baltimore, MD: Williams & Wilkins, 1996.
19. Gerber GS, Thisted RA, Scardino PT, et al. Results of radical prostatectomy in men with clinically localized prostate cancer: Multi-institutional analysis. *JAMA* 1996;276:615–619.

20. Moon TD, Brawer MK, Wilt TJ. Prostate intervention versus observation trial (PIVOT): A randomized trial comparing radical prostatectomy with palliative expectant management for treatment of localized prostate cancer. *J Natl Cancer Inst* 1995; 19:69–71.

21. Wilt TJ, Brawer MK. Early intervention or expectant management for prostate cancer: The prostate cancer intervention versus observation trial (PIVOT): A randomized trial comparing radical prostatectomy with expectant management for the treatment of clinically localized prostate cancer. *Semin Urol* 1995;13:130–136.

22. Hanks GE. The Wilt et al article reviewed. PIVOT: The radiation oncologist's friend. *Oncology* 1997; 11:1139–1140.

23. Wilt TJ, Brawer MK. The prostate cancer intervention versus observation trial (PIVOT). *Oncology* 1997;11:1133–1139.

24. Small EJ. Prostate cancer. *Curr Opin Oncol* 1997; 9:277–286.

25. Brausi M, Palladin PD, Latini A. "Watchful waiting" for clinically localized prostate cancer: Long term results [abstract]. *Eur Oncol* 1996;30(Suppl 2):225.

26. McLaren DB, McKenzie M, Duncan G, Pickles T. Watchful waiting or watchful progression? Prostate specific antigen doubling times and clinical behavior in patients with early untreated prostate carcinoma. *Cancer* 1998;82:342–348.

27. Hugosson J, Aus G, Norlen L. Surveillance is not a viable and appropriate treatment option in the management of localized prostate cancer. *Urol Clin North Am* 1996;23:557–573.

28. Litwin MS, Hays RD, Fink A, et al. Quality of life and treatment outcomes in men treated for localized prostate cancer. *JAMA* 1995;273:129–135.

29. Yarbro CH, Ferrans CE. Quality of life of patients with prostate cancer treated with surgery or radiation. *Oncol Nurs Forum* 1998;25:685–693.

30. Nam R, Klotz IH, Jewett MAS, et al. Prostate specific antigen velocity as a measure of the natural history of prostate cancer: Identification of a rapid riser subset. *Br J Urol* 1998;81:100–104.

31. Walsh PC, Brooks, JD. The Swedish cancer paradox. *JAMA* 1997;277:497–498.

32. Williams TR, Love N. Treatment of localized prostate cancer. *Postgrad Med* 1996;100(3):105–120.

33. Middleton RG, Thompson I, Austenfeld MS, et al. Prostate Cancer Clinical Guidelines Panel summary report on the management of clinically localized prostate cancer. *J Urol* 1995;154:2144–2148.

34. Mazur DJ, Merz JF. How older patients' treatment preferences are influenced by disclosures about therapeutic uncertainty: Surgery versus expectant management for localized prostate cancer. *J Am Geriatr Soc* 1996;44(8):934–937.

35. O'Rourke ME. *Prostate cancer treatment selection: The family decision process.* Unpublished doctoral dissertation, University of North Carolina, Chapel Hill, 1997.

36. O'Rourke ME, Germino BB. Spousal caregiving across the prostate cancer trajectory. *Quality Life: Nurs Challenge* 1998;6:66–72.

37. Volk RJ, Cantor SB, Spann SJ, et al. Preferences of husbands and wives for prostate cancer screening. *Arch Fam Med* 1997;6:72–76.

38. Weeks JC, Cook EF, O'Day SJ, et al. Relationship between cancer patients' predictions of prognosis and their treatment preferences. *JAMA* 1998;279: 1709–1714.

39. Mazur DJ, Merz JF. Older patients' willingness to trade off urologic adverse outcomes for a better chance at five-year survival in the clinical setting of prostate cancer. *J Am Geriatr Soc* 1995;43:979–984.

40. Nattinger AB, Hoffman RG, Howell-Pelz A, Goodwin JS. Effect of Nancy Reagan's mastectomy on choice of surgery for breast cancer by US women. *JAMA* 1998;279:762–766.

41. Kirby R. Treatment options for early prostate cancer. *Urology* 1998;52:948–962.

42. Boccon-Gibod L. The management of localised [sic] cancer of the prostate. *Eur Urol* 1996;29(Suppl): 62–68.

43. Carter HB, Morrell CH, Pearson JD, et al. Estimation of prostatic growth using serial prostate-specific antigen measurements in men with and without prostate disease. *Cancer Res* 1992;52: 3323–3328.

44. Herr HW. Quality of life in prostate cancer patients. *CA Cancer J Clin* 1995;47:207–217.

45. Shrader-Bogen CL, Kjellberr JL, McPherson CP, Murray CL. Quality of life and treatment outcomes. Prostate carcinoma patients' perspectives after prostatectomy or radiation. *Cancer* 1997;79: 1977–1986.

46. Fossa SD, Aass N, Opjordsmoen S. Assessment of quality of life in patients with prostate cancer. *Semin Oncol* 1994;21:657–661.

47. Esper P, Mo F, Chodak G, et al. Measuring quality of life in men using the Functional Assessment of Cancer Therapy-Prostate instrument. *Urology* 1997; 50:920–928.

48. Warnecke RB, Ferrns CE, Johnson TP, et al. Measuring quality of life in culturally diverse populations. *J Natl Cancer Inst Mong* 1996;20:29–38.

49. Ferrans CE. Development of a quality of life index for patients with cancer. *Oncol Nurs Forum* 1990; 17(Suppl 3):15–19.

50. Christman NJ. Uncertainty and adjustment during radiotherapy. *Nurs Res* 1990;39:17–20.

51. Mishel MH, Hostetter T, King B, Granham V. Predictors of psychosocial adjustment in patients newly diagnosed with gynecological cancer. *Cancer Nurs* 1984;7:291–299.

52. Mishel MH, Sorenson DS. Uncertainty in gynecological cancer: A test of the mediating functions of mastery and coping. *Nurs Res* 1991;40:236–230.

53. Bailey DE, Mishel MH. Uncertainty management strategies for men electing watchful waiting as a treatment option for prostate cancer [abstract 156]. *Oncolo Nurs Forum* 1997;24:326.

54. Taylor SE, Bunk BP, Collins RL, Reed GM. Social comparison and affiliation under threat. In: Montada L, Fillip SH, Lerner MJ (eds). *Life Crises and Experiences of Loss in Adulthood.* Hillsdale, NJ: Erlbaum,1992:213–227.

55. Jenkins RA, Pargament KI. Religion and spirituality as resources for coping with cancer. *J Psychosoc Oncol* 1995;13:51–74.

56. Walls CT, Zarit SH. Informal support from black churches and the well-being of elderly blacks. *Gerontologist* 1991;31:490–495.

57. Brown-Saltzman K. Replenishing the spirit by meditative prayer and guided imagery. *Semin Oncol Nurs* 1997;13:255–259.

58. Germino BB, Mishel MH, Belyea M, et al. Uncertainty in prostate cancer. Ethnic and family patterns. *Cancer Prac* 1998;6:107–113. .

Chapter 8

SURGICAL CARE OF THE PATIENT WITH PROSTATE CANCER

DAWN M. OSBORNE

OVERVIEW

INTRODUCTION

TRANSURETHRAL RESECTION OF THE PROSTATE

RADICAL RETROPUBIC PROSTATECTOMY

CRYOABLATION OF THE PROSTATE

BILATERAL ORCHIECTOMY

SUMMARY

INTRODUCTION

Surgery has long been an accepted standard of care for men with prostate cancer. Men diagnosed with prostate cancer may undergo various surgeries to assist in the staging of prostate cancer, to cure them of prostate cancer, or to relieve symptoms of the disease. Surgery may include transurethral resection of the prostate (TURP) to alleviate symptoms of bladder outlet obstruction caused by tumor bulk. Radical retropubic or perineal prostatectomy is usually performed for cure of prostate cancer or as salvage treatment after other treatment modalities have failed. Cryoablation of the prostate is offered as a cure for prostate cancer or for palliation of disease. Bilateral orchiectomy is offered as an option for hormonal control of metastatic prostate cancer. It is essential that nurses caring for these patients understand the physical and emotional needs of this specific population. (Table 8-1 lists care guidelines for patients undergoing surgery for treatment of prostate cancer.)

TRANSURETHRAL RESECTION OF THE PROSTATE

TURP is not a cure for prostate cancer.[1] TURP is usually performed on elderly men with prostate cancer exhibiting signs and symptoms of bladder outlet obstruction caused by

TABLE 8-1. Standard of Care for Patient's Undergoing Surgery for Treatment of Prostate Cancer [37–39]

NURSING DIAGNOSIS: *Knowledge deficit regarding surgery*
EXPECTED OUTCOME: Patient will verbalize understanding of preoperative and postoperative course.
NURSING INTERVENTIONS:
1. Assess the patient's knowledge of prostate cancer and planned procedure.
2. Educate the patient regarding the following: • Need for bowel preparation • NPO after midnight • Coughing and deep breathing • Incentive spirometry • Antiembolism or compression stockings • Early ambulation • Presence of catheters and drains • Bladder spasms • Pain management • Incision • Increased fluid intake after TURP • No straining with bowel movement

NURSING DIAGNOSIS: *Altered urinary elimination*
EXPECTED OUTCOME: Catheter will remain patent, and patient will maintain urinary output of at least 30 cc/hour.
NURSING INTERVENTIONS:
1. Assess bladder for distention by palpating bladder above pubic bone.
2. Assess patency of catheter.
3. Keep catheter taped securely at all times.
4. Maintain accurate intake and output every shift.
5. Empty urinary drainage bag when two-thirds full to keep bladder from becoming distended.
6. Adjust rate of CBI as needed to keep urine clear.
7. Do not allow CBI bags to become empty.
8. Manually irrigate catheter with NSS as needed to remove clots, but do not forcefully irrigate.
9. Encourage fluid intake to 2–3 L/day.
10. Maintain IV therapy at prescribed rate.
11. Teach patient the following: • Care for Foley catheter. • Manage leg and overnight drainage bags. • Secure catheter at all times • Keep drainage bag below level of bladder. • Monitor for signs and symptoms of obstruction and urinary tract infection and notify physician if they occur.

NURSING DIAGNOSIS: *Risk for fluid and electrolyte imbalance*
EXPECTED OUTCOME: Patient will maintain a urinary output of at least 30 cc/hour. Electrolytes will be within normal parameters.
NURSING INTERVENTIONS:
1. Monitor electrolytes and report abnormal values to physician.
2. Monitor intake and output.
3. Maintain IV therapy as prescribed.
4. Report decrease in urinary output to physician.
5. Report any changes in mental status to physician.

NURSING DIAGNOSIS: *Bleeding related to surgery*
EXPECTED OUTCOME: Patient will remain hemodynamically stable, as evidenced by no overt signs of bleeding and stable vital signs.
NURSING INTERVENTIONS:
1. Monitor hemoglobin and hematocrit. Notify physician of decrease in hemoglobin of 1 g or greater.
2. Assess dressings for signs of bleeding.
3. Monitor vital signs for tachycardia and hypotension.
4. Assess catheter, drains, and nasogastric tube for signs of bleeding.

5. Assess for signs of hypoxia: • Pulse oximetry • Lethargy • Anxiety • Restlessness • Change in mental status
6. If in use, maintain traction on catheter to control venous bleeding.

NURSING DIAGNOSIS: *Risk for thrombophlebitis and pulmonary embolism*
EXPECTED OUTCOME: Patient will not experience thrombophlebitis or pulmonary embolism.
NURSING INTERVENTIONS:
1. Assess patient for shortness of breath.
2. Assess patient's calf for: • Pain • Redness • Edema • Warmth
3. Patient wears antiembolism or compression stockings when in bed.
4. Reinforce leg exercises as instructed preoperatively.
5. Ambulate patient on Postoperative Day 1.
6. Administer anticoagulants as prescribed.

NURSING DIAGNOSIS: *Altered comfort related to pain and bladder spasm*
EXPECTED OUTCOME: Patient will verbalize acceptable level of comfort.
NURSING INTERVENTIONS:
1. Assess quantity, quality, and duration of pain.
2. Assess for bladder distention, kinked tubing, and free flow of urine.
3. Assess security of catheter and retape as needed.
4. Administer narcotics for pain as prescribed.
5. Administer antispasmodics as prescribed.
6. Teach patient to: • Splint incision when getting in and out of bed and coughing and deep breathing • Wear scrotal supporter if indicated • Take sitz bath if indicated

NURSING DIAGNOSIS: *Risk of infection related to surgery and indwelling catheter*
EXPECTED OUTCOME: Patient will not experience a fever or other signs of infection.
NURSING INTERVENTIONS:
1. Assess for signs of infection: • Fever • Redness, pain, swelling, and drainage from incision and drain sites • Cloudy or foul-smelling urine • Increase in white blood cell count • Tachycardia • Diaphoresis • Mental status changes • Change in breath sounds
2. Encourage coughing, deep breathing, and incentive spirometry every hour.
3. Perform indwelling urinary catheter care bid with soap and water.
4. Use aseptic technique when emptying or changing drainage bag.
5. Notify physician of temperature ≥ 38.5°C.
6. Obtain urine, blood, or other cultures as prescribed.

NURSING DIAGNOSIS: *Risk of constipation as a result of narcotics and antispasmodics*
EXPECTED OUTCOME: Patient will have easy bowel movement.
NURSING INTERVENTIONS:
1. Administer stool softeners and laxatives as prescribed.
2. Encourage patient to drink at least 2–3 L of fluid a day.
3. Educate patient not to strain when moving bowels.
4. Ambulate once on Postoperative Day 1 and then at least bid.

NURSING DIAGNOSIS: *Incontinence resulting from surgery*
EXPECTED OUTCOME: Patient will be able to manage incontinence.

(Continued on next page)

TABLE 8-1. *Continued*

NURSING INTERVENTIONS:
1. After removal of indwelling catheter, instruct patient regarding measures to assist in alleviating incontinence. • Modification in dietary habits and fluid intake • Timed voiding • Kegel exercises • Behavior modification • Incontinence devices • Possible surgical interventions

NURSING DIAGNOSIS: *Body image disturbance related to cancer diagnosis and surgery*
EXPECTED OUTCOME: Patient and family will adapt to altered body image.
NURSING INTERVENTIONS:
1. Assess ability to adjust to altered body image.
2. Provide opportunities for patient-family to discuss feelings of altered body image.
3. Emphasize that disease and surgery have no affect on patient's masculinity.
4. Reassure patient of ability to continue roles and relationships with family and friends.
5. If patient wishes, arrange for him to talk with someone who has had surgery for prostate cancer.
6. Refer patient and family to support or self-help group if appropriate.

NPO, nothing by mouth; TURP, transurethral resection of the prostate; CBI, continuous bladder irrigation; NSS, normal saline solution; IV, intravenous; bid, twice a day.　　　　Courtesy of Dawn M. Osborne.

tumor bulk. The tumor may press on the prostatic urethra, causing bladder outlet obstruction and urinary retention. By removing some of this tissue, the symptoms can be relieved. The symptoms of bladder outlet obstruction include urgency, frequency of urination, nocturia (waking up at night to urinate), and urinary retention. Men who undergo a TURP for benign prostatic hyperplasia (BPH), who have not been previously diagnosed with prostate cancer may, postoperatively, have a previously unknown positive pathology on examination of the prostatic tissue (T1a and T1b disease). Depending on the patient's age, comorbidities, and the stage of the disease, these men may be offered definitive treatment for the cancer.

TURP is performed under general or spinal anesthesia. Patients are placed in the lithotomy position and, with a transurethral resectoscope and electrocautery, the anterior, posterior, and lateral portions of the prostate are resected. All resected tissue removed is sent for pathologic analysis. Continuous bladder irrigation (CBI) is used during resection to assist debris washout and help minimize bleeding. After completion of the resection, a urinary catheter is placed in the bladder, and CBI may be continued for 24 hours postoperatively.[2]

Preoperative education must include the need for coughing, deep breathing, and early ambulation postoperatively to minimize the effects of anesthesia and prevent possible embolism. Ambulation is also important to help reduce the side effects of constipation resulting from the use of antispasmotics. Patients should be informed that they will have a urinary catheter until the urine is clear enough for removal. Removal of the catheter will depend on the practices of the attending physician. The need to increase fluid intake to at least 2 L/day must be stressed. Patients should be instructed not to strain when having a bowel movement because this increases the risk for urinary bleeding and clot retention. An over-the-counter stool softener should be taken once a day for at least 6 weeks postoperatively to prevent constipation. These instructions should be reinforced on discharge.

Immediate postoperative complications can include bleeding, clot retention, urinary tract infection, and transurethral resection syndrome (TUR syndrome). TUR syndrome can occur when patients absorb large quantities (greater than 2 L) of CBI fluid. This absorption can result in hypervolemia and hyponatremia, which can cause changes in mental status and visual disturbances. Therefore, it is important that, during the procedure, in addition to the usual parameters, the anesthesiologist monitor oxygen saturation, electrocardiogram, and serum sodium levels.[3]

To reduce the risk of postoperative bleeding and clot retention, the CBI should be closely monitored. The flow of the CBI and the patient's bladder should be assessed at least every 30 minutes to ensure that the patient is not experiencing urinary retention. To reduce the risk of retention and the discomfort of bladder spasm, the nurse should assess the drainage tubing for kinks and keep it secured to the upper thigh at all times. If clot retention occurs, the nurse should manually irrigate the catheter with normal saline solution and a piston syringe. If one is unable to clear the clots or if heavy bleeding occurs, the urologist should be contacted immediately.

Urinary tract infection can be caused by the surgery itself, insertion of the urinary catheter, or a break in aseptic technique when dealing with the catheter postoperatively. Whenever the nurse finds it necessary to interrupt the closed urinary drainage system, strict aseptic technique must be used. It is important that antibiotics prescribed to prevent urinary tract infection are administered.

Postoperatively, the patient may experience bladder spasms caused by irritation to the bladder mucosa from the urinary catheter. Bladder spasms may cause the patient to feel the urge to urinate or to move his bowels. Spasm can also cause the continuous flow of the CBI to be interrupted. Bladder spasms can be controlled with rectal and oral medications, such as belladonna and opium suppositories, and oxybutynin.[4] These medications relax the bladder mucosa and help alleviate the irritation. If the spasms are unrelieved by antispasmotics and suppositories, meperidine may be administered intravenously or intramuscularly.

The patient usually has intravenous fluids administered immediately postoperatively. Oral intake can begin immediately after surgery if the patient is stable and not nauseous. If not contraindicated for medical reasons, the patient's total intake should be at least 2 L of liquid a day to decrease bleeding, the chance of clot retention, and urinary tract infection.[5] Close monitoring of intake and urinary output is extremely important. The nurse must evaluate the patient to ensure he has a urinary output of at least 30 cc/h and that intake does not far exceed output. A noticeable increase of intake over output may be a sign of urinary retention. Intravenous therapy can be discontinued when the patient is orally taking the required 2 L of fluid a day.

The indwelling urinary catheter is removed once the patient has minimal hematuria (when the urine color is yellow to light pink), and the attending physician deems it time

TABLE 8-2. Clinical Pathway: Transurethral Prostatectomy (Expected LOS: 2 Days)

PREADMISSION TESTING: OUTPATIENT • OUTCOME: MEDICALLY STABLE	DAY 1 ADMISSION • OUTCOME: MEDICALLY STABLE	DAY 2 POSTOP. DAY 1 • OUTCOME: CBI DISCONTINUED	DAY 3 DISCHARGE DAY • OUTCOME: NO GROSS HEMATURIA DISCHARGE
Transitional activities: Precert arranged • Consents signed	*Transitional activities:* Admit • Obtain referrals • Review pathway • Obtain copay	*Transitional activities:* Review pathway	*Transitional activities:* Discharge • Complete transfer form, if needed • Implement transportation arrangements
Assessment-consult: History and physical • Medical consult, if needed • Medical clearance	*Assessment-consult:* Assess allergies • Focus genitourinary assessment • Nursing care history • Home needs assessment • Social service • Initiate nursing discharge plan • Assess pain-anxiety level • Screen for nutrition risk • Assess learning needs	*Assessment-consult:* Focus genitourinary assessment • Nursing assessment per guidelines • Assess pain-anxiety level	*Assessment-consult:* Focus genitourinary assessment • Assess pain-anxiety level • Nursing assessment per guidelines
Tests-diagnostics: Preadmission testing as per anesthesia with results to chart	*Procedures and treatments:* IV therapy • Vital signs	*Procedures and treatments:* Discontinue CBI • Discontinue IV • Foley catheter to straight drainage	*Procedures and treatments:* Remove Foley catheter • If catheter not removed, connect to leg bag
Education: Preop instructions • Provide and review timeline	*Education:* Review timeline • Signs and symptoms of bladder spasm • Foley catheter care instructions • Elimination instructions	*Tests-diagnostics:* CBC/screen 7 if indicated	*Education:* Elimination precautions • Monitor voiding • Reinforce medication instructions • Reinforce discharge instructions
Medication-pain management: Current patient meds as per anesthesia on morning of surgery	*Medication-pain management:* Current patient meds • Antibiotic • Stool softener • Antispasmotic • Laxative PRN	*Education:* Reinforce Foley catheter care instructions • Elimination precautions • Leg bag instructions, if needed • Medication instructions • Discharge instructions	*Medication-pain management:* Current patient meds • Antibiotics • Stool softener • Antispasmotic • Laxative PRN
Psychological and spiritual: Provide supportive measures as needed	*Activity-mobility safety:* Bed rest, if spinal anesthesia • Meet safety needs	*Medication-pain management:* Current patient meds • Antibiotics • Stool softener • Antispasmotic • Laxative PRN	*Activity-mobility safety:* OOB ambulating as per baseline
Nutrition and elimination: NPO after midnight	*Psychological and spiritual:* Orient to room • Advanced directives • Provide supportive measures as needed	*Activity-mobility safety:* OOB ambulating as per baseline	*Psychological and spiritual:* Provide supportive measures as needed
	Nutrition and elimination: Foley catheter with-without CBI • Medically appropriate diet	*Psychological and spiritual:* Provide supportive measures as needed	*Nutrition and elimination:* Medically appropriate diet • Encourage PO fluids • Maintain I&O • Document bowel movements
		Nutrition and elimination: Medically appropriate diet • Encourage PO fluids • Maintain I&O • Document bowel movements	

LOS, length of stay; Precert, precertification; preop, preoperative; meds, medications; IV, intravenous; PRN, as occasion requires; NPO, nothing by mouth; CBI, continuous bladder irrigation; CBC, complete blood cell count; OOB, out of bed; PO, oral; I&O, intake and output.

Courtesy of Dawn M. Osborne

to remove the catheter. The patient may experience urinary retention after the catheter is removed because of retained debris from surgery or bladder atony from relaxation of the bladder caused by prolonged catheter drainage. The urinary catheter may need to be reinserted temporarily until the problem is resolved.

If the patient is discharged with a catheter in place, home care should be arranged to monitor the level of hematuria and assist with catheter care. Home care nurses should ensure that the patient is cleaning the catheter twice a day with soap and water and can change from a leg bag to an overnight urinary drainage bag.

The patient usually remains in the hospital 1 to 3 days after TURP. Table 8-2 is an example of a clinical pathway that a patient having this procedure may follow. Clinical pathways are guidelines that can be used by physicians and nurses in the care of patients undergoing a certain procedure. It is important that each patient be treated on an individual basis. Clinical pathways can reduce costs and decrease length of stay in the uncomplicated patient. Table 8-3 is an example of the instructions for the patient and family that accompany the pathway. These instructions are given to the patient before admission so that he will know what to expect over the course of his hospital stay.

Long-term complications of TURP can include incontinence, impotence, urethral strictures, and bladder neck contracture.[4, 6] The patient should be informed that such complications may occur and he needs to inform his physician of any symptoms. The patient also needs to realize that there is a high probability that he will experience retrograde ejaculation after TURP.[7] Retrograde ejaculation occurs because, during the course of surgery, the bladder neck is often enlarged and not able to close completely as it normally does during orgasm and ejaculation. The semen flows in a backward direction through the incompletely closed bladder neck and then into the bladder. Retrograde ejaculation is not harmful, but the patient should be informed that his first voided urine after ejaculation will be cloudy. Approximately 5% of men who undergo TURP for bladder outlet obstruction will need repeat resection within 5 years.[6]

RADICAL RETROPUBIC PROSTATECTOMY

Although radical prostatectomy has long been accepted as a cure for localized prostate cancer, the number of radical prostatectomies being performed has risen significantly in the past 10 years.[8] In a study conducted from 1989 to 1991 in Wisconsin, the number of reported prostate cancer cases increased by 33%; during the same period, the number of radical prostatectomies increased by 226%.[9] The reason for the increase in the number of radical prostatectomies is unclear, but it is believed that the increased use of prostate-specific antigen (PSA) as a screening tool for prostate cancer is a factor. With the increased use of PSA, more and earlier stage prostate cancers are being found, triggering an increase in surgery.

The patient's cancer stage, age, general medical condition, and life expectancy all play a role in the physician's decision to perform radical surgery. Generally, men with localized disease (T1, T2) who are 70 years old or younger and in good medical condition with life

TABLE 8-3. Transurethral Resection of the Prostate (TURP) Patient Family Timeline

BEFORE YOUR HOSPITAL STAY	**DAY 2**
	Urinary catheter irrigation is discontinued
7–10 DAYS BEFORE SURGERY	Intravenous fluid discontinued
History and physical exam	Possible blood work
Anesthesia evaluation	Out of bed, ambulating
Testing, including blood and radiographs	Drink at least 2 quarts of liquid a day
Primary care physician provides written	Discharge instructions
clearance for surgery	Arrange transportation
Obtain referrals from primary care physician if	
needed	**DAY 3**
	Urinary catheter may or may not be removed
DAY BEFORE SURGERY	Instruction on physical activity, elimination, diet,
Nothing to eat or drink after midnight	and medications
	Instructed to make follow-up appointment with
MORNING OF SURGERY	urologist
Take current medications if instructed by	Information and telephone numbers for
anesthesia	questions provided
Report to the hospital Short Procedure Unit	
	AFTER YOUR HOSPITAL STAY
DURING YOUR HOSPITAL STAY	
	1-2 DAYS
ADMISSION TO THE HOSPITAL DAY 1	Call for follow-up appointment with urologist
Go to the Short Procedure Unit	
Provide referrals and arrange any payments	**1 WEEK IF DISCHARGED WITH CATHETER**
Intravenous catheter inserted	See physician for removal
To Operating Room	
TURP is completed, and a urinary catheter	**10 DAYS – 2 WEEKS**
inserted	See urologist to determine activity level
To Recovery Room, vital signs monitored	
To room on Nursing Unit, vital signs are	**3 – 6 MONTHS**
monitored	Maintain regular check-ups
Urinary catheter continuously irrigated	
Bed rest	**These are suggested guidelines only. Your care**
Abdomen checked by nurse	**will depend on your rate of recovery and your**
Antibiotics and routine medication	**physician's orders.**

Courtesy of Dawn M. Osborne.

expectancy of 10 to 20 years are offered the option of radical prostatectomy.[10, 11] These men are considered ideal candidates because, if the disease is organ-confined, they are considered cured of disease if there are no signs of recurrence 5 years after surgery. Unfortunately, not all patients who undergo radical prostatectomy have organ-confined disease. Pathologic upstaging of disease after radical prostatectomy ranges from 20 to 60%.[12] These patients may undergo further treatment for their disease after surgery.

Radical prostatectomy involves the removal of the entire prostate, including the prostatic capsule, the seminal vesicles, and a portion of the bladder neck. The procedure is performed under general or spinal anesthesia. The prostate can be approached by either a retropubic or a perineal incision (Figure 8-1). The retropubic approach allows for open pelvic lymph node dissection, gives better exposure to certain anatomic landmarks, and allows for dissection of the neurovascular bundles if the nerve-sparing technique is to be

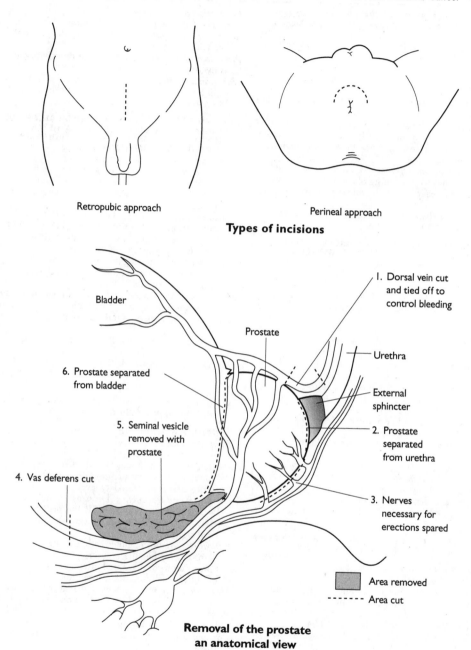

Retropubic approach   Perineal approach

Types of incisions

Bladder

Prostate

6. Prostate separated
from bladder

5. Seminal vesicle
removed with
prostate

4. Vas deferens cut

1. Dorsal vein cut
and tied off to
control bleeding

Urethra

External
sphincter

2. Prostate
separated
from urethra

3. Nerves
necessary for
erections spared

▨ Area removed

------ Area cut

**Removal of the prostate
an anatomical view**

FIGURE 8-1. Removal of the Prostate: An Anatomical View

Source: From JE Oesterling and MA Moyad (1997), *The ABC's of Prostate Cancer: The Book That Could Save Your Life.* Lanham, MD: Madison Books, p. 117. Used with permission from Madison Books.

Table 8-4 Clinical Pathway: Radical Prostatectomy (Expected LOS: 3 Days)

PREADMISSION TESTING: OUTPATIENT • OUTCOMES: MEDICALLY STABLE • UNDERSTANDS ADMISSION PROCESS

Transitional activities: Precert arranged • Consents signed

Assessment-consult: History and physical • Medical consult, if needed • Medical clearance • Screen for nutrition risk

Procedures and treatments: GoLYTELY ½ to 1 gallon day before surgery

Tests-diagnostics: Preadmission testing as per anesthesia with results to chart • Autologous blood donation

Education: Preop instructions • Provide and review timeline

Medication-pain management: Current patient meds as per anesthesia on morning of surgery • Antibiotics

Psychological and spiritual: Provide supportive measures as needed

Nutrition and elimination: Clear liquids day before surgery • NPO after midnight

DAY 1 ADMISSION •OUTCOMES: MEDICALLY STABLE • MINIMAL HEMATURIA VIA FOLEY CATHETER • MINIMAL PAIN

Transitional activities: Admit • Obtain referrals • Review pathway • Obtain co-pay

Assessment-consult: Assess allergies • Focus GU and GI assessment • Nursing care history • Home needs assessment • Social service • Initiate nursing discharge plan • Assess pain-anxiety level • Screen for nutrition risk • Assess learning needs

Procedures and treatments: IV therapy • Vital signs • Transfuse, if necessary • External drains to collection device • Reinforce dressing PRN • Pneumatic compression stockings • Incentive spirometry • Postop instruction sign posted

Tests-diagnostics: CBC • Screen 7

Education: Signs and symptoms of bladder spasm • Instruct in incentive spirometry

Medication-pain management: Pain medication • Antibiotics

Activity-mobility safety: Bed rest • Meet safety needs

Psychological and spiritual: Orient to room • Advanced directives • Provide supportive measures as needed

Nutrition and elimination: Foley catheter to straight drainage • NPO • NGT to low intermittent suction • I&O

DAY 2: POSTOP DAY 1 • OUTCOMES: MEDICALLY STABLE • MINIMAL HEMATURIA VIA FOLEY CATHETER • MINIMAL PAIN • MINIMAL OUTPUT FROM DRAINS • INCISION WITHOUT INDURATION

Transitional activities: Review pathway

Assessment-consult: Focus GU and GI assessment • Nursing assessment per guidelines • Wound assessment • Assess pain-anxiety level • Assess learning needs • Social service consult for VNA

Procedures and treatments: JP to bulb suction • Dressing change PRN • Pneumatic compression stockings while in bed • IV therapy • Vital signs • Incentive spirometry

Tests-diagnostics: CBC

Education: Foley catheter care instructions • Leg bag instructions • Elimination precautions

Medication-pain management: Current patient medications • Antibiotics • Pain medication • Antispasmotic

Activity-mobility safety: OOB to chair in AM • Ambulate with assistance in PM

Psychological and spiritual: Provide supportive measures as needed

Nutrition and elimination: Discontinue NGT • Clear liquid diet • Foley catheter to straight drainage • Maintain I&O

DAY 3: POSTOP DAY 2 • OUTCOMES: MEDICALLY STABLE • MINIMAL HEMATURIA VIA FOLEY CATHETER • MINIMAL PAIN • MINIMAL OUTPUT FROM DRAINS • INCISION WITHOUT INDURATION

Transitional activities: Review pathway

Assessment-consult: Focus GU and GI assessment • Nursing assessment per guidelines • Wound assessment • Assess pain-anxiety level • Arrange transportation home

Procedures and treatments: IV therapy • Possible discontinuation of JP drain • Dressing change PRN • Pneumatic compression stockings while in bed • Incentive spirometry • Vital signs

Education: Reinforce leg bag instructions • Discharge instructions • Elimination precautions • Reinforce discharge instructions

Medication-pain management: Current patient medications • Antibiotics • Pain medication • Antispasmotic

Activity-mobility safety: OOB ambulating as per baseline

Psychological and spiritual: Provide supportive measures as needed

Nutrition and elimination: Medically appropriate diet • Encourage PO fluids • Foley catheter to straight drainage • Maintain I&O

DAY 4: POSTOP DAY 3 • OUTCOMES: MEDICALLY STABLE • MINIMAL HEMATURIA VIA FOLEY CATHETER • MINIMAL PAIN • MINIMAL OUTPUT FROM DRAINS • INCISION WITHOUT INDURATION

Transitional activities: Review pathway • Complete VNA form • Discharge

Assessment-consult: Focus GU and GI assessment • Nursing assessment per guidelines • Wound assessment • Assess pain/anxiety level

Procedures and treatments: Dressing change PRN • Possible discontinuation of JP and/or Penrose drain • Discontinue IV therapy • Incentive spirometry • Vital signs

Education: Reinforce Foley catheter care instructions • Reinforce leg bag instructions • Medication instruction • Reinforce discharge instructions • Encourage PO fluids • Elimination precautions

Medication-pain management: Current patient medications • Antibiotics • Pain medication • Antispasmotic

Activity-mobility safety: OOB ambulating as per baseline • No heavy lifting or strenuous activity

Psychological and spiritual: Provide supportive measures as needed

Nutrition and elimination: Medically appropriate diet • Encourage PO fluids • Foley catheter to straight drainage • Maintain I&O

LOS, length of stay; Precert, precertification; preop, preoperative; NPO, nothing by mouth; GU, genitourinary; GI, gastrointestinal; IV, intravenous; PRN, as occasion requires; postop, postoperative; CBC, complete blood cell count; NGT, nasogastric tube; I&O, intake and output; VNA, Visting Nurse Association; JP, Jackson-Pratt; OOB, out of bed; AM, morning; PM, evening; PO, oral.

Courtesy of Dawn M. Osborne

used. Pelvic lymph node sampling is important in the staging of the disease. If there is positive lymph node involvement, the prostatectomy is aborted, and the patient is treated with another modality. Studies have shown that patient selection for the nerve-sparing procedure is extremely important. Recovery of sexual function depends on the patient's age, preoperative sexual function, stage of the disease, and whether there is unilateral or bilateral nerve preservation.[13, 14] Potency rates associated with the bilateral nerve-sparing technique range from 31 to 76%, whereas those for the unilateral nerve-sparing technique range from 13 to 56%.

The perineal approach is associated with less blood loss and less postoperative pain and allows for facilitation of the reconstruction of the bladder and vesicourethral anastomosis.[15] With the perineal approach, if a staging pelvic lymph node dissection is indicated, a separate open or laparoscopic procedure must be done. The approach used usually depends on the surgeon's preference and expertise.

Preoperative teaching should include the need for a clear liquid diet and bowel preparation such as polyethylene glycol-electrolyte solution (GoLYTELY, Braintree Laboratories Inc., Braintree, MA) the day before surgery.[16] The importance of coughing, deep breathing, incentive spirometry, use of compression stockings, and early ambulation should be stressed preoperatively because thrombophlebitis and pulmonary embolism are two of the most common complications of pelvic surgery.[17] Patients should also be told that postoperatively they will have an indwelling urinary catheter, nasogastric tube, and some form of drain at the surgical site.

An indwelling urinary catheter will be placed during radical prostatectomy. The bladder should be assessed frequently for distention. The catheter should be secured to the patient's upper thigh or abdomen at all times so that there is no pressure on the urethral-bladder anastomosis. The catheter should not be manipulated in any way except by the surgeon. Patients need to be instructed to wash the catheter at the meatus twice daily to decrease the risk of infection and irritation. Patients should also be instructed in how to change from a leg bag to an overnight drainage bag using clean technique. The nurse should encourage the patient to use the overnight drainage bag while sleeping. This will ensure that the bladder does not become distended from urine backflow. Patient's intake and output should be closely monitored to watch fluid balance. The catheter will remain in place for 2 to 4 weeks postoperatively to allow for adequate healing of the urethral anastomosis.

The average length of stay for radical prostatectomy has decreased from 5 days to 2 to 3 days.[17, 18, 19] (See Table 8-4 for a clinical pathway for patients undergoing radical prostatectomy.) Table 8-5 presents a schedule for patients and families, given preoperatively, informing them of what to expect during the course of hospitalization. Because the patient's length of stay is so short, there is not much time for education; therefore, every available opportunity must be used to enhance the learning process. Patients are often overwhelmed with everything they must learn. It is vital that home care be arranged at discharge for monitoring of the surgical wound and indwelling urinary catheter. Home

TABLE 8-5. Radical Prostatectomy: Patient Family Timeline

BEFORE YOUR HOSPITAL STAY

7–10 DAYS BEFORE SURGERY

History and physical exam

Anesthesia evaluation

Testing, including blood and radiograph

Autologous blood donation if needed

Primary care physician provides written
clearance for surgery

Obtain referrals from primary care physician if
needed

DAY BEFORE SURGERY

Drink GoLYTELY as instructed

Nothing to eat or drink after midnight

MORNING OF SURGERY

Take current medications if instructed by
anesthesia

DURING YOUR HOSPITAL STAY

ADMISSION TO THE HOSPITAL DAY I

Go to the Short Procedure Unit

Provide referrals and arrange any payments

Intravenous catheter inserted

To Operating Room

Surgery is completed, and a urinary catheter,
drains, and nasogastric tube are inserted

To Recovery Room, vital signs monitored

To room on Nursing Unit, vital signs are
monitored

Dressings and drains checked by nurse

Bed rest with compression stockings

Antibiotics and routine medication

DAY 2

Intravenous fluid discontinued

Possible blood work

Out of bed, ambulating

Nasogastric tube removed

Clear liquid diet

Discharge instructions

Social work to arrange for home care nursing

DAY 3

Possible removal of drains

Diet advanced to solid food

Instruction on physical activity, elimination, diet,
and medications

Discharge instructions

Arrange transportation home

DAY 4

Urinary catheter care instructions reinforced

Instructed to make follow-up appointment with
urologist

Information and telephone numbers for
questions provided

AFTER YOUR HOSPITAL STAY

1-2 DAYS

Call for follow-up appointment with urologist

10 DAYS – 2 WEEKS

See urologist to have catheter removed and to
determine activity level

3 – 6 MONTHS

Maintain regular check-ups

These are suggested guidelines only. Your care will depend on your rate of recovery and your physician's orders.

Courtesy of Dawn M. Osborne.

care nurses will be able to continue patient education and be available to answer questions and deal with any problems patients may have.

Short-term complications after radical prostatectomy include bleeding, thrombophlebitis, pulmonary embolism, urinary tract infection, and wound infection. In the immediate postoperative period, vital signs, intake and output, and dressings should be assessed hourly. Vital signs should be monitored to ensure that the temperature, blood pressure, pulse, and respiration rate remain stable. An increase in heart rate and a decrease in blood pressure can be signs of internal bleeding. Hypotension may also be an indication of hypovolemia. An increase in respiration rate can indicate pulmonary embolism or fluid overload. An increase in temperature may be caused by a wound infection, urinary tract infection, or pneumonia. Intake and output should be assessed hourly. Urine output should be at least 30 cc/hr. The nurse should notify the physician if the urine output falls below this rate. If a Penrose drain is in place, there may be a large amount of drainage, and dressings should be reinforced or changed as needed. Pulmonary status should also be closely monitored. The nurse should have the patient cough and deep breathe and perform leg exercises once an hour to help prevent thrombophlebitis and pneumonia. Antiembolism or compression stockings are used to help prevent deep vein thrombosis.

Patient-controlled analgesia (PCA) is administered using a basal rate to manage postoperative pain. A constant dose of narcotic is administered so that the patient is as comfortable as possible. A patient experiencing pain is not as likely to cough and deep breathe or perform the required leg exercises. On the first postoperative day, the PCA can be adjusted so that the patient can administer his own pain medication as needed by intravenous bolus. If the patient has an abdominal incision, he should be given a pillow to hold against the incision when coughing and deep breathing and moving in and out of bed. The splint will help decrease the incisional pain that these exercises can cause. Antispasmotics may help alleviate bladder spasm induced by the indwelling urinary catheter. Belladonna and opium suppositories are not routinely given unless ordered by the attending physician. Rectal manipulation should be avoided after radical prostatectomy because the prostate that was removed sits on the rectum, and injury to the surgical site is a possibility. To help prevent constipation from narcotics, an oral laxative should be given once a day as soon as the patient is taking things by mouth. Stool softeners may also be administered twice daily to prevent constipation.

On the first postoperative day, the nasogastric tube is removed and the patient is started on a clear liquid diet. Solid food is added when bowel sounds return. The patient should ambulate with assistance at least twice a day. When the patient is in bed or sitting in a chair, compression stockings should be worn to decrease the risk of deep vein thrombosis and embolism. Coughing, deep breathing, and use of incentive spirometry should continue to be performed hourly.

Urinary incontinence is one of the major long-term complications of radical prostatectomy. Most patients have some form of incontinence immediately after catheter removal. Approximately 5 to 8% of men will remain incontinent 1 year after surgery.[20, 21] Age has been shown to be a factor in regaining continence. Older men have a higher incontinence rate than younger men.[22] After the catheter is removed, patients should be instructed in timed voiding. With timed voiding, at set intervals, the patient empties his bladder whether he feels the urge to urinate or not. Timed voiding keeps the bladder from overfilling and causing overflow incontinence. Kegel exercises can be performed to help strengthen the pelvic floor muscles that were weakened by surgery. Kegel exercises are done by squeezing or contracting the pubococcygeal muscle. This exercise must be performed repeatedly throughout the day. The patient will receive no benefit if the exercises are not done consistently. If after 1 year a patient remains severely incontinent, the urologist may recommend an artificial urinary sphincter for continence.

Fecal incontinence has been reported in 10% of radical retropubic patients and in 15% of perineal prostatectomy patients.[23] The exact mechanism of injury leading to fecal incontinence is unknown. However, at present, it is believed that contributing factors include damage to the rectal sphincter with the perineal approach, and prolonged retraction of tissue may lead to neurologic compromise with the retropubic approach. Fecal incontinence is not yet a well-recognized complication of radical prostatectomy.

During radical prostatectomy, the nerves that control sexual function may be damaged or severed. Damage to these nerves can cause impotency. If there is no evidence of tumor invasion or spread, surgeons will attempt to preserve the neurovascular bundles during radical prostatectomy. In a study of 503 men who were potent preoperatively, 76% who had both neurovascular bundles preserved were potent compared with 60% who had unilateral neurovascular preservation.[24] A correlation between age and return of sexual function does exist. In men younger than 50 years, at least 91% maintain potency after surgery. Men must be told that, although potency may be maintained, there will be no prostatic fluid, and therefore, no emission or ejaculation. Various treatment options are available to men with impotency, including medications, vacuum devices, and penile prosthesis.

Bladder neck contractures and urethral strictures are another common complication of radical prostatectomy. In a Medicare study, 20% of the men stated that they had treatment for strictures within 4 years of radical prostatectomy.[25] Strictures can be caused by scar tissue at the site of the urethral anastomosis. Strictures are relieved by simple dilatation of the urethra or by cutting out the scar tissue. It is not uncommon for strictures to recur.

A study involving men who had a radical prostatectomy as primary treatment for localized disease between 1985 and 1992 found that 34.9% of the patients required follow-up cancer treatment within 5 years of the initial surgery.[26] These findings were in line with those of a national survey of Medicare patients who underwent a radical prostatectomy between 1988 and 1990. The Medicare study reported that 28% of these men had some form of follow-up treatment within 4 years of the initial surgery. As previously noted, often a patient's disease is upstaged on pathologic examination. The likelihood of both local and systemic relapse increases in cancers that have penetrated the prostatic capsule or have positive inked margins or if cancer is present at the urethral margin at pathologic review.[27] The chance of recurrence increases even more so if there is seminal vesicle or lymph node involvement. The management of patients with positive surgical margins is controversial. Treatment options include adjuvant external beam radiation therapy, adjuvant androgen deprivation, and surveillance with delayed treatment.[28] Treatment decision should be made by the patient and his urologist.

CRYOABLATION OF THE PROSTATE

Cryoablation, or cryosurgery, of the prostate has been in existence since the 1960s.[29] Because of the high complication rate, the procedure was all but abandoned until the late

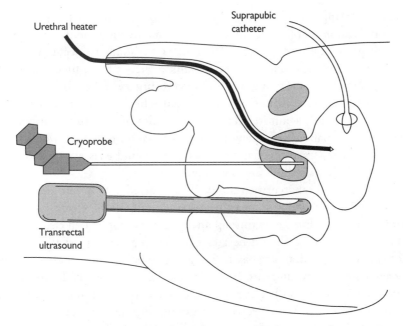

FIGURE 8-2. Schematic sagittal view of prostate cryoablation procedure

Source: From JD Schmidt, J Doyle, and S Larson. Prostate cryoablation: Update 1998. *CA: A Cancer Journal for Clinicians*, 1998;48:239–252. Used with permission from *CA: Cancer Journal for Clinicians*.

1980s. As a result of improvements in cryosurgical instrumentation, the introduction of transrectal ultrasonography, and increased patient demand for new treatment options, cryosurgery is once again a treatment option for men with prostate cancer. Cryoablation is being used to treat clinically localized prostate cancer (T1-T3), as salvage therapy for local failures of prior treatment, and to debulk large primary tumors.[30, 31]

The technique of transrectal ultrasound-guided percutaneous transperineal prostate cryoablation can vary among institutions. Patients are usually administered general anesthesia and placed in the lithotomy position. A suprapubic tube (SPT) is inserted in the bladder, and a urethral warming device is placed to prevent damage to the urethra caused by the freezing procedure. Under transrectal ultrasound guidance, probes are placed through the perineum into the prostate (Figure 8-2). Liquid nitrogen is run through the probes, and the prostate is frozen. The tips of the probes in the prostate are frozen to a temperature of -180°C to -190°C. Freezing of the prostate tissue causes stasis of blood, which leads to thrombosis and necrosis, or death, of the cancerous tissue. Over time the necrotic tissue sloughs and is eliminated from the body via the urethra.

Preoperative instructions include the need for a bowel preparation to clear the intestinal tract. Patients should also be given routine preoperative instructions as described in Table 8-1. Further instructions include care of the perineal wound and SPT care. Patients may be hospitalized for 1 to 4 days and discharged with an SPT in place.

Immediate postoperative nursing care consists of monitoring the pulse and blood pressure for indications of bleeding. Intake and output are monitored to ensure fluid balance and adequate drainage of the SPT. The SPT should be securely taped to the patient's abdomen and the tubing assessed for kinks. Patency of the tube is also monitored because sloughing of prostate tissue occurs after cryosurgery. If the tube becomes blocked, the nurse gently irrigates the catheter with normal saline solution until the blockage is cleared and urine is once again free flowing. The color of the urine is also assessed for heavy bleeding. The patient's temperature is monitored for elevation, which could indicate wound or urinary tract infection. The perineal wound is assessed for bleeding and signs of infection such as redness and swelling.

In preparation for discharge, men should be instructed in SPT care and in the clamping and unclamping of the tube to measure postvoid residuals. SPT care consists of washing around the tube once a day with soap and water and applying a clean, dry dressing around the tube. The tube should be attached to a leg bag during the day and then switched to an overnight drainage bag before going to bed at night. Patients should also be instructed in perineal wound care, including local care and sitz baths, to help alleviate discomfort and aid in wound healing. Home care should be arranged for patients discharged with a SPT in place to assist with the monitoring and care of the catheter and the perineal wounds. Depending on the postvoid residual, the SPT generally can be removed in 7 days. Sloughing of necrotic tissue may cause urinary tract obstruction once the SPT is removed. Patients should be instructed to contact their physician if they have any difficulty urinating once the tube is removed.

The most common complication after cryosurgery is urethral sloughing. This is a result of necrosis of the prostatic urethra. Mild to moderate sloughing is generally treated with watchful waiting and catheterization. Severe sloughs may be treated with transurethral prostatectomy.[32] Other complications from cryosurgery include urinary tract obstruction, fistulas, incontinence, impotence, and bladder neck contractors. Penile numbness has also been reported. This appears to be a temporary condition but can last for several months.[32, 33]

Positive biopsy rates vary from 7.7 to 23% after cryosurgery as the primary treatment for prostate cancer. The apex of the prostate and the seminal vesicles are the most likely sites for residual cancer.[34] This is possible because temperatures low enough to destroy cancer cells in these areas are not realized during treatment. Treatment options for cryosurgery failure are salvage radical prostatectomy, salvage radiation therapy, endocrine therapy, repeat cryosurgery, and observation.

BILATERAL ORCHIECTOMY

Bilateral orchiectomy (removal of the testicles or surgical castration) is still considered the gold standard for hormonal manipulation in patients with metastatic prostate cancer.[35] Orchiectomy can be performed on an outpatient basis under local anesthesia. The advantages of orchiectomy are that it is immediately effective in decreasing testosterone levels, there is no difficulty with patient compliance, and it is cost effective. After orchiectomy, castration levels of plasma testosterone are reached in 3 to 12 hours.

Complications of orchiectomy are the same as those associated with any surgical procedure and include bleeding and wound infection. Postoperative pain can be controlled with oral analgesics, scrotal elevation, and ice. Sitz baths, when allowed by the physician, may also aid in relieving discomfort. Patients should be instructed in recognizing signs and symptoms of wound infection and also in using some type of scrotal supporter until wound healing is complete and discomfort is eliminated.

Long-term side effects of orchiectomy include loss of libido and potency, hot flashes, osteoporosis, fatigue, and loss of muscle mass.[36] In some men, endocrine therapy has been successful in combating some of these side effects.

Men may be reluctant to undergo orchiectomy because they may see it as a loss of manhood. Patients' fears may be reduced by meeting and talking with other patients who have successfully undergone this procedure. Encourage the patient to attend a prostate cancer support group where he can meet others and voice his concerns. Men also need to be informed that scrotal cosmesis can be maintained by the implantation of a testicular prosthesis. Because of the psychological impact of surgical castration, these patients need a great deal of education and support.

SUMMARY

Surgical treatments for prostate cancer can have good outcomes for cure or palliation. However, complications and side effects can be associated with any surgical intervention. The patient should discuss at length all options with his family and physician before making any decisions.

REFERENCES

1. El-Mahdi A, Kuban D. Treatment of carcinoma of the prostate in the 1990's. *Compr Ther* 1992;18: 10–15.
2. Eddins CW, Heitkemper M, Power D. Management of men with reproductive problems. In: Phipps WJ, Cassmeyer VL, Sands JK, Lehman M (eds). *Medical-Surgical Nursing Concepts and Clinical Practice*, 5th ed. St. Louis, MO: CV Mosby, 1995:1779–1813.
3. Mebust WK. Transurethral surgery. In: Walsh PC, Retik, AB, Vaughan ED, Wein AJ (eds). *Campbell's Urology*, 7th ed. Philadelphia: WB Saunders, 1998:1511–1528.
4. Kozlowski JM, Grayhack JT. Carcinoma of the prostate. In: Gillenwater JY, Grayhack JT, Howards SS, Duckett JW (eds). *Adult and Pediatric Urology*, 3rd ed. St. Louis, MO: CV Mosby; 1996:1541–1574.
5. Swiger KI, Warner JP. Nursing care of men with reproductive and urinary disorders. In: Polaski AL, Tatro SE (eds). *Luckmann's Core Principles and Practice of Medical-Surgical Nursing*. Philadelphia: WB Saunders, 1996:1444–1468.
6. Narayan P. Neoplasms of the prostate gland. In: Tanagho EA, McAninch JW (eds). *Smith's General Urology*, 13th ed. Norwalk, CT: Appleton & Lange, 1992:378–412.
7. Matassarin-Jacobs E. Nursing care of men with reproductive disorders. In: Black JM, Matassarin-Jacobs E (eds). *Medical-Surgical Nursing: Clinical Management for Continuity of Care*, 5th ed. Philadelphia: WB Saunders, 1997:2343–2385
8. Karakiewicz PI, Zini A, Meshref AW, et al. Population-based patterns of radical retropubic prostatectomy use. *Urology* 1998;52:219–223.
9. Pezzino G, Remington PL, Anderson HA, et al. Trends in the surgical treatment of prostate cancer

in Wisconsin, 1989–1991. *Natl Cancer Inst* 1994;86: 1083–1086.

10. Fowler FJ, Bin L, Collins M, et al. Prostate cancer screening and beliefs about treatment efficacy: A national survey of primary care physicians and urologists. *Am J Med* 1998;104:526–532.

11. Desch CE, Penberthy L, Newschaffer CJ, et al. Factors that determine the treatment for local and regional prostate cancer. *Med Care* 1996;34:152–162.

12. Lassen PM, Thompson IM. Treatment options for prostate cancer. *Urol Nurs* 1994;14:12–15.

13. Talcott JA, Rieker P, Clark JA, et al. Patient-reported symptoms after primary therapy for early prostate cancer: Results of a prospective cohort study. *J Clin Oncol* 1998;15:275–283.

14. Van Erps P, Van Den Weyngaert D, Denis L. Surgery or radiation: Is there really a choice for early prostate cancer. *Crit Rev Oncol Hematol* 1998; 27:11–27.

15. Resnick MI, Schellhammer PF. Radical perineal or retropubic prostatectomy? *Contemp Urol* 1996;8: 40–46.

16. Harris MJ, Thompson IM. The anatomic radical perineal prostatectomy: A contemporary and anatomic approach. *Urology* 1996;48:762–768.

17. Christie F. Clinical snapshot pulmonary embolism. *Am J Nurs* 1998;98:36–37.

18. Gaylis FD, Frieedel WE, Armas OA. Radical retropubic prostatectomy outcomes at a community hospital. *J Urol* 1998;159:167–171.

19. Naitoh J, Zeiner RL, Dekernion JB. Diagnosis and treatment of prostate cancer. *Am Fam Physician* 1998; 57:1531–1539.

20. Weldon VE, Tavel FR, Heuwirth H. Continence, potency and morbidity after radical perineal prostatectomy. *J Urol* 1997;158:1470–1475.

21. Richie JP. Localized prostate cancer: Overview of surgical management. *Urology* 1997;49:35–37.

22. Naitoh J, Zeiner RL, Dekernion, JB. Diagnosis and treatment of prostate cancer. *Am Fam Physician* 1998; 57:1531–1539.

23. Bishoff JT, Motley G, Optenberg SA, et al. Incidence of fecal and urinary incontinence following radical perineal and retropubic prostatectomy in a national population. *J Urol* 1998;160:454–458.

24. Walsh PC, Partin AW, Epstein JI. Cancer control and quality of life following anatomical radical retropubic prostatectomy: Results at 10 years. *J Urol* 1994;152:1831–1836.

25. Altwein J, Ekman P, Barry M, et al. How is quality of life in prostate cancer patients influenced by

modern treatment? The Wallenberg symposium. *Urology* 1997;49:66–76.

26. Lu-Yao GL, Potosky AL, Albertsen PC, et al. Follow-up prostate cancer treatments after radical prostatectomy: A population-based study. *J Natl Cancer Inst* 1996;88:166–172.

27. Garnick MB, Fair WR. Prostate cancer: Emerging concepts. *Ann Intern Med* 1996;125:118–125.

28. Wieder JA, Soloway MS. Incidence, etiology, location, prevention and treatment of positive surgical margins after radical prostatectomy for prostate cancer. *J Urol* 1998;160:299–315.

29. Porter MP, Ahaghotu CA, Loening SA, See WA. Disease-free and overall survival after cryosurgical monotherapy for clinical stages B and C carcinoma of the prostate: A 20-year followup. *J Urol* 1997;158: 1466–1469.

30. Schmidt JD, Doyle J, Larison, S. Prostate cryoablation: Update 1998. *Cancer J Clin* 1998;48:239–253.

31. Zippe CD. Cryosurgery of the prostate techniques and pitfalls. *Urol Clin North Am* 1996;23:147–163.

32. Wong WS, Chinn DO, et al. Cryosurgery as a treatment for prostate carcinoma. *Cancer* 1997;79: 963–974.

33. Shinohara K, Connolly JA, Presti JC, Carroll PR. Cryosurgical treatment of localized prostate cancer (stages T1 to T4): Preliminary results. *J Urol* 1996; 156:115–121.

34. Shinohara K, Rhee B, Presti JR, Carroll PR. Cryosurgical ablation of prostate cancer: Patterns of cancer recurrence. *J Urol* 1997;158:2206–2210.

35. Schroder FH. Endocrine treatment of prostate cancer. In Walsh PC, Retil AB, Vaughan ED, Wein AJ (eds). *Campbell's Urology,* 7th ed. Philadelphia: WB Saunders, 1996:2627–2644

36. Fellows GJ, Clark PB, Beynon LL, et al. Treatment of advanced localised prostatic cancer by orchiectomy, radiotherapy, or combined treatment. *Br J Urol* 1992;70:304–309.

37. Held-Warmkessel J. Prostate cancer. In: Groenwald SL, Frogge M, Goodman M, Yarbro C (eds). *Cancer Nursing Principles and Practice,* 4th ed. Sudbury, MA: Jones and Bartlett, 1997:1334–1354.

38. Held JL, Osborne DM, Volpe H, Waldman AR. Cancer of the prostate: Treatment and nursing implications. *Oncol Nurs Forum* 1994;21:1517–1529.

39. Klimaszewski AD, Karlowicz KA. Cancer of the male genitalia. In: Karlowicz KA (ed). *Urologic Nursing Principles and Practice.* Philadelphia: WB Saunders, 1995:271–308.

Chapter 9

A PATIENT'S PERSPECTIVE ON THE DIAGNOSIS AND TREATMENT OF PROSTATE CANCER WITH RADIATION THERAPY

EDGAR HERBERT, JR.

Because prostate-specific antigen (PSA) tests clearly showed the strong probability that cancer was present, it was not a great surprise when biopsies proved, in fact, that it did exist in my prostate gland. My immediate reaction was "Here I go again!"

This was in stark contrast to the news a few years before that I had only 6 to 9 months to live if I didn't have open heart surgery soon to replace my aortic valve, which had slowly calcified over many years. The only warnings I had were a few near-blackouts that occurred over a 1-week period, which led me to consult a cardiologist. His findings were such a devastating blow that I had a hard time keeping my composure. I think that going through heart surgery in good shape and recovering in a short time made the fact that I now had cancer anticlimactic. Accordingly, the cancer finding didn't bother me very much. I went about my daily activities as usual, slept well, and so on. Neither did it bother my wife. My children are all older and it wasn't any great shock to them.

When the urologist broke the news, he mentioned treatment options, surgery and radiology. He said he did not recommend surgery because of my age (79) and the nature of the cancer, but he highly recommended radiation treatment. I asked him what the cure rate is for this treatment. He replied "good." It took me only a few moments to reply, "Okay, go ahead and set it up." He then called a nearby oncologist, and I was in his office 2 days later.

The oncologist advised that radioactive treatment would be scheduled 5 days a week for 6 weeks less 2 days set aside for internal treatment. Internal treatment involved insertion of 11 catheters directly into the prostate, and the procedure required hospitalization. He further advised that I could go back and forth from home for the exterior treatments. In response to my inquiry about side effects, he replied that a lot depends on the individual; some experience diarrhea, nausea, and impotence. Then he showed me the treatment room and explained that I would come in, lie flat on a movable bed, be positioned by technicians directly under that radiation equipment, be given the dose, be moved out, get up, and then go home. The time involved amounted to mere minutes for the whole procedure. It certainly didn't sound hard to take, and later experience proved it wasn't. He also briefed me on the internal treatments. Frankly, I don't recall losing any sleep over the matter but just continued my normal daily activities. I think one has to have confidence and trust in specialists to maintain peace of mind.

Exterior treatments commenced the following week and were precisely as the oncologist described. I had no sensations while undergoing them and no side effects. Later on, in the fifth week, the interior treatments began, which was a different story.

This procedure involved hospitalization. On Day 1, while I was under anesthesia, the urologist, assisted by the oncologist, embedded the 11 catheters into my prostate. On completion of this phase, I was taken to my room, where I woke with no feeling of pain but I did sense the catheters. The nurse in attendance stressed the importance of lying flat on my back with no turning whatsoever until after the catheters were removed. The afternoon of Day 1 was no problem. However, as night went on, I became increasingly restless and found it very difficult to sleep. It seemed that when I did doze off, a nurse would come in to check body functions, draw blood, and so on. Consequently, I got very little sleep. Not being able to turn in any direction was mild torture. I knew I could have called a nurse to administer an opiate; however, I'm inclined to be stoic and did not want it because I had no pain per se.

About 9 AM on Day 2, nurses managed to transfer me from the bed to a gurney without disturbing the catheters and then to a waiting ambulance for the three-block ride to the oncology center. Here I was moved directly into the radiation room, where technicians connected electrodes from the equipment to the catheters and administered the dose into the tumor. This process went smoothly and seemed to take only a few minutes. On disconnecting the electrodes, I was then returned to my hospital bed. Five hours later, the whole process was repeated, culminating with removal of the catheters. What a relief it was to be able to move finally. After this last treatment, I was taken back to my hospital bed by gurney and ambulance. Here I finally got some sleep, interrupted, of course, by nurses making their nightly rounds. I was released about 9 AM of Day 3. Daily treatments followed until the sixth week was completed.

I must emphasize that at no time did I have any side effects such as pain or bleeding, except for discomfort during the internal procedure. I went about my usual daily activities at home, including golfing or walking 2 miles every morning. In general, I kept busy. My advice to anyone who has to go through what I did is "Don't let it get you down. Try to keep from worrying about it, and above all, don't be a 'couch potato.' " If impotence becomes a problem, be sure to let your urologist know because he or she can best advise you on the most helpful course of action to correct that matter.

One thing that helped ease any anxieties I may have experienced was the demeanor of the doctors, nurses, and support staff. Nothing could have made me feel better than their helpful, cheerful attitude.

Chapter 10

RADIATION THERAPY

HEIDI M. VOLPE

OVERVIEW

INTRODUCTION
PRETREATMENT WORKUP
SIMULATION-TREATMENT PLANNING
EXTERNAL BEAM RADIATION
  Treatment Volume and Technique
  Treatment Field
  Stages T1a and T1b
  Stage T1c
  Lymph Node Treatment
  Control Rate
  Stages T3 and T4
  Total Androgen Suppression
  Postprostatectomy Treatment
  Management of Advanced Disease

THREE-DIMENSIONAL CONFORMAL
  RADIATION THERAPY
EXTERNAL BEAM SIDE EFFECTS
  Bowel
  Skin
  Urinary Tract
  Sexual Functioning
  Fatigue
  Myelosuppression
INTERSTITIAL IMPLANTATION
  (BRACHYTHERAPY)
  Patient Preparation
  Procedure
  Postimplant Side Effects and Nursing Care
COMBINATION THERAPY
PSYCHOSOCIAL ISSUES
CONCLUSION

INTRODUCTION

The management of prostate carcinoma is controversial in almost all disease stages. The treatment decision should be based on patient factors, including general health, age, tolerance of expected side effects, and tumor-specific factors such as prostate-specific antigen (PSA) level, clinical stage, and histologic factors such as the Gleason score. Radiation therapy is a treatment modality useful in the management of prostate cancer. This chapter describes treatment of the patient using radiation therapy, both external and brachytherapy, and the associated nursing management.

Radiation oncology is a discipline that uses radiation therapy as a treatment modality to deliver a therapeutic dose of ionizing radiation. The radiation oncology team consists of a physician, radiation therapist, and physicist who are educated and specially trained in the principles of radiation physics and the biologic effects of ionizing radiation. This team may include other professionals such as nurses, dietitians, researchers, and social workers to aid in the care, education, and support of patients and their families.

Therapeutic radiation can be either particulate or electromagnetic in nature with the capability of ionizing matter. Radiation therapy is a technique used to kill or inactivate cancer cells. Cell death occurs when the ionizing radiation directly affects the DNA by breaking or damaging the molecule. A goal of radiation treatments is not only to eradicate areas of tumor but also to preserve the integrity of surrounding normal tissue and organs.

The radiosensitivity of a cell is greatest just before and during cell division. Cell differentiation is also a factor in cell radiosensitivity. Undifferentiated cell populations are generally the most sensitive to radiation, and well-differentiated cells are relatively radioresistant.[1] The radiosensitivity of a tumor differs from its radiocurability (ability to be eradicated). Adenocarcinoma can differ in cell differentiation from well to poor. Therefore, high doses of radiation are given to patients with adenocarcinoma of the prostate. Even though the prostate tumor may take several months to regress after treatment, it is considered radiocurable.

Radiation therapy kills a certain percentage of cancer cells per unit of time of treatment.[2] Radiation doses are given in individual treatments, a process known as a *fractionation*. Cumulative fractions will ultimately achieve a predetermined total radiation dose. Patients can be treated with single or multiple daily fractions (hyperfractionation). The unit or quantity of the absorbed radiation dose is the gray (Gy). Cells not completely destroyed may be able to recover between 4 and 24 hours after a radiation treatment. Patients need to be educated regarding cell recovery so they understand the importance of keeping scheduled daily appointments for their radiation treatments. Radiation treatments are based on the concept that malignant cells do not efficiently repair themselves from radiation injury as normal cells do. Therefore, most malignant tumors can be destroyed by certain amounts of radiation while sparing normal tissue. Some normal cells will die, but the body is able to replace damaged cells through normal cell growth and replacement.[3]

Patients with early-stage, organ-confined prostate cancer (T1-T2, N0) are generally managed by radical prostatectomy, radiation therapy, or watchful waiting. Radiation therapy may be given with conventional or conformal external beam radiation, or brachytherapy (interstitial implantation). Because of a lack of randomized trials, there is no evidence of one modality's superiority over another. In older, less healthy patients with higher grade or more advanced tumors, treatment with radiation therapy is preferred. Although the controversy over prostatectomy versus radiation continues, the National Institutes of Health Consensus Conference concluded that, in early-stage prostate cancer, the 10-year survival rates for radical prostatectomy and radiation therapy were similar.[4] Comparing outcomes of radiation therapy and surgery is also limited because the regional lymph node status of patients treated with radiation therapy is usually unknown at diagnosis. Surgical findings are generally reported on the basis of pathologic findings. The classic radical prostatectomy has a sexual impotence rate of almost 100%; because radiation therapy has been shown to be as effective in the treatment of these patients, some will opt for radiation instead of surgery.[5] In addition, a nerve-sparing radical prostatectomy technique, with lower impotency rates, may be an option for some patients (See Chapter 8).

Patients with surgically staged T1-T2 tumors treated with radiation therapy have survival rates comparable to those treated with radical prostatectomy.[6] The Radiation Therapy Oncology Group (RTOG) study 77-06, involving 104 patients with stage T1b-2, N0 tumors treated with radiation, found that the clinical tumor-free survival was 96% at 5 years and 86% at 10 years, and locoregional tumor control was 93% and 84%, respectively. These results are comparable to those reported with radical prostatectomy.[7]

Patients with Clinical Stages T3 and T4 are considered to have locally advanced tumors and are generally treated with external beam radiation alone or in combination with androgen ablation.[8] The timing of hormonal intervention is controversial. Total androgen suppression (TAS) can be initiated as a neoadjuvant and adjuvant treatment or at the completion of radiation therapy (see Combination Therapy discussion).

PRETREATMENT WORKUP

Most patients arrive at the radiation oncology department with a preliminary workup already completed. Tests may include an ultrasonogram with needle biopsy or transurethral resection of the prostate (TURP), confirming pathologic confirmation.

Diagnostic workup includes a detailed clinical history and general physical assessment that involves a rectal examination to evaluate disease status. Radiographic imaging studies generally include a computed tomography (CT) scan of the abdomen and pelvis or magnetic resonance imaging (MRI), radioisotope bone scan, and chest radiography. Renal function is commonly evaluated either by an intravenous pyelogram or the contrast material used during the CT scan. There is, however, a current trend to omit these studies in patients with low-stage, low-grade tumors; Gleason scores of 3 or less; and PSA values less than 10 because the risk of metastasis is low.

Helpful laboratory tests include a current PSA level, complete blood cell count, and serum chemistry panel. If hormonal therapy is to be added, baseline liver function tests and testosterone levels are warranted.

SIMULATION-TREATMENT PLANNING

CT scans are useful in all patients who are to receive radiotherapy. Imaging studies allow more exact definition of tumor volume and can even provide differences in tissue densities that aid in dosimetric calculations.

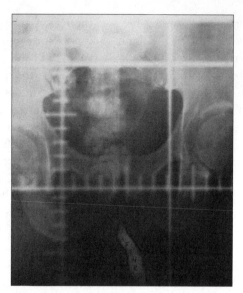

FIGURE 10-1. Simulation film (urethrogram) with contrast dye
Courtesy of the Radiation Oncology Department, Albert Einstein Medical Center, Philadelphia, PA.

Advances in computers and software have allowed the introduction of three-dimensional (3-D) conformal radiation therapy (3D CRT). CT is necessary for 3-D treatment planning in which multiple beams are used to help decrease the dose to any one organ while maximizing the tumor dose. In treatment planning, it allows more precise delineation of the prostate tumor and enables a higher dose of radiation to be given to the prostate while reducing the volume of normal tissue in the treatment field. Lower radiation doses to normal tissue may result in fewer side effects such as bowel and bladder complications.

Simulation is a treatment planning process using a machine that replicates the beam arrangement, couch-gantry position, and beam geometry of the treatment machine. Most modern simulation machines use fluoroscopy to outline field borders defined by the radiation oncologist. Diagnostic quality films are obtained at simulation. CT scans may be performed at the same time, or a newer technique allows the simulation to be performed using a CT scanner. On average, the prostate simulation takes approximately 1 hour and is generally performed by a registered radiation therapist under the guidance of a radiation oncologist. Patients are required to lie on a narrow table for the duration of the simulation.

Various methods are used to help define the location and size of the prostate. This may be achieved by fluoroscopy, in which contrast dye is often used to perform a urethrogram to define the prostate apex. Contrast dye is instilled into the bladder or balloon of an indwelling urinary catheter, helping to delineate the prostate base (Figure 10-1).

A second indwelling urinary catheter or rectal tube is inserted into the rectum. Contrast dye or a rectal marker is used to outline the contours of the rectum, a critical area of normal tissue that is in the treatment field.

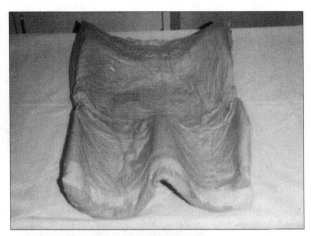

FIGURE 10-2. Rigid, patient immobilization device
Courtesy of the Radiation Oncology Department, Albert Einstein Medical Center, Philadelphia, PA.

During simulation, either nonpermanent marks or small, permanent tattoos are placed to aid in the daily positioning of patients. Techniques can vary among institutions, because some radiation oncologists require filming on the treatment machine before the final tattoos are placed. Tattoos are the size of a freckle and are placed by pricking the skin with a small needle containing India ink. Tattoo placement usually is performed by the radiation therapist. Until permanent marks are placed, patients need to be instructed not to shower or wash off temporary markings.

To ensure that the daily positioning of the patient is consistent and to define leg position, an individually fabricated, rigid immobilization device (alpha cradle, thermoplastics) may be constructed during this simulation session (Figure 10-2).

Radiographs taken during the simulation are used by the dosimetry and physics departments to outline and reconstruct the exact tumor volume specific to the treatment area (Figures 10-3 and 10-4). A computer is used to produce a drawing of the prostate from different angles. This diagram (isodose curve) shows the exact doses of radiation that will be given to the prostate and surrounding tissue (Figure 10-5). Reconstruction of the prostate and radiation field borders are drawn out by the dosimetrist onto the simulation films as per the treatment specifications of the radiation oncologist. The borders outlined will include the initial treatment field and cone-down (boost) areas if there is to be a field reduction during the course of treatment. The initial plan may not actually be the final approved boost area, because additional portal or radiographs are taken closer to the time the cone-down will be given. Fields may also be modified at any time during treatment at the radiation oncologist's discretion.

Portal films are x-rays that depict the actual treatment area receiving radiation. The initial portal films are taken at simulation and are used for treatment planning. Additional portal films (verification films) are taken at regular intervals during the course of

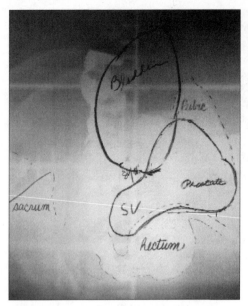

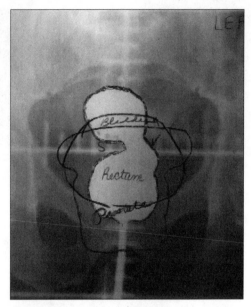

FIGURE 10-3. Anterior/posterior simulation film with treatment volumes

FIGURE 10-4. Laterally opposed simulation film

Courtesy of the Radiation Oncology Department, Albert Einstein Medical Center, Philadelphia, PA.

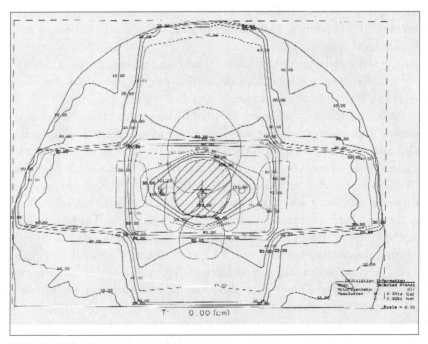

FIGURE 10-5. Computerized isodose curve

Courtesy of the Radiation Oncology Department, Albert Einstein Medical Center, Philadelphia, PA.

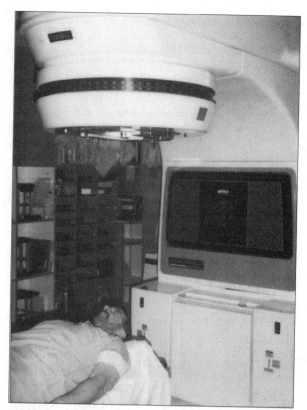

FIGURE 10-6. Linear accelerator radiation treatment machine
Courtesy of the Radiation Oncology Department, Albert Einstein Medical Center, Philadelphia, PA. Photo by Heidi M. Volpe.

radiation so that each field can be assessed by the radiation oncologist for accuracy and changes can be made, as necessary. Some institutions take verification films on a weekly basis, but this can vary. The number of portal films, in most instances, will correspond to the number of fields being treated.

EXTERNAL BEAM RADIATION

External beam radiation (teletherapy, radiotherapy, irradiation) is currently the most widely used method of delivering radiation treatments. Radiation is produced from a radioactive source or electromagnetic energy from within a machine and is then delivered to a target site on a patient from a specified distance. This technique was initiated at Stanford University in the 1950s as a curative modality[5] (Figure 10-6).

Various types of radiation-producing machines exist, each capable of generating different energies and treating at different depths. Currently, the linear accelerator is the most commonly used type for treating externally with high-energy photons (6–25 MV).[9]

TREATMENT VOLUME AND TECHNIQUE

Field size is described as width times the length, measured in centimeters. The radiation technique, used to treat prostate cancer, is most commonly derived from a four-field box plan. This technique uses an anteroposterior field and laterally opposed fields. With a linear accelerator, each field is treated once daily, generally on a Monday-through-Friday schedule. The daily radiation dose typically ranges from 1.8 to 2.0 Gy. Field size will differ on the basis of inclusion of pelvic lymph nodes and tumor volume. There is much controversy in the literature regarding whether pelvic lymph nodes should be included in the treatment field.

High-risk patients may benefit from receiving whole pelvic irradiation followed by a prostate boost. To define the high-risk population, the following calculation of risk of lymph node positivity can be used:

$$2/3 \text{ (initial PSA)} + 10 \text{ (Gleason score} - 6)$$

The risk of lymph node involvement using this equation is defined as intermediate risk falling between 15 and 35% and the highest risk as greater than 35%.[10] Tumor stage may also be considered in this calculation.

A study of 506 patients with clinically localized prostate cancer treated with or without whole pelvic irradiation concluded that intermediate-risk patients who received whole pelvic irradiation had significantly improved PSA failure-free survivals. This study also concluded that high-risk patients had no significant benefit from receiving whole pelvic irradiation.[10]

Currently, the RTOG is conducting a four-arm Phase III trial (Study 94-13) examining the effect of whole pelvic radiation in conjunction with TAS for high-risk patients. These patients are considered high risk if the risk of lymph node involvement is greater than 15%. The whole pelvis receives a dose of 50.4 Gy followed by a 19.8-Gy boost, to a total dose of 70.2 Gy to the prostate. Patients randomized to prostate-only radiation receive a total dose of 70.2 Gy.[5, 10, 15]

TREATMENT FIELD

When the whole pelvis is treated followed by a field reduction (boost) focused on the prostate, the treatment area commonly encompasses an initial field, approximately 15 x 15 cm, that includes the prostate, periprostatic tissue, seminal vesicles, external iliac, and pelvic and presacral lymph nodes. For patients with D1 tumors, the field size is increased to 15 x 18 cm to include the common iliac lymph nodes.[5] Field sizes will vary depending upon patient anatomy.

Treatment borders are derived from simulation and CT films. For large-field radiation, the superior margin is generally at the level of L5, S1, and the inferior border is at the lower aspect of the ischial tuberosities. The right and left field edges are 1 to 2 cm to the widest diameter of the pelvic side walls. From the lateral direction, the anterior field margin is at the posterior cortex of the pubic bone, and the posterior portion of the field extends to include pelvic and presacral lymph nodes (Figures 10-7 and 10-8).

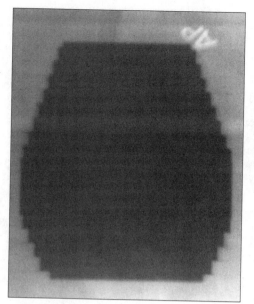 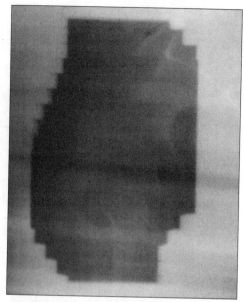

FIGURE 10-7. Large anterior and posterior radiation treatment field, to the prostate including pelvic lymph nodes, using a four-field box technique

FIGURE 10-8. Large laterally opposed radiation treatment field, using a four-field box technique

Courtesy of the Radiation Oncology Department, Albert Einstein Medical Center, Philadelphia, PA.

For small-field radiation, borders of the superior margin are reduced to 1 cm above the seminal vesicles or 2 cm above the indwelling urinary catheter balloon. The inferior border can remain the same. Laterals are designed to encompass only prostate and periprostatic tissue.[8] Field reduction of the prostate (cone down) and for those patients receiving small-field radiation only, the volume ranges from 8 x 10 for T1 and T2 to 10 x 12 or 12 x 14 for T3 and T4[5] (Figures 10-9 and 10-10).

The initial large radiation field is treated so that the regional lymphatics commonly receive 45 to 50 Gy. Field reduction, or small (boost) fields, allows the prostate to receive a total dose between 65 and 74 Gy while sparing critical structures; shielding of the posterior rectal wall, anal canal and sphincter, uninvolved urethra, pubic bone, and small bowel is common.[9]

STAGES T1a and T1b

T1a and T1b tumors are small, and aggressive treatment may not be necessary in all patients unless the tumor is not organ-confined.[12] Management includes hormonal therapy, watchful waiting, prostatectomy, and radiation therapy. Watchful waiting, in these low-stage patients, is usually only recommended in those with Gleason scores of 4 or less and PSA values less than 10.

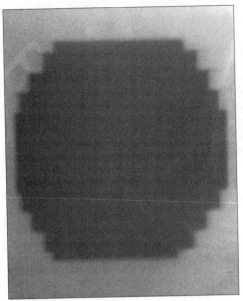

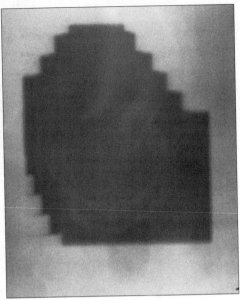

FIGURE 10-9. Small (anterior/posterior) field pelvic radiation treatment portal using a four-field box technique

FIGURE 10-10. Small, opposed lateral fields using a four-field box technique

Courtesy of the Radiation Oncology Department, Albert Einstein Medical Center, Philadelphia, PA.

STAGE T1c

In patients with Clinical Stage T1c, a broad spectrum of findings exists. These patients are found to have the disease by needle biopsy after PSA elevation. Although rectal examination is clinically negative, pathologically these patients may have positive biopsies from one or both prostatic lobes. For patients with Stage T1 disease, the overall rate of survival with radiation therapy is equal to that of the general population.[4] Current data do not support whole pelvic radiation for early-stage cancer; however, patients with undetected micrometastases may benefit from this approach.[13]

LYMPH NODE TREATMENT

Pelvic lymph node inclusion in the treatment portal should be considered in patients younger than 71 with Stage T1c-T2a tumors and Gleason scores of 6 or more or PSA of 20 ng/mL or more and in patients with Stages T2b-T3. These criteria are followed at Washington University.[5]

CONTROL RATE

In patients with T1 and T2 tumors, clinical local control rates of 80% at 10 years have been observed.[14] The survival rate for Stage T2 patients treated with radiation therapy ranges from equivalent to 20% below that of the general population.[4]

STAGES T3 AND T4

Radiation therapy is also used in Stages T3 and T4 because of difficulty in surgical prostate removal and the concern that gross and microscopic disease may remain in the lymph nodes.[15] Clinical local control for Stages T3 and T4 have been reported at 50 to 70%.[11] These outcomes are now being reconsidered as the measurement of the serum marker; PSA has shown that active prostate cancer persists in many patients who formerly would have been considered cured by conventional radiotherapy.[16] Multiple publications have reported positive second biopsies in the range of 14 to 91% at 18+ months after radiation in clinically negative prostate glands. The rate of positive biopsies was higher in patients with initially staged T2c-T3 tumors and those with elevated PSA levels at the time of biopsy. This supports the fact that radiation success cannot be adequately measured by clinical local control, as determined by rectal exam.[11] These findings also emphasize the need to improve local control rates because radiation, as a single modality, is less effective than once thought. This is particularly true for patients with Stages T2c-T4, Gleason grades of 4 or more, and initial PSA levels greater than 15 ng/mL.[11]

Recommendations for improving local control include dose escalation through the use of 3-D CRT and the administration of hormonal therapy before and during radiation (neoadjuvant cytoreduction). (See Three-Dimensional Conformal Radiation Therapy discussion.)

TOTAL ANDROGEN SUPPRESSION

An alternative to dose escalation, when attempting to improve local control, is TAS (cytoreduction). Neoadjuvant cytoreduction may decrease tumor volume before radiation treatments with the goal of increasing tumor control. Refer to the Combination Therapy discussion for further information.

POSTPROSTATECTOMY TREATMENT

Radiation, when used as adjuvant postprostatectomy therapy in Stages T3 and T4 disease, significantly improves local control compared with radical prostatectomy alone.[17]

Patients offered radical prostatectomy as a definitive treatment option usually have clinically organ-confined disease (Clinical Stages T1a-T2c). If postoperatively more extensive disease is noted pathologically, the risk of systemic spread is increased. Patients with positive margins or seminal vesicle involvement at prostatectomy have local relapse rates between 20% and 50%.[18] Patients receiving radiation postprostatectomy usually start 6 to 12 weeks postoperatively. Patients found to have a more advanced stage of disease at surgery but negative pelvic lymph node dissections may be treated with limited pelvic irradiation. Other patients may require whole pelvic irradiation. Radiation therapy can be administered to postprostatectomy patients who have positive surgical margins, seminal vesicle involvement, or detectable PSA after surgery and in patients who develop local disease recurrence.

Correlation among the patient's clinical stage, PSA, and Gleason score also appears to be a predictor for seminal vesicle and pelvic lymph node involvement. Using PSA values as a determinant to define tumor recurrence varies. After radiation, remaining nonmalignant epithelial tissue can continue to produce detectable PSA even when no cancer is present. In contrast, PSA levels should be undetectable in patients after prostatectomy, if successful, because both the malignancy and normal prostate tissue were removed.[19] Assignment of a predetermined value as the number that reflects where a post-treatment PSA level should be is difficult and controversial. In response to this dilemma, the American Society of Therapeutic Radiology and Oncology (ASTRO) Consensus Conference suggested the definition be based not on an absolute number value but on serial rising PSA values as the indicator of failure.[20]

MANAGEMENT OF ADVANCED DISEASE

Patients with complications associated with advanced prostate cancer, such as urinary obstruction, hematuria, pelvic pain, spinal cord compression, and pain from soft tissue or osseous metastases, may also benefit from palliative radiation treatments. The treatment goal is to reduce the tumor directly causing these symptoms.

Spinal cord compression, from direct tumor extension or metastases, is considered an oncologic emergency. Signs and symptoms can vary but usually include loss of muscle strength and tone, urinary or bowel changes, incontinence, diarrhea or constipation, motor weakness, numbness, pain, and paresthesias. Frequently, an MRI is done to confirm the diagnosis. Compression of the spinal cord must be relieved quickly to prevent permanent neurologic damage. High-dose corticosteroids are usually administered, and surgical decompression may be necessary if the compression is rapidly progressive, in patients who have undergone previous spinal radiation, and in those with spinal instability[4] (see Chapter 14).

THREE-DIMENSIONAL CONFORMAL RADIATION THERAPY

Three-dimensional CRT is a variation of standard external beam radiation, the goal of which is to increase the radiation dose to the tumor by sharply defining the treatment volume of the prostate while sparing critical structures from side effects. Standard external beam radiation therapy doses are limited because of the proximity of critical structures, including the bladder and rectum. For local tumor control, doses in excess of 65 Gy (to the tumor) are needed to eradicate even early-stage disease. Higher doses are necessary for more advanced disease. Local tumor control is directly related to the radiation dose being accurately delivered to the treatment area. The enhanced high-performance computer technology of today has enabled the 3-D CRT era.

Three-dimensional treatment planning is a complex, detailed process whereby CT images are used to generate high-resolution 3-D reconstructions of the prostate and surrounding structures. Patients undergo standard simulation procedures to determine reference points. The simulation films are used in conjunction with the 3-D reconstructions in planning and calculating treatment volume and isodose distributions (Figure 10-11). Immobilization casts are required for reproducing daily patient positioning. Dose escala-

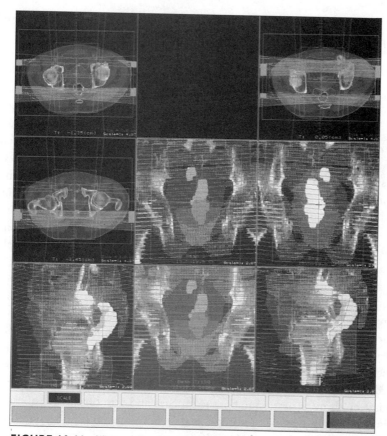

FIGURE 10-11. 3D treatment planning representation
Courtesy of the Radiation Oncology Department, Albert Einstein Medical Center, Philadelphia, PA.

tion studies with dose rate ranges between 68.4 and 79.2 Gy are currently being analyzed in clinical trials through RTOG Study 94-06.[16]

EXTERNAL BEAM SIDE EFFECTS

Radiation therapy side effects can be categorized into acute and late toxicities. Acute side effects are those symptoms occurring during treatment and within the first 90 days after radiation. Late or delayed effects encompass the time period after 90 days, may occur many months to years after treatment completion, and may be progressive and persistent. The severity of side effects can be correlated to treatment volume, daily and total radiation doses, type of treatment, anatomic site of treatment, and individual tolerance. Patients should be instructed that side effects are site specific and occur within the treatment field. The nurse needs to individualize care based on assessment findings. Interventions should be in place before treatment initiation to prevent or minimize occurrence of possible side effects. Patient education and direct care can assist with symptom relief.

BOWEL

Alterations in bowel elimination are one of the most common acute manifestations of radiation therapy to the abdomen and pelvis. Radiation treatments cause inflammation of the mucosa of the small and large bowels. Radiation enteritis is directly related to the dose rate and the volume of small bowel within the treatment field. Onset generally occurs during the second to third week of treatment or at a dose rate between 15 and 30 Gy. Acute gastrointestinal side effects most commonly include diarrhea, abdominal cramping, tenesmus, proctalgia, and occasionally rectal bleeding. Patients with hemorrhoids may experience discomfort earlier than other patients. This is because of preexisting irritation. Diarrhea severity can vary from mild (two to four stools per day) to severe (eight or more stools in a 24-hour period) and requires prompt intervention to prevent dehydration and electrolyte imbalance.[21] Diarrhea, with or without tenesmus, can be controlled with the administration of atropine and diphenoxylate hydrochloride (Lomotil, Searle, Chicago, IL), loperamide (Imodium, Jannsen, Titusville, NJ), opium preparations such as paregoric, and emollients such as kaolin and pectin[5] (Table 10-1).

The nurse needs to assess the patient for diarrhea, including amount and frequency, and needs to inspect the perianal tissues for signs of excoriation (Table 10-2). Patients should be instructed on following a low-residue diet, increasing fluid intake, and using antidiarrheal medication (see Table 10-3, pages 154–155). It is important to monitor the patient for dehydration through assessment of the mucosa and skin turgor and questioning him about fluid intake and urinary output (I&O). The volume of liquid stool should also be measured and calculated into the I&O. If the patient is hospitalized, I&O monitoring is easier. Proctitis and rectal discomfort may be alleviated by warm sitz baths several times a day, hydrocortisone-based treatments (ProctoFoam, Schwartz, Milwaukee, WI; Cortifoam, Schwartz, Milwaukee, WI), or anti-inflammatory suppositories (Anusol, Warner-Lambert Consumer, Morris Plains, NJ; Rowasa, Solvay, Marietta, GA). Each patient's tolerance and development of side effects will differ. Interventions should be tailored to individual patient needs based on severity.

Radiation therapy may cause late bowel sequelae in 1 to 3% of irradiated patients.[5] Toxicities include persistent bowel changes, diarrhea, fistula formation, perforation, and bleeding. The onset and duration may be related to slow or incomplete healing of the bowel mucosa and chronic changes related to edema, fibrosis, and vascular insufficiency. More severe reactions such as chronic intermittent bleeding usually can be conservatively treated with laser or fulguration, but intestinal obstruction may necessitate surgery.

SKIN

Skin tolerance to radiation is dose dependent, and toxicity results from a loss of cells in the epidermis, dermis, and microvasculature endothelium.[22] Skin reactions such as erythema, pain, and dry or moist desquamation may develop in the perineum or intergluteal

TABLE 10-1. Antidiarrheal Agents

Drug	Dose	Frequency	Partial List of Potential Side Effects	Contra-indications	Patient Education
Diphenoxylate hydrochloride with atropine sulfate	5 mg for initial control, then reduce to meet individual needs; control may be maintained with 5 mg daily	2 tablets qid	Paresthesia, lethargy, sedation, drowsiness, restlessness, headache, paralytic ileus, vomiting, nausea, anorexia, abdominal discomfort, urinary retention, flushing, dryness of skin and mucous membranes, blurred vision, rash	Hypersensitivity Obstructive jaundice, Cirrhosis, Pseudomembranous enterocolitis MAO inhibitors	Increase fluid intake to at least 3,000 mL/day Keep record of frequency of bowel movements and be alert for constipation Report if diarrhea does not improve after a few days, if blood is noted in stool, or if fever is present
Loperamide	2 mg (5 mL/tsp)	4 tsp or 2 capsules after first loose bowel movement, then 2 tsp or 1 capsule after each subsequent loose bowel movement	Abdominal pain, distention, or discomfort; nausea, vomiting, constipation, drowsiness or dizziness, dry mouth, rash	History of liver disease Pseudomembranous colitis	Patients instructed to report any of the following symptoms: muscle weakness, anorexia, vomiting, drowsiness, irritability
Paregoric	0.3–1 mL; mix with sufficient water to ensure passage to the stomach	qd-qid	Nausea, vomiting, physical dependency with long-term use, dizziness, lightheadedness	None significant	
Kaolin-pectin	60–120 mL	After each loose bowel movement	None significant	Suspected obstructive bowel lesions; may reduce absorption of other PO drugs	

Source: Data compiled from Wilkes et al,[35] Nursing '98 Books,[36] and Wilkes et al.[37]
qid, four times daily; qd, every day; MAOIs, monoamine oxidase inhibitors; PO, oral.

TABLE 10-2. Diarrhea and Foods to Avoid

DIARRHEA*

Some chemotherapy drugs, radiation, and infection may cause diarrhea. This happens when food passes quickly through the bowel before the body gets enough vitamins, minerals, and water. Diarrhea can cause dehydration and electrolyte imbalances. The following instruction is a guide to use if diarrhea occurs:

- Notify your physician or nurse if you are experiencing three or more watery stools per day.
- Drink 6–8 glasses of liquids per day. Drink fluids such as fruit juice, tea, Gatorade, and soup. Avoid carbonated beverages, which can aggravate diarrhea.
- Eat plenty of foods and drink liquids that contain salt (sodium) and potassium. These are minerals, important to the body, and are lost when you have diarrhea.
- Avoid extremely hot or cold foods.
- Avoid milk or milk products.
- Avoid spicy or fatty foods and foods high in fiber such as whole-grain bread and cereal, fresh fruit, raw vegetables, and popcorn. Also avoid rich pastries, caffeine, alcohol, and tobacco.
- Eat small amounts of food and liquids throughout the day instead of three large meals. Suggested are eggs, rice, yogurt, broth, applesauce, broiled or baked chicken and fish, pasta, canned fruit, and cooked vegetables.
- If diarrhea is severe, a clear liquid diet for 12–24 hours may be advised by the physician or nurse.
- Keep rectal area clean and dry using mild soap and water. If experiencing discomfort, soaking in a tub of warm water and using a topical cream (i.e., Desitin) may be helpful.
- Over the counter anti-diarrheal products, such as Immodium A-D, may be used according to package directions. Ask your physician or nurse for further information.
- Call your physician or nurse if the following symptoms occur with the diarrhea:
  - Lightheadedness
  - Fever
  - Inability to urinate for 6 hours or more
  - Diarrhea continues despite measures taken

FOODS TO AVOID WHEN DIARRHEA OCCURS†

- Milk and milk drinks—limit to 2 cups per day
- Meats with large amounts of tough connective tissue
- Raw vegetables with tough skins or seeds
- Dried beans and peas
- Corn
- Pumpkin, squash
- Gas-forming vegetables such as broccoli, brussels sprouts, cabbage, onions, cauliflower, cucumbers, green peppers, rutabagas, turnips, sauerkraut
- Olives, pickles
- Tough skins on fruits
- Dried fruit
- Berries
- Figs
- Very coarse cereals such as bran, bran flakes, shredded wheat, granola, wheat germ
- All whole-grain rye and wheat products
- Seeds in or on breads, rolls, or crackers
- Breads or bread products made with nuts or dried fruit
- Potato chips or other snack chips
- Popcorn
- Chunky peanut butter
- Nuts
- Coconut
- Sweets and desserts containing nuts, coconut, or fruits that are not allowed
- Cloudy juices

From SN DiLima (ed), *Oncology Patient Education Manual.* Gaithersburg, MD: Aspen, 1994.

*Used with permission from Ireland Cancer Center, University Hospitals of Cleveland, Case Western Reserve University, Cleveland, Ohio.

†Used with permission from Sherry Page, RN, BSN, OCN, Radiation Oncology, Allison Cancer Center, Midland, Texas.

fold. Reactions are increased when skinfolds are in the treatment area because of uneven distribution of the radiation dose and the warm, moist environment produced in these areas.

Erythema is caused by inflammation from an increase in blood volume beneath the epidermis. Dry desquamation (erythema and inflammation) is caused by a loss of the epidermal cells. Moist desquamation occurs when there is serosanguineous drainage with open dermal areas. This usually results in pain and frequently requires a break in treatment for healing.[22]

Patients should be assessed for evidence of alteration in skin integrity and instructed in proper skin hygiene. The perineal area should be washed, without rubbing and using tepid water (avoid extreme temperatures), and patted dry. Patients should be instructed to avoid soaps, deodorants, perfumes, powders, cosmetics, and lotions. Frequent daily sitz baths are helpful in providing comfort and keeping the perineum clean. The importance of cleanliness should be reinforced to prevent infection. Cotton undergarments and loose-fitting clothing can enhance comfort. Management goals are to minimize discomfort, promote healing, and prevent infection. Topical use of skin preparations such as petroleum jelly, lanolin, zinc oxide, Desitin (Pfizer, New York), Aquaphor (Beiersodorf, Norwalk, CT), or Proctofoam (Schwartz, Milwaukee, WI) may be indicated for moist or dry desquamation. These preparations can be applied to the area of skin reaction as frequently as needed, except just before the radiation treatment. Cornstarch can be used on dry desquamation.

Edema of the leg, scrotum, and penis can occur but is extremely rare in patients treated with radiation alone. It is most often associated with a prior lymphadenectomy and is not seen with implant or small-field external beam radiation therapy (Chapter 14).

URINARY TRACT

Genitourinary symptoms such as dysuria, frequency, hesitancy, urgency, and nocturia are common during radiation treatments. The pathophysiology of radiation-induced bladder injury is not fully understood.[23]

Radiation treatments can cause irritation, edema, inflammation, and vascular changes of the bladder urothelium, vasculature, and smooth muscle. Reduction in bladder capacity may result from functional and anatomic changes caused by vascular damage with fibroblast and collagen deposits of the bladder smooth muscle.[23] These changes lead to irritating voiding symptoms (frequency, urgency, dysuria, decreased flow). Acute or chronic radiation cystitis with or without microscopic or gross hematuria may occur months to years after treatment completion if the bladder mucosa remains with areas of inflammation or telangiectasia. Cystoscopy is useful in determining the cause of bladder symptoms; if necessary, cauterization can be performed during this procedure to prevent further bleeding. Incomplete bladder emptying, or the need for catheterization, can predispose patients to infection. Urinary tract infections need to be ruled out for patients with persistent symptoms (Chapter 13).

TABLE 10.3. Low-Residue Diet for Pelvic-Abdominal Radiation Therapy

PURPOSE

The low-residue diet provides foods that are not stimulating to the lower gastrointestinal tract and are almost completely digestible. The goal of the diet is to control the diarrhea associated with pelvic and abdominal radiation. Follow this diet closely if you have loose stools, cramping, or frequent bowel movements.

RECOMMENDATIONS

- Good nutrition is especially important for the person receiving radiation treatments. A balanced diet can help maintain strength, protect the body's nutrient stores, and help rebuild normal tissue affected by radiation.
- Fiber, also called bulk or roughage, is the portion of food that is not digested and is passed in bowel movements. If your intestines are irritated by radiation, the normal amount of fiber may be too much for your body to handle. Increased cramping and diarrhea may result.
- Milk and milk products should be eliminated from your diet if they worsen diarrhea.
- Although it is important to eat well, do not make yourself eat more than you can. Try small meals with several snacks daily.
- Take advantage of the "up times." On good days, eat when you feel hungry, even if it isn't meal time.
- Foods should be prepared and served attractively to increase the appetite and make meal times more pleasant.
- Stay away from any food that causes you problems. You may tolerate fried foods, spicy foods, and sweets less well than other people. Carbonated drinks, beers, and chewing gum may encourage cramps.
- If you have diarrhea, drink plenty of fluids to replace those you have lost. Also eat foods high in potassium such as bananas, nectars, meats, and potatoes, since potassium is lost when you have diarrhea.
- If you are nauseated, try eating cold food with little aroma, such as cold meats, cheese, and crackers. Eat slowly and rest after eating. Eat dry foods such as toast or crackers. Avoid liquids at mealtime and take them 30–60 minutes before eating.
- Get some fresh air.
- When in doubt, use common sense and rely on your past experiences. Be aware of foods not recommended on your diet and those you don't tolerate, but don't be afraid to eat!

A NOTE TO THE DIABETIC:

- Your usual meal plan can be adapted to accommodate the residue-restricted diet.
- Continue to avoid concentrated sweets and other foods not allowed on your diet.
- Starch, fruit, and vegetable exchanges should be selected from low-residue foods.
- Continue your medication and blood sugar monitoring. Since fiber tends to lower blood sugar, your insulin or hypoglycemic drug may have to be adjusted. Discuss this with your physician.

(Continued on next page)

Symptoms of acute cystitis generally occur 3 to 5 weeks into therapy and gradually subside 2 to 8 weeks after treatment completion when mucosal healing occurs. Medications such as methenamine mandelate (Mandelamine, Warner Chilcott Professional Products, Rockaway, NJ), urinary anesthetics such as phenazopyridine hydrochloride (Pyridium, Warner Chilcott Professional Products, Rockaway, NJ), and smooth muscle antispasmodics such as flavoxate hydrochloride (Urispas, SmithKline Beecham, Pittsburgh, PA), hyoscyamine sulfate (Cystospaz, PolyMedica, Woburn, WA), and oxybutynin chloride (Ditropan, Alza, Palo Alto, CA) may relieve symptoms of acute cystitis by inhibiting the muscarinic effects of acetylcholine. Patients need to be instructed that phenazopyridine will cause the urine to turn orange or red and will stain clothing and other surfaces. Patients taking antispasmodic medications need to be monitored for side effects, including palpitations, hypertension, arrhythmias, and central nervous system stimulation.

Alpha$_1$ blocker therapy can also be used to treat urethral irritative symptoms. The action of these drugs (terazosin, doxazosin mesylate, and tamsulosin hydrochloride) are to block prostate α-receptors, resulting in relaxation of the smooth muscle of the urinary

TABLE 10.3. (continued)

FOOD	RECOMMENDED	NOT RECOMMENDED
Beverages	Carbonated drinks, coffee, tea (limit caffeine-containing beverages to 2–3 glasses daily), milk (limit to 2 cups per day including that used in cooking)	Milk in excess of 2 cups, tea, colas in excess of 3 cups
Breads	White bread, seedless rye, rusk saltines, soda crackers, Zwieback, pancakes, muffins, waffles, French toast	Whole-grain breads; graham crackers; cornbread; breads containing nuts, seeds, or bran; doughnuts, pastries
Cereals	Cooked cereals, such as cream of wheat, grits, Malt-o-Meal, strained oatmeal, dry cereals from corn, oat, or rice	Whole-grain cereals, such as granola cereals, bran flakes, Grape-Nuts
Desserts	Plain cakes, cookies, gelatin, sherbet, ice cream, and puddings prepared with milk allowance, whipped toppings, popsicles, pies made with allowed foods	Desserts prepared with coconut, fruits, or nuts
Eggs	Soft scrambled, lightly poached, boiled, soufflé, omelet	Raw eggs
Fats	Butter, cream, cream substitutes, margarine, mayonnaise, gravies, oils, crisp bacon, plain salad dressing	Fried foods, salad dressings with seeds, such as poppyseed dressing
Fruits and juices	Ripe bananas, baked apple (without skin); cooked or canned fruits without seeds; white grapes, cherries, plums, applesauce, peaches, apricots, mandarin oranges; jellied cranberry sauce; all fruit juices that are clear; strained orange juice	All other fruits, especially those with skins and seeds; prune juice
Meats, fish, and poultry	Baked, broiled, creamed, or stewed; very tender beef, chicken, lamb, liver, fish, sweetbreads, tuna, turkey, salmon, veal, lean pork, crisp bacon, canned ham, shellfish	Tough meats with gristle, smoked meats or fish, corned beef, frankfurters, luncheon meats, sausage
Potatoes	White potatoes: boiled, baked, creamed, scalloped, mashed; grits, macaroni, rice, spaghetti, strained sweet potatoes, i.e., commercial baby food	Potato skins; sweet potatoes unless strained; brown or whole-grain rice; wild rice
Salads	Gelatin; fruits and vegetables prepared from allowed foods	All others
Soups	Broth, bouillon soups, cream soups prepared from allowed foods and milk allowance	Highly seasoned soups
Sweets	Sugar, clear jelly, honey, syrup, hard candies, milk chocolate, gumdrops, marshmallows	Candies made with coconut, dried fruit, or nuts
Vegetables	Cooked, canned, or frozen vegetables; beets, asparagus tips, wax or green beans, acorn squash (no seeds), cooked or peeled tomatoes, vegetable juices	All other vegetables, dried beans, peas, legumes, corn
Miscellaneous	Salt, cream sauce, catsup, flavoring extracts, lemon juice, paprika, vinegar, smooth peanut butter, chocolate, cocoa, mild herbs and spices	Pepper, mustard, nuts, olives, pickles, popcorn, raisins, spices, other herbs and seeds such as sesame, caraway, celery, poppy

From SN DiLima (ed), *Oncology Patient Education Manual.* Gaithersburg, MD: Aspen, 1994.
Used with permission from Sherry Page, RN, BSN, OCN, Radiation Oncology, Allison Cancer Center, Midland, Texas.

sphincter and thereby improving urinary symptoms.[24] Patients taking terazosin (Hytrin, Abbott, Abbott Park, IL) and doxazosin mesylate (Cardura, Pfizer, New York) must be assessed closely for hypotension. Tamsulosin (Flomax, Boehringer Ingelheim, Ridgefield, CT) has fewer side effects and does not have the same degree of effect on blood pressure.

For all patients, unless contraindicated, daily fluid intake of 2,000 to 2,500 mL should be encouraged. The avoidance of bladder-irritating products, such as coffee, tea, alcohol, spices, and tobacco, may help to decrease symptoms.

Rarely, incontinence or severe reactions (urethral stricture) occur if there is scarring and injury to the muscle fibers located at the bladder neck or sphincter.[3] Urethral strictures may be improved by periodic urethral dilatation. In more severe cases, surgery (TURP) may be indicated. Patients with incontinence should always undergo urodynamic testing by a urologist. It is important to diagnose the type of incontinence (urge vs. stress) to treat and manage it effectively (see Chapter 13).

SEXUAL FUNCTIONING

Erectile dysfunction is a significant side effect that affects the quality of life of many patients. Alterations in sexual functioning can occur from one factor or a combination, including psychological factors, cardiovascular disease, diabetes, medications, alcohol or drug intake, and cancer therapy. Patients who are potent before external beam radiation treatments have a 30 to 50% risk of experiencing erectile dysfunction (decreased libido and erections to total impotence) from possible radiation damage to the small blood vessels and the nerves responsible for erections.[3] Changes in sexual functioning may take a year or longer to occur.

The rates of patients maintaining potency after brachytherapy are 90% for those younger than 60 years, 80% for those 60 to 70 years old, and 50% for those older than 70.[25]

Impotence precipitated by hormonal ablation is usually temporary. Some patients may defer certain treatment options because of the potential for impotence. Nurses need to be involved in educating patients on temporary and possible permanent impotence risk from different therapy options and in supporting the patient's decisions and sexual rehabilitation. It is vital that the nursing assessment of and patient involvement with pertinent sexuality issues begins before treatment. Developing a trusting relationship with the patient will encourage openness when discussing sensitive issues. The nurse must be aware of cultural barriers and use terms familiar to the individual patient. He or she must initiate frequent conversations regarding the topic of sexual functioning and encourage the patient and their significant others to be involved and ask questions. This should be done in a quiet, private location.

Patient assessment and evaluation needs to be ongoing, at regular intervals, during and after treatment. If sexual dysfunction occurs, treatment options need to be explained, and the nurse should assist the patient in obtaining appointments with the appropriate professional. Treatment options may include psychotherapy alone or with spouse participation, insertion of penile implants (semirigid silicone rods or inflatable devices), vacuum erection devices, intrapenile injections with vasoactive agents (papaverine, phentolamine, or prostaglandin E), or use of the newly approved drug sildenafil (Viagra) (see Chapter 13).

FATIGUE

Complaints of mild to moderate fatigue are common during radiation and occur most commonly at about the fourth week of treatment, continuing and increasing slightly through the end of the therapy course. For most patients, fatigue resolves within the month after radiation is completed. The acute fatigue effect from radiation may be related to alterations in the patient's relative serum interleukin-1 levels.[21]

Fatigue is often viewed as a side effect that is inevitable and untreatable. Those providing health care are usually inadequately prepared to deal with the fatigue symptoms arising from cancer treatment.[26] Nurses need to be able to differentiate between tiredness and acute and chronic fatigue. This distinction will help the nurse and patient deduce the cause and make intervention easier.

Fatigue can be attributed to any number of factors, including anemia, infection, depression, anxiety, sleep deprivation, malnutrition, diarrhea, pain, medications, or the waste products resulting from tumor breakdown.[27] As with any cancer patient, the prostate cancer patient may experience several or many of these symptoms. Fatigue may be enhanced in those patients receiving combination radiation and hormonal ablation secondary to a lowering of the hemoglobin level[28] (see Combination Therapy discussion). Sleep deprivation may lend to fatigue because side effects of treatment (urinary frequency, nocturia, diarrhea, hot flashes) can interfere with normal sleep patterns.

The nurse should assess fatigue levels and assist patients in identifying those activities that increase fatigue. Energy conservation techniques may include incorporation of rest periods throughout the day. Although patients may be adhering to a low-residue diet, adding complex carbohydrates may provide increased energy. Nursing roles include educating and assisting patients and their families in locating and using available resources for needs such as transportation options or home care help. These types of interventions can relieve burden and decrease fatigue.

To help patients effectively manage the symptoms associated with fatigue, as with all side effects, nursing assessments should be frequent and interventions planned on an individual basis.

MYELOSUPPRESSION

Myelosuppression occurs when areas with large amounts of active bone marrow are irradiated. This side effect in prostate cancer patients can be exacerbated by adjuvant hormonal therapy and in those with compromised marrow, as in the elderly and those with metastatic disease. With approximately 40% of active marrow located in the pelvis, those receiving large-field external beam radiation are at a relatively high risk for bone marrow depression. However, overall, these patients rarely have myelosuppression of significance that requires intervention or treatment breaks.[21] Radiation to the pelvis generally does not decrease the hemoglobin level more than 0.5 g/dL; however, 80 to 90% of patients treated with a combination of radiation and androgen suppression show decreased hemoglobin levels up to 4 g/dL[28] (see Combination Therapy discussion).

Nursing assessment before radiation or hormonal induction will establish a baseline that can be used during treatment for comparison. Identification of the cause of myelo-suppression is key because the treatment options can be very different. Oncology nurses are vital in assessing and educating patients regarding the signs and symptoms of anemia and monitoring lab values. Patients may be asymptomatic or may complain of fatigue, dyspnea alone or with exertion, headaches, chest pain, and paresthesias.[29]

INTERSTITIAL IMPLANTATION (BRACHYTHERAPY)

Brachytherapy derives from *brachy,* a Greek word meaning "near to." In this treatment modality, radioactive material is placed near or in a tumor. The concept of using radioactive implantation is not new, dating back almost 100 years. Novel transperineal insertion of radium needles via digital rectal palpation led to uneven placement and poor response rates. Despite further attempts to improve the procedure, prostate brachytherapy was soon abandoned.

Although previously primitive in technique, today significant advances have occurred in areas of treatment planning and placement technique, thereby improving local control rates and reducing bowel and bladder toxicity. Prostate visualization with transrectal ultrasonography or CT guidance and the perineal templates aid in guiding radioisotope placement. Computer advances have assisted physics departments in improved configuration (algorithm) plans for optimal seed placement.

Patients eligible for implantation are typically those with organ-confined disease (T1 and T2) and a life expectancy of 5 years or more. Larger T2 and T3 lesions, if implanted, should receive a portion of the total implant dose from external beam radiation therapy. Those patients with very large prostates or a history of TURP may not be good candidates.

Prostate brachytherapy can be performed alone before or after completion of external beam radiation therapy. Prostate brachytherapy results have been as favorable as those of radical prostatectomy.[24] The advantage of implant is the ability to provide a higher confined radiation dose with toxicity reduction to normal surrounding tissue. Technical improvements have come at a time of increasing use of the serum PSA as a screening tool for discovering increasing numbers of clinically organ-confined tumors. The use of routine posttreatment PSA measurements have provided a previously unavailable mechanism for assessing treatment efficacy.[30] Common isotopes used are permanently implanted iodine-125, palladium-103, and temporary iridium-192. However, temporary iodine-125, palladium-103, and permanently implanted gold-198 are also used. The choice of isotope is primarily based on the radiation it emits and the grade of the lesion. Iodine-125 has a 60-day half-life and is commonly used to treat patients with Gleason scores between 2 and 6. Palladium-103 has a shorter half-life of 17 days, but at a higher initial dose rate, it is used to treat patients with Gleason scores of 7 or greater.

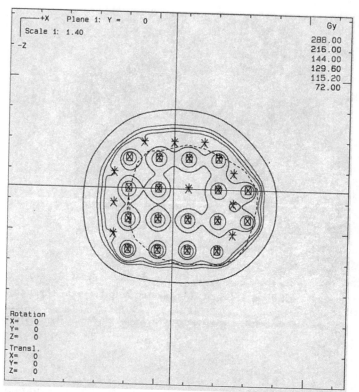

FIGURE 10-12. Prebrachytherapy treatment plan depicting plan of prostate seed placement
Courtesy of the Radiation Oncology Department, West Virginia University Hospital, Morgantown, West Virginia.

Temporary implants, if used, are generally removed after 24 to 72 hours, the length of time determined by the prescribed dose.[21] Prostate brachytherapy treatment is based on the different tumor parameters, and patients may require both external beam radiation and implantation to achieve optimal results. Some physicians recommend external beam radiation before implantation, and others reverse this order.

Patients with Clinical Stages T1 and T2 treated first with permanently implanted iodine-125 seeds followed 21 days later with a simultaneous course of external beam radiation were able to have reduced daily fraction doses because of the combined effect. Disease freedom was defined as a PSA value of 0.5 ng/mL or less. The 10-year disease-free survival rate was comparable to the 10-year results of patients who underwent radical prostatectomy.[31]

Ten-year brachytherapy results from 152 patients with T1-T3 prostate carcinoma treated with an iodine-125 implant with or without external beam radiation showed a 65% 10-year survival rate. Sixty-four percent of the patients at 10 years remained clinically and biochemically free of disease.[30]

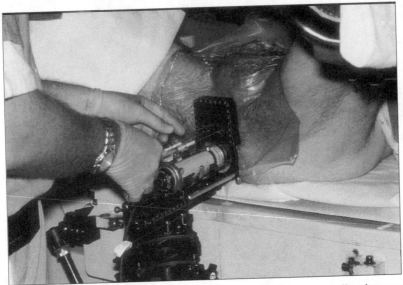

FIGURE 10-13. Transperineal technique of brachytherapy needle placement through table mounting template
Courtesy of the Radiation Oncology Department, West Virginia University Hospital, Morgantown, West Virginia. Photo courtesy of Scott V. Watkins.

PATIENT PREPARATION

Preimplant patient preparation includes a volume study. A prostatic ultrasonogram is performed to calculate prostate volume and symphysis pubis proximity. This study provides the picture measurement of the prostate that enables the physics department to calculate, in advance, the number of radioactive seeds needed and the plan for their placement (see Figure 10-12, page 159). Patients may be required to maintain a clear liquid diet 24 hours before the exam, followed by a Fleet (Fleet, Lynchburg, VA) enema the day of the exam. Bowel preparations may vary among institutions.

PROCEDURE

Needle placement is performed on an outpatient basis under spinal or general anesthesia with the patient in a lithotomy position. A customized mounting apparatus attaches to the operating room table and stabilizes the template and ultrasound probe. Needles are then placed through the template guide (Figure 10-13). The radioactive seeds are implanted through the placed needles directly into the prostate tissue via a perineal approach (Figure 10-14). After all seeds are placed, the needles are removed.[2] An alternative approach is to position needles singly, deposit the seeds, and then withdraw that needle before moving to the next (Figure 10-15).

After implantation, a cystourethroscopy may be performed to assess for bleeding of the urethra or bladder and to retrieve any seeds that may have been inadvertently placed there.[24] An indwelling urinary catheter may be placed postoperatively to assess urine amount and color and clot presence. Once the urine is free of clots, 200 cc of sterile water

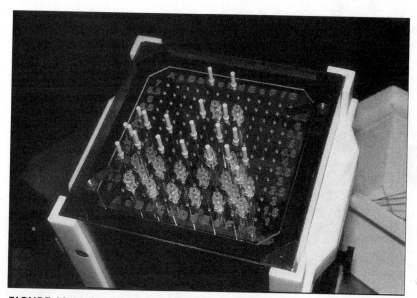

FIGURE 10-14. Needle safe holding loaded brachytherapy needles that are arranged on a grid representing placement through the table-mounted template
Courtesy of the Radiation Oncology Department, West Virginia University Hospital, Morgantown, West Virginia. Photo courtesy of Scott V. Watkins.

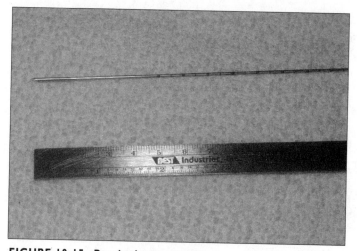

FIGURE 10-15. Brachytherapy needle
Courtesy of the Radiation Oncology Department, West Virginia University Hospital, Morgantown, West Virginia. Photo courtesy of Scott V. Watkins.

is instilled in the bladder, and then the catheter is removed. The fluid in the bladder will decrease the time interval to evaluate whether the patient is able to void spontaneously.[24] The patient is usually discharged the same day. Postimplant studies can also include a follow-up CT scan the next day to confirm accurate isotope placement (Figures 10-16 and 10-17).

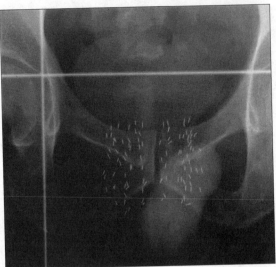

FIGURE 10-16. Postimplant x-ray. Seeds can be visualized in the prostate

Courtesy of the Radiation Oncology Department, West Virginia University Hospital, Morgantown, West Virginia. Photo courtesy of Scott V. Watkins.

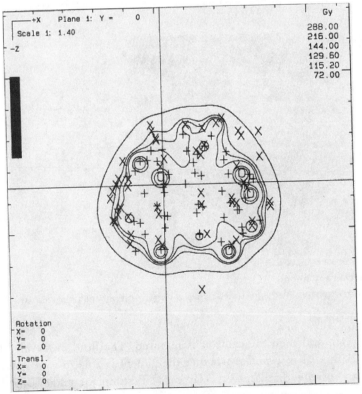

FIGURE 10-17. Postbrachytherapy treatment plan depicting radioactive seed placement

Courtesy of the Radiation Oncology Department, West Virginia University Hospital, Morgantown, West Virginia.

POSTIMPLANT SIDE EFFECTS AND NURSING CARE

Side effects are usually minimal and may include minor dysuria, frequent urination, mild pain, or a feeling of inability to pass urine freely. These symptoms are common and usually will stop in 1 to 4 months. Hematuria, caused by the trauma of needle insertion, is common during the first 24 hours and usually resolves within 72 hours. Patients need to be instructed on signs and symptoms of urinary retention from clot formation as well as measures that can help prevent this potentially serious occurrence. Increased fluid intake is encouraged, and a course of prophylactic antibiotic coverage is given to prevent infection. Although uncommon, in some cases, urinary side effects can be severe (urinary retention) and prolonged (as a result of edema), requiring an indwelling urinary catheter or patient self-catheterization for a period of time. The patient can be instructed on catheter care at home. (See Table 10-4 and Chapter 14.)

Recent changes have been made in the instructions regarding straining of urine and retrieval of any seeds passed postimplantation. After implantation, urine straining is no longer required. Patients are asked to watch for any seeds that may be passed when urinating. Seed retrieval is no longer advisable because of concerns of additional, unnecessary radiation exposure. Any seeds eliminated while voiding can safely be flushed into the sewage system.

Additional side effects may include slight bleeding beneath the scrotum with local ecchymosis and tenderness of the perineum. Patients should be instructed about skin care, including daily cleansing of the perineum with soap and water and the importance of keeping the perineum clean and dry to prevent infection. Ice packs can be used during the first 24 hours to reduce edema and ecchymosis. Sitz baths can be used as needed. Pain is usually minimal, and mild analgesics such as acetaminophen and ibuprofen should be adequate to alleviate discomfort.

Sexual intercourse may resume within 2 weeks, but a condom should be used for 2 months because a seed could be expelled through urination or ejaculation. Semen initially may be bloody, black, or dark brown. This discoloration is a normal result of bleeding that may have occurred during the implant and released into the ejaculate.

Diet should not need to be altered unless proctitis occurs, and then, if necessary, a low-residue diet can be followed. Inflammation of the rectum can occur after implantation because of small amounts of radiation that are given off from the prostate to the rectum. Iodine-125 and palladium-103 are low-energy radioactive materials, and, when implanted, most of the radiation is contained within the prostate gland. However, small amounts of the radiation are given off to structures in very close proximity, such as the rectum. Patients should be advised that their urine and stool are not radioactive, nor are objects that they handle.

Other radiation safety precautions are followed to reduce or eliminate the chances of others being unnecessarily exposed to radioactivity. A six-foot distance is a safe zone between the patient and others. Special attention should be given to avoid prolonged, close-proximity contact with pregnant women, possibly pregnant women, and children for the first 2 months after the implant. If desired, the patient may purchase a lead-lined

TABLE 10-4. Nursing Management of Side Effects Related to Prostatic Brachytherapy

SIDE EFFECT	SYMPTOMS	NURSING INTERVENTIONS
Skin impairment	• Bruising of scrotum/perineum • Tenderness • Hematoma (rare)	• Cleanse perineum with soap and water twice daily. • Apply ice pack to perineum for 24 hours.
URINARY DYSFUNCTION	**DYSURIA** • Increased nocturia • Urgency • Frequency • Difficulty starting stream • Interrupted stream	• Send urinalysis to lab/culture as needed. • Administer ibuprofen, 400 mg, three times daily. • Titrate alpha$_1$ blockers. • Administer phenazopyridine hydrochloride if dysuria is present beyond 1 month. • Decrease oral liquid intake after 8 PM. • Curtail caffeine, tea, and alcoholic beverages.
	URINARY RETENTION • Unable to spontaneously urinate • Not emptying bladder completely	• Perform voiding trial in recovery room. • If voiding trial is unsuccessful, insert indwelling urinary catheter and repeat trial within 48 hours. • If voiding trial is still unsuccessful, teach intermittent self-catheterization. • Record time and amount of voids. • Insert suprapubic catheter if patient is unable to perform intermittent self-catheterization.
	HEMATURIA • Blood tinged urine • Gross hematuria with clots	• Encourage patient to increase oral fluid intake. • Administer IV hydration if needed. • Provide continuous bladder irrigation until urine clears.
PERINEAL PAIN	Pain in scrotum/perineum	• Encourage patient to take pain medication as needed. • Apply ice to perineum for first 24 hours. • Encourage patient to take warm sitz baths as needed.
PROCTITIS	Small "gassy" bowel movements Soft stool Painless rectal bleeding Rectal irritation Diarrhea	• Provide information about a low-residue diet if patient moves bowels more than three times daily. • Encourage patient to use cortisone preparation as suppositories or apply topical preparations to perianal area. • Encourage patient to take warm sitz baths as needed. • Suggest the use of loperamide hydrochloride.

IV, intravenous.

Source: From Abel LJ, Blatt HJ, Stipetich RL, et al. Nursing management of patients receiving brachytherapy for early stage prostate cancer. *Clinical Journal of Oncology Nursing,* 1999;3:10. Copyright 1999 by Oncology Nursing Press, Inc. Used with permission.

undergarment. This can be worn to protect others from almost all emitted radiation.[24] If hospitalization is needed after implantation, the patient may be placed in a private or semiprivate room depending on the institutional policy.

Nursing care of the prostate implant patient begins at the preimplant stage through the postimplant. Nurses can manage many aspects of the patient's care, ranging from coordinating initial testing, educating patients and families on procedures, side effects, and symptom management, to providing direct patient care during the operative procedure.[2]

COMBINATION THERAPY

The addition of hormonal therapy, either before (neoadjuvant) and during or after definitive radiation therapy, is increasing in popularity. Reducing or eliminating the amount of circulating male hormone has long been established as the standard of treatment for metastatic prostate cancer and today is standard in selected patients with disease that is regionally advanced in the prostate capsule.[32] Patients diagnosed with early-stage disease (low stage, PSA, and Gleason scores) generally have an excellent prognosis, whereas those with moderate- to high-grade disease often have poor PSA responses without combined therapy.[32] The combination of radiation therapy and TAS shows potential for improving the outcome in patients with locally advanced prostate cancer. Several clinical trials have demonstrated improved PSA and local failure rates with combination therapy.[16, 33] The results of a RTOG 86-10 Phase III trial, in which patients with T2b-T4 tumors were randomized to radiation with or without neoadjuvant hormonal therapy, showed that at 4 years the risk of local failure was reduced by almost half and the risk of biochemical failure reduced by a factor of nearly 2.5 in patients who received total androgen suppression and radiation.[16]

RTOG Phase III trial 85-31 evaluated adjuvant goserelin acetate implant (gonadotropin-releasing hormone agonist) given monthly after definitive radiation and continuing until relapse. All patients had locally advanced disease. Reported local failure rates among the 950 patients were 17% versus 32% in the radiation-alone group.[33] No clear overall survival benefits have yet been demonstrated. Patient survival is still being monitored.

Further RTOG trials such as 92-02, in which patients received neoadjuvant hormonal therapy with or without adjuvant goserelin, accrued more than 1,500 patients. Results are still being analyzed and are not yet available.

The ability to achieve complete tumor eradication with radiotherapy for bulky prostatic cancers is a challenge. For such patients, neoadjuvant hormonal therapy can effectively "debulk" the local disease and minimize the volume of normal tissue exposed to higher radiation doses.[34] Additional reasons for using combination androgen ablation and radiation includes synergism in programmed cell death and reduced local failure and biochemical rates, as demonstrated in clinical trials. The most common treatment with hormonal intervention includes bilateral orchiectomy, leuprolide acetate, goserelin acetate, flutamide, megestrol acetate, ketoconazole, and diethylstilbestrol (DES). There is decreasing use of DES because of the risk of multiple toxicities, including thromboembolism, and fluid retention, leading to congestive heart failure.

Side effects of lowered testosterone levels include decreased libido, impotence, and hot flashes. Patients can also experience breast enlargement and tenderness and loss of body hair. Patients who receive combination therapy (hormonal therapy and concurrent radiation therapy) have an increased incidence of diarrhea because certain hormones may increase the risk of this side effect. Antiandrogens (flutamide and ketoconazole) have been associated with abnormalities in liver function studies, specifically the aspartate aminotransferase (AST) and alanine aminotransferase (ALT). Patients should be closely monitored with blood studies because unrecognized elevation can lead to irreversible liver damage and, in rare cases, death. The neoadjuvant and adjuvant combination of the LHRH agonist (goserelin acetate) and the antiandrogen (flutamide) has been associated with anemia. Anemia develops before radiation and frequently is associated with fatigue. Hemoglobin decreases may be as large as 4 g/dL to levels that fall below 10 g/dL and is especially pronounced in African-American males. Recognition of this side effect may eliminate diagnostic tests (endoscopy or bleeding studies), avoiding discomfort, inconvenience, and expense.[28] Although poorly documented in the medical literature, decreased hemoglobin levels occur in almost all patients receiving combined hormonal (especially goserelin acetate and flutamide) and radiation therapy, as seen at Albert Einstein Medical Center. Because the hemoglobin decrease may not always cause a decrease below the institutional low normal range, it can go unrecognized.

Substantial issues and uncertainties, such as timing of usage and duration, still surround combination hormonal therapy with other treatment modalities because information is lacking in long-term overall survival and cancer-specific survival. The optimal duration of neoadjuvant treatment remains unknown.[32]

PSYCHOSOCIAL ISSUES

Psychosocial issues arise from the disruptive nature of a cancer diagnosis. These issues and stressors affect almost every area of a patient's life and also involve the family. Stress and anxiety can be related to the fear produced by the prostate cancer diagnosis and impending treatment, but it also extends throughout the patient's life as a fear of relapse and death. Those issues can disturb the balance of the entire family, and coping with life changes can be a challenge.

For the prostate cancer patient receiving radiation therapy, stressors arise initially from "fear of the unknown" with regard to treatment planning, the treatment itself, and the need to alter one's schedule to go to the radiation center daily for treatment.

The patient should be educated regarding the treatment planning process, and the nurse should allay fears that the treatment is painful or that the patient will remain "radioactive" when the treatment is over. The nurse should provide stress and coping skills with education and available resources such as area support groups and pertinent literature. If a patient wants to continue working through treatment, he may be concerned about fitting his radiation treatment into his work schedule; the nurse should make reasonable attempts to facilitate transition and accommodate patient needs. An individualized approach with concern and support of self-esteem can help reduce patient anxiety. The patient's emotional risk factors, current level of functioning, and amount of social support should be assessed.

Treatment side effects and altered sexual health may be a major concern for the prostate cancer patient before, during, and after treatment with regard to potential late side effects. Before treatment, the nurse should initiate conversation with patients to discuss concerns and encourage those who are reluctant to open up by providing a quiet, private area to discuss issues.

Generally, for prostate cancer patients, the radiation therapy treatments are fairly well tolerated. Although many patients will go through therapy appearing to need minimal psychosocial support, it is important to remember to assess their needs frequently and be available to discuss concerns privately. The nurse plays a vital role in helping patients and their families maintain psychosocial well-being.

CONCLUSION

As the incidence and prevalence of prostate cancer increases, promising multimodality treatments continue to improve the encouraging survival statistics. Screening mechanisms with PSA has allowed prompt, early treatment to patients frequently before the disease is clinically detectable. It is vital that patients and their families understand the nature, treatment options, and scope of prostate cancer. The ultimate goal is to return the patient to as healthy and normal a lifestyle as possible. The nurse has opportunities in all aspects of the patient's care for clinical practice, education, and research.

I thank S. Watkins, MD, interim section chief, Section of Radiation Oncology, West Virginia University Hospitals, for his helpful review and critique of the final versions of this chapter. I also thank Shirley Johnston, chief medical dosimetrist, and S. O. Asbell, MD, chair of the Department of Radiation Oncology, Albert Einstein Medical Center, Philadelphia, for their help with this chapter.

REFERENCES

1. Hilderley LJ. Radiotherapy. In: Groenwald SL, Frogge MH, Goodman M, Yarbro CH (eds). *Cancer Nursing Principles and Practice,* 4th ed. Sudbury, MA: Jones and Bartlett, 1997:247–282.
2. Cash JC, Dattoli MJ. Management of patients receiving transperineal palladium-103 prostate implants. *Oncol Nurs Forum* 1997;24:1361–1366.
3. Marks S. *Prostate and Cancer: A Family Guide to Diagnosis, Treatment and Survival.* Tucson, AZ: Fisher Books, 1997.
4. Catalona WJ. Management of cancer of the prostate [review]. *N Engl J Med* 1994;331:996–1004.
5. Perez CA. Prostate. In: Perez CA, Brady LW (eds). *Principles and Practice of Radiation Oncology,* 3rd ed. Philadelphia: Lippincott-Raven, 1998:1583–1694.
6. Asbell SO, Krall JM, Pilepich MV, et al. Elective pelvic irradiation in stages A2, B carcinoma of the prostate: Analysis of RTOG 77-06. *Int J Radiat Oncol Biol Phys* 1988;15:1307–1316.
7. Hanks GE, Asbell SO, Krall JM, et al. Outcome for lymph node dissection negative T1b, T2 (A-2, B) prostate cancer treated with external beam radia-

tion therapy in RTOG 77-06. *Int J Radiat Oncol Biol Phys* 1991;21:1099–1103.

8. Oesterling J, Fuks Z, Lee CT, Scher HI. Cancer of the prostate. In: DeVita VT, Hellman S, Rosenberg SA (eds). *Cancer: Principles and Practice of Oncology,* 5th ed. Philadelphia: Lippincott-Raven, 1997: 1322–1386.

9. Bagshaw MA, Kaplan ID, Cox RC. Radiation therapy for localized disease. *Cancer* 1993;71(Suppl): 939–952.

10. Seaward SA, Weinberg V, Lewis P, et al. Identification of a high-risk clinically localized prostate cancer subgroup receiving maximum benefit from whole-pelvic irradiation. *Cancer J Sci Am* 1998;4: 370–377.

11. Zeitman AL, Westgeest JCM, Shipley WU. Radiation-based approaches to the management of T3 prostate cancer. *Semin Urol Oncol* 1997;15:230–238.

12. Lowe BA. Management of stage T1a prostate cancer. *Semin Urol Oncol* 1996;14:178–182.

13. Ben-Josef E, Porter AT. Radiotherapy of T1c prostate cancer. *Semin Urol Oncol* 1995;13:191–196.

14. Zeitman AL, Prince EA, Nakfoor BM, Shipley WU. Neoadjuvant androgen suppression with radiation in the management of locally advanced adenocarcinoma of the prostate: Experimental and clinical results. *Urology* 1997;49:74–83.

15. Garnick MB. Prostate cancer: Screening, diagnosis, and management. *Ann Intern Med* 1993;118:804–818.

16. Roach M. Neoadjuvant total androgen suppression and radiotherapy in the management of locally advanced prostate cancer. *Semin Urol Oncol* 1996; 14:32–38.

17. Anscher MS, Robertson CN, Prosnitz LR. Adjuvant radiotherapy for pathologic stage T3/4 adenocarcinoma of the prostate: Ten-year update. *Int J Radiat Oncol Biol Phys* 1995;33:37–43.

18. Anscher MS, Prosnitz LR. Multivariate analysis of factors predicting local relapse after radical prostatectomy—Possible indications for postoperative radiotherapy. *Int J Radiat Oncol Biol Phys* 1991;21: 941–947.

19. Sandler HM. Prostate cancer: Patient's dilemma? *Cancer J Sci Am* 1998;4:347–348.

20. American Society for Therapeutic Radiology and Oncology Consensus Panel. Consensus statement guidelines for PSA following radiation therapy. *Int J Radiat Oncol Biol Phys* 1997;37:1035–1041.

21. Maher KE. Male genitourinary cancers. In: Dow KH, Bucholtz JD, Iwamoto R, et al (eds). *Nursing Care in Radiation Oncology,* 2nd ed. Philadelphia: WB Saunders, 1997:184–219.

22. Sitton E. Managing side effects of skin changes and fatigue. In: Dow KH, Bucholtz JD, Iwamoto R, et al (eds). *Nursing Care in Radiation Oncology,* 2nd ed. Philadelphia: WB Saunders, 1997:79–100.

23. Marks LB, Carroll PR, Dugan TC, Anscher MS. The response of the urinary bladder, urethra, and ureter to radiation and chemotherapy. *Int J Radiat Oncol Biol Phys* 1995;31:1257–1280.

24. Abel LJ, Blatt HJ, Stipetich RL, et al. Nursing management of patients receiving brachytherapy for early stage prostate cancer. *Clin J Oncol Nurs* 1999;3:7–15.

25. Ragde H, Blasko JC, Grimm PD, et al. Interstitial iodine-125 radiation without adjuvant therapy in the treatment of clinically localized prostate carcinoma. *Cancer* 1997;80:442–453.

26. Nail LM. Interventions for Cancer Treatment-Related Fatigue. Newtown, PA: Associates in Medical Marketing, 1998. *Anemia and Fatigue in Cancer Patients: Nursing Care Management.* Philadelphia: Nursing symposium, April 1997, Ruth McCorkle, moderator.

27. DuPen AR, Panke JT. Common clinical problems. In: Varricchio C, Pierce M, Walker CL, Ades TB (eds). *A Cancer Source Book for Nurses,* 7th ed. Sudbury, MA: Jones and Bartlett, 1997:174–184.

28. Asbell SO, Leon SA, Tester WJ, et al. Development of anemia and recovery in prostate cancer patients treated with combined androgen blockade and radiotherapy. *Prostate* 1996;29:243–248.

29. Lynch MP, Jacobs LA. The assessment and diagnosis of anemia in the patient with cancer. Newtown, PA: Associates in Medical Marketing, 1998. *Anemia and Fatigue in Cancer Patients: Nursing Care Management.* Philadelphia: Nursing symposium, April 1997, Ruth McCorkle, moderator.

30. Ragde H, Elgamal AAA, Snow PB, et al. Ten-year disease free survival after transperineal sonography-guided iodine-125 brachytherapy with or without 45-gray external beam irradiation in the treatment of patients with clinically localized, low to high Gleason grade prostate carcinoma. *Cancer* 1998;83:989–1001.

31. Critz FA, Levinson AK, Williams WH, et al. Simultaneous radiotherapy for prostate cancer:

125-I prostate implant followed by external-beam radiation. *Cancer J Sci Am* 1998;4:359–363.

32. Garnick MB. Hormonal therapy in the management of prostate cancer: From Huggins to the present. *Urology* 1997;49(Suppl 3A):5–15.

33. Pilepich MV, Caplan R, Byhardt RW, et al. Phase III trial of adjuvant androgen suppression using goserelin in patients with carcinoma of the prostate treated with definitive radiotherapy: Results of 85–31 [abstract]. *Int J Radiat Oncol Biol Phys* 1995; 32:188.

34. Zelefsky MJ, Harrison A. Neoadjuvant androgen ablation prior to radiotherapy for prostate cancer: Reducing the potential morbidity of therapy. *Urology* 1997;49:38–45.

35. Wilkes GM, Ingwersen K, Burke MB. *1997-1998 Oncology Nursing Drug Handbook*. Sudbury, MA: Jones and Bartlett, 1997:601–607.

36. Nursing '98 Books, *Nursing '98 Drug Handbook*. Springhouse, PA: Springhouse Books, 1998: 656–661.

37. Wilkes GM, Ingwersen K, Burke MB. *Oncology Nursing Drug Reference*. Sudbury, MA: Jones and Bartlett, 1994:575–581.

Chapter 11

HORMONAL THERAPY

LAURA STEMPKOWSKI

OVERVIEW

RATIONALE FOR HORMONAL MANIPULATION
PRIMARY HORMONAL MANIPULATION
   Medical Castration
   Surgical Castration
   Pure Antiandrogens
   Steroidal Antiandrogens
   Total Androgen Blockade
INDICATIONS FOR HORMONAL
   MANIPULATION
   Metastatic Prostate Cancer
   Neoadjuvant Hormonal Therapy
     Before Surgery
     Before Radiation Therapy
   Adjuvant Therapy
SIDE EFFECT MANAGEMENT

   Hot Flashes
   Fatigue
   Impotence
   Osteoporosis
HORMONE-REFRACTORY DISEASE–ANDROGEN
   INDEPENDENCE
   Antiandrogen Withdrawal Response
   Secondary Hormonal Manipulation
   Chemotherapy
NOVEL APPROACHES TO HORMONAL
   MANIPULATION
   Sequential Androgen Blockade
   Intermittent Androgen Suppression
   Monotherapy
CONCLUSION

Over the last decade, we have seen a paradigm shift in the use of hormonal manipulation in the treatment of prostate cancer. With the widespread use of prostate-specific antigen (PSA) as a screening tool and the advent of transrectal ultrasonography (TRUS), a large number of men are now being diagnosed with earlier Stage (A or B) disease. Before these improved methods of early detection, 40 to 60% of men were found to have locally advanced (Stage C) or metastatic (Stage D) disease at the time of diagnosis.[1] Hormonal manipulation became and continues to be the gold standard of treatment for metastatic prostate cancer.[2]

    Although many prostate cancers are now diagnosed and treated while still localized, a significant number will show progression after definitive therapy (radiation therapy or radical prostatectomy). About 50% of men are understaged clinically and are then found

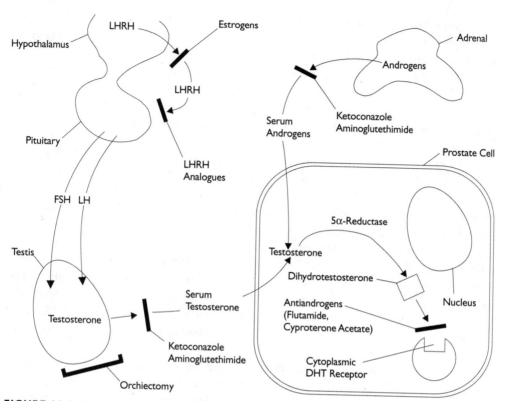

FIGURE 11-1. Scheme of achieving castrate androgen levels

LHRH, luteinizing hormone–releasing hormone; FSH, follicle-stimulating hormone; LH, luteinizing hormone; DHT, dihydrotestosterone.
Source: From Garnick MB. Urologic Cancer. In: Rubenstein E, Federman DD (eds). *Scientific American Medicine.* New York: Scientific American. Section 12, IX:1–17, with permission.

to have tumors that extend beyond the prostatic capsule (pT3) at surgery.[2] Because of these findings, hormonal manipulation may be initiated earlier as neoadjuvant or adjuvant therapy.

This chapter examines the scientific basis for hormonal manipulation and reviews its use in early prostate cancer as well as in advanced disease. The effects of androgen ablation on quality of life are recognized, and side effect management is discussed. Finally, newer approaches to hormonal manipulation, currently under investigation, are explored.

RATIONALE FOR HORMONAL MANIPULATION

Prostate cell growth is under the hormonal control of the hypothalamic-pituitary-testicular axis[1] (Figure 11-1). The hormones involved in the axis are released by the body in a pulse-like manner. Luteinizing hormone–releasing hormone (LHRH) is produced by the cells of the arcuate nucleus of the hypothalmus. The effect of LHRH is the stimulation of pituitary gonadotroph receptors with production and release of luteinizing hormone

(LH) and follicle-stimulating hormone (FSH). Both the hypothalamus and the pituitary are sensitive to hormonal feedback. High levels of testosterone or low levels of estrogens result in a reduced frequency of the pulse-like release of LH.

LH stimulates production of the androgen, testosterone, by the Leydig cells of the testicles through a series of enzymes that convert cholesterol to testosterone. Within the prostate gland, testosterone is converted to dihydrotestosterone (DHT), a more potent form of testosterone, by the enzyme 5 α-reductase.[3] The prostate requires DHT for normal growth and function.[1]

The androgen receptor is responsible for the effect of DHT on the cell. DHT has significantly more affinity for the androgen receptor than to testosterone.[3] Once bound by DHT, the androgen receptor enters the cell nucleus and binds to specific DNA sequences in the nucleus.[4, 5] This results in the expression of genes responsible for prostate cell androgen-responsive growth.[1]

The impact of adrenal steroids on intraprostatic DHT levels has only recently been understood.[6] Weak sex steroids, delta-4-androstenedione, dihydroepiandrosterone (DHEA), and DHEA sulfate (DHEA-S), are produced by the adrenal gland.[6–10] The enzymes required to convert these steroid precursors to DHT are found within the prostate.[6, 10, 11] As a result, it is estimated that 10 to 40% of intraprostatic DHT is of adrenal origin, although adrenal steroid synthesis accounts for only 5 to 10% of circulating serum testosterone.[6–10]

The goal of hormonal manipulation is to halt the growth of androgen-dependent prostate cancer cells and to induce apoptosis through androgen deprivation. Apoptosis, or programmed cell death (PCD), is a process initiated by many types of cells in response to environmental stress or toxic damage.[12, 13] This is a genetically programmed process requiring the expression of specialized genes responsible for the death of the cell and its ability to avoid immune inflammatory responses. By eliminating damaged cells and thereby preventing their proliferation, apoptosis is nature's way of maintaining the integrity of the species.

The loss of androgens promoting the survival of carcinoma cells results in cellular death within 24 hours.[14] This process does not appear to require new DNA synthesis or the presence of tumor suppressor gene p53, which is necessary for apoptosis to occur in other systems such as radiation- or chemotherapy-induced PCD.[15] Regardless of the method of hormonal manipulation, the end result is inhibition of the DHT–androgen receptor interaction, promoting PCD of the prostate cancer cell.[1]

PRIMARY HORMONAL MANIPULATION

Hormonal therapy remains the first-line treatment for metastatic prostate cancer and can be accomplished medically or surgically. Either approach will stop the production of the androgen, testosterone, in the testicles. Side effects are the result of testosterone suppression and are the same whether testicular androgen suppression is achieved medically or surgically. Decreased libido, impotence, fatigue, hot flashes, weight redistribution, and muscle atrophy may occur and have an impact on quality of life. Side effect management is discussed later and is summarized in the nursing standard of care provided in Table 11-1.

MEDICAL CASTRATION

By eliminating pulsatile LHRH stimulation, the LHRH agonists inhibit LH secretion from the pituitary.[1] The intermittent release of LHRH stimulates LH production, but continuous LHRH stimulation results in desensitization of the pituitary gland and inhibits LH production.[1] After administration of the first dose of LHRH agonist, there is an initial increase in testosterone levels resulting from the increased LH production induced by the LHRH agonist. This occurs during the first few days of treatment, lasting 5 to 8 days until complete desensitization of the pituitary occurs and serum testosterone subsequently falls to castrate levels. When LHRH agonists are used as monotherapy, this initial increase in testosterone has been associated with a disease flare. Patients who are symptomatic with metastatic bone pain or obstructive urinary symptoms may experience an increase in bone pain or urinary obstruction. These effects are the result of the transient increase in testosterone and can be completely eliminated by administering flutamide, an antiandrogen that blocks testosterone at the androgen receptor, before the adminstration of the LHRH agonist.[16]

In monotherapy with LHRH agonists, it is also important to confirm that castrate levels of testosterone have been achieved. If serum testosterone levels are not reduced to castrate levels (< 20 mg/dL), it has been recommended that the addition of an antiandrogen be considered.[17]

LHRH agonists are given by injection on a regular basis, with the frequency dependent on the preparation used (Table 11-2). Although they are covered by Medicare and most insurers, LHRH agonists are very costly (about $3,300/year). Medicare, however, will not reimburse for self-administration of the drug. Both leuprolide and goserelin are now available in longer acting depot formulations, which provide a more convenient dosing regimen for the patient.

SURGICAL CASTRATION

Bilateral orchiectomy removes the source of the production of testicular androgen. Although surgery is more cost effective and associated with minimal risk, the choice between medical or surgical androgen suppression is a very personal one. Bilateral orchiectomy may not be acceptable to some men concerned about their body image and self-perception of masculinity. Its permanence may be an advantage in that frequent visits for injections will not be necessary. Its irreversibility may be a disadvantage if side effects are associated with significant morbidity. Orchiectomy eliminates the choice of potential alternatives currently under investigation, such as intermittent androgen deprivation.

Although there has been debate as to the equivalency of LHRH agonist therapy and orchiectomy, data have not shown a difference when evaluated as part of total androgen blockade (TAB).[18]

TABLE 11-1. Hormonal Therapy Standard of Care

NURSING DIAGNOSIS: *Testosterone suppression related to hormonal therapy*

OUTCOME: Serum testosterone level falls to castrate level (< 20 mg/dL). • PSA level will be decreased. • Pt will verbalize reduction in symptoms.

NURSING INTERVENTION: Monitor serum testosterone levels. • Educate patient as to need to adhere to plan of follow-up surveillance as recommended by physician such as PSA, physical exam with DRE, and diagnostic studies such as bone scan.

NURSING DIAGNOSIS: *Knowledge deficit related to hormonal therapy*

OUTCOME: Pt will verbalize understanding of rationale for treatment with hormonal manipulation, goals of treatment, potential side effects, and interventions to minimize side effects.

NURSING INTERVENTION: Assess pt's understanding of goals of hormonal therapy and potential side effects and their management. • Educate as appropriate, providing repetition and clarification as needed. • Provide additional informational support and other resources such as National Cancer Institute (1-800-4-CANCER) and American Cancer Society, Prostate Cancer Support Groups.

NURSING DIAGNOSIS: *Altered body image related to side effects of therapy such as hot flashes, fatigue, altered sexual functioning*

OUTCOME: Pt will verbalize an acceptable level of self-esteem and self-image.

NURSING INTERVENTION: Assess pt's response to effects of treatment that affect body image. • Encourage verbalization of feelings. • Encourage pt to participate in support groups, if appropriate.

OUTCOME: Pt will have tolerable level of discomfort related to hot flashes.

NURSING INTERVENTION: Assess pt for incidence, frequency, and intensity of hot flashes. • Educate pt as to treatment options available. • Assess effectiveness of intervention and need to try alternative interventions.

OUTCOME: Pt will verbalize understanding of management of fatigue.

NURSING INTERVENTION: Assess pt for causes of fatigue such as anemia, pain, inadequate nutrition, weight loss, inadequate rest or sleep, depression, or anxiety. • Educate pt as to cause of fatigue. • Encourage pt to keep a diary of fatigue and evaluate diary for patterns of fatigue. • Assist pt in identifying activities that can be performed by other people. • Encourage pt to participate in preferred/favorite activities and delegate others. • Encourage program of regular exercise such as walking.

OUTCOME: Pt will describe methods personally acceptable for management of erectile dysfunction.

NURSING INTERVENTION: Assess pt for decreased libido and erectile dysfunction. • Educate pt and significant other in treatment options for erectile dysfunction. • Recognize that sexual dysfunction may be multifactorial and refer as appropriate.

NURSING DIAGNOSIS: *Risk for fracture related to osteoporosis*

OUTCOME: Pt will not sustain a fracture.

NURSING INTERVENTION: Consider bone mineral density determination at beginning of hormonal therapy and at periodic intervals. • Consider concurrent administration of bisphosphonate to inhibit bone resorption. • Encourage lifestyle modifications that reduce other risk factors associated with osteoporosis; maintain normal weight for height, regular exercise, and no smoking.

NURSING DIAGNOSIS: *Potential for side effects related to drug therapy such as diarrhea, interstitial lung disease, or risk for injury resulting from alcohol interaction with nilutamide*

OUTCOME: Pt will verbalize understanding of diarrhea management.

NURSING INTERVENTION: Educate pt as to potential drug side effects. • Reduce dose of flutamide by 50% if diarrhea develops. If diarrhea does not resolve, stop flutamide and use another agent on trial basis. • Educate pt to take flutamide q8h and not tid.

OUTCOME: Pt will have prompt recognition of breathing problems.

NURSING INTERVENTION: Assess pt for shortness of breath, cough, chest pain, or fever, and teach pt to notify nurse or physician immediately if they occur. • Monitor pt during first 3 mo of nilutamide therapy for respiratory problems. If they develop, obtain chest radiograph and monitor pt for interstitial changes. Stop drug if changes develop. • Monitor pt to ascertain that symptoms improve.

OUTCOME: Pt will not drink alcohol while taking nilutamide.

NURSING INTERVENTION: Educate pt as to danger of consuming alcohol while taking nilutamide.

OUTCOME: Pt will not sustain injury while taking nilutamide.

NURSING INTERVENTION: Educate pt to avoid night driving while taking nilutamide.

PSA, prostate-specific antigen; Pt, patient; DRE, digital rectal exam; q, every; tid, three times a day.
Data compiled from Millikan et al,[17] Bennett,[21] Harris et al,[22] Portenoy and Miaskowski,[46] Stepan et al,[49] Townsend et al,[50] Sisson de Castro,[51] and Daniell.[52]

TABLE 11-2. LHRH Agonists

Drug	Formulation	Dosage
Leuprolide (Lupron)*	Lyophilized particles for reconstitution to suspension f or IM injection	Equivalent of 7.5 mg/mo Available in the following injections: 7.5 mg/mo 22.5 mg/3 mo 30 mg/4 mo
Goserelin (Zoladex)†	Prepared syringe with implant for SC injection in upper abdomen	Equivalent of 3.6 mg/mo Available in the following injections: 3.6 mg/mo 10.8 mg/3 mo

IM, intramuscular; SC, subcutaneous; mo, month.
*Product information, TAP Pharmaceuticals, 1995.
†Product information, Zeneca Pharmaceuticals, 1996.

TABLE 11-3. Pure Antiandrogens

Drug	Dosage	Financial Assistance
Flutamide (Eulexin)*	750 mg/day; 125-mg capsules, 2 capsules q8h	Commitment to Care: 1-800-521-7157
Bilcalutamide (Casodex)†	50 mg qd	Financial assistance program: 1-800-424-3727
Nilutamide‡ (Nilandron, Anandron)	1st month: 300 mg/day (50 mg, 6 tablets/day) Maintenance: 150 mg/day (50 mg, 3 tablets/day)	Financial assistance program: 1-800-221-4025

*Product Information, Schering Corporation, 1996. †Product Information, Zeneca Pharmaceuticals, 1995.
‡Product Information, Hoechst Marion Roussel, 1996. qd, every day, q, every; h, hour.

PURE ANTIANDROGENS

Pure antiandrogens are nonsteroidal compounds that directly bind to the androgen receptor with high affinity and specificity but do not have intrinsic hormonal activity.[1] Because they block androgens only at the receptor level (see Figure 11-1), peripheral testosterone is maintained at a normal to supernormal level.[19] Currently, three such preparations are available (Table 11-3), which continue to undergo clinical study. Flutamide is the oldest of the three and has been the most extensively studied.

Side effects common to the pure antiandrogens are breast tenderness, gynecomastia, hot flashes, anemia, and asthenia. Gynecomastia may be due to an imbalance between estrogens and testosterone, particularly when the testosterone level is high as when antiandrogens are given alone. Levels of serum estradiol, necessary for the aromatization of testosterone to estrogens, rise when pure antiandrogens are administered, which may lend further explanation.[20] Interestingly, breast tenderness and gynecomastia are seen less frequently when a pure antiandrogen is given in combination with an LHRH agonist.

Liver dysfunction has been reported with all three of the drugs. The incidence has been low (< 2%) and is usually evidenced by elevated liver enzymes (aspartate transaminase, alanine aminotransferase). Cholestatic jaundice, hepatic necrosis, and hepatic encephalopathy have also been reported. At the first sign of liver injury, which most often is an elevation in liver enzymes, the antiandrogen should be discontinued. Hepatic injury is usually reversible after discontinuation of therapy. Liver function tests (LFTs) should be monitored at baseline and 1 month into therapy, and it has been suggested that they should continue to be monitored at 3-month intervals.[21]

Other side effects vary depending on the drug used. Flutamide has been associated with diarrhea; varying incidences have been reported, the highest being 16%.[21] This often resolves by decreasing the dose by 50% to one capsule every 8 hours (375 mg/day).

Reversible interstitial lung disease has been reported in 2.4% of patients treated with nilutamide.[22] Patients experiencing this side effect typically present with progressive exertional dyspnea, which may be associated with cough, chest pain, or fever. These symptoms most often occur within the first 3 months of treatment, and interstitial changes are confirmed by chest radiograph. Discontinuing nilutamide has resulted in resolution of pulmonary symptoms. Nilutamide has also been associated with alcohol intolerance in 5% of patients and visual disturbances in the form of delayed adaptation to darkness. These potential side effects have implications for patient teaching and safety.

Antiandrogens are not covered by Medicare and are expensive. The costs vary, averaging about $300/month. Nilutamide monographs quote a cost of $233.58 for a 1-month prescription. All three of the pharmaceutical companies manufacturing the antiandrogens have excellent financial assistance programs and will provide the drug free of charge or at a reduced cost for patients who are financially eligible. Telephone numbers to access these programs can be found in Table 11-3.

STEROIDAL ANTIANDROGENS

Steroidal antiandrogens inhibit LH secretion from the pituitary and also block androgens at the receptor level. Because of this double effect, they are associated with side effects not seen with the pure antiandrogens. Sexual dysfunction can occur; most patients experience decreased libido and erectile dysfunction. Thrombotic incidents have been reported in a significant number of patients.[19]

Gynecomastia is not seen with the steroidal antiandrogens because they lower the testosterone without an estrogenic effect. Another advantage of the steroidal antiandrogens is the lack of hot flashes.[23]

TABLE 11-4. Biochemical Effects of Primary Hormonal Therapy

Biochemical Effect	THERAPY				
	Orchiectomy	LHRH Agonists	Pure Antiandrogens	Steroid Antiandrogens	Total Androgen Blockade*
Removes source of testosterone	Yes				
Inhibits LHRH secretion by the hypothalamus		Yes			Yes
Inhibits LH secretion by the pituitary		Yes		Yes	Yes
Blocks binding of DHT to androgen receptor			Yes	Yes	Yes

LHRH, luteinizing hormone–releasing hormone; LH, luteinizing hormone; DHT, dihydrotestosterone.
Data compiled from Brufsky and Kantoff,[1] and Boccon-Gibod.[19] *Orchiectomy or LHRH agonist plus antiandrogen.

Of the steroidal antiandrogens, cyproterone acetate (CPA) is the best studied.[1] It is used widely in Canada and Europe but is not approved for use in the United States. Megestrol acetate (Megace) is used in the United States.

TOTAL ANDROGEN BLOCKADE

Despite initial responses to monotherapy with medical or surgical castration, in most patients, distant metastatic disease will progress within 12 to 16 months.[1, 24] At the time of hormonal failure, serum levels of testosterone are often within castrate levels; however, levels of intraprostatic DHT may be as high as 25 to 40% of baseline.[6, 25] Weak adrenal sex steroids are converted into testosterone and DHT in the prostate.

The goal of TAB is to maximize androgen suppression. Orchiectomy or an LHRH agonist is combined with an antiandrogen to reduce testicular androgen levels and to block the action of adrenal androgens (Table 11-4).

INDICATIONS FOR HORMONAL MANIPULATION

METASTATIC PROSTATE CANCER

Each year about 45,000 patients present with metastatic prostate cancer. Metastatic disease will later develop in at least the same number of patients who have had prior definitive treatment with surgery or radiotherapy.[26] The most common sites of metastatic prostate cancer are the bones and retroperitoneal lymph nodes. When prostate cancer has metastasized, the focus of treatment becomes palliation and prolonged survival rather

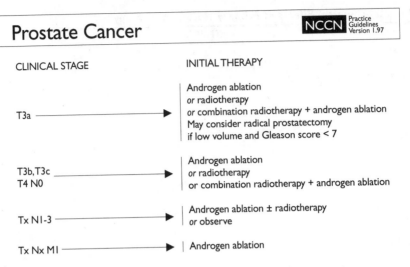

FIGURE 11-2. Initial therapy

The NCCN guidelines are a statement of consensus of its authors regarding their views of currently accepted approaches to treatment. Any clinician seeking to apply or consult any NCCN guideline is expected to use independent medical judgement in the context of individual clinical circumstances to determine any patient's care or treatment. The National Comprehensive Cancer Network makes no warranties of any kind whatsoever regarding their content, use, or application and disclaims any responsibility for their application or use in any way.

From *Oncology*, November 1997, pp. 190, 192, and 193. Copyrighted by the National Comprehensive Cancer Network. All rights reserved. These guidelines and illustrations may not be reproduced in any form without the express written permission of the NCCN.

than cure. Androgen blockade is the most well-established treatment of metastatic disease and has remained the standard of care (Figures 11-2 and 11-3). With initiation of hormonal therapy, about 80% of men with symptomatic metastatic disease will demonstrate a response. Objective responses include a decrease in tumor size, lower serum PSA levels, reduced urinary obstructive symptoms, reduced bone pain, improved appetite, or improved sense of well-being.[27]

TAB has become a widely accepted treatment approach to the management of metastatic disease. Clinical trials have shown a survival advantage with TAB compared with medical or surgical castration alone. In a National Cancer Institute study,[24] 603 patients with untreated Stage D2 prostate cancer were randomized to either leuprolide and flutamide or leuprolide and placebo. In the combination therapy group, both progression-free survival (16.5 months vs. 13.9 months) and overall survival (35.6 months vs. 28.3 months) were greater (P = .039; P = .035, respectively).

In Canada, Beland and associates[28] conducted a multicenter, randomized, double-blind trial that compared nilutamide with placebo in 194 men with untreated Stage D2 prostate cancer who had undergone orchiectomy. Results showed a significant difference (P = .001) in the percentage of patients who demonstrated a complete or partial regression of disease (46% in the nilutamide group vs. 20% in the placebo group). The median

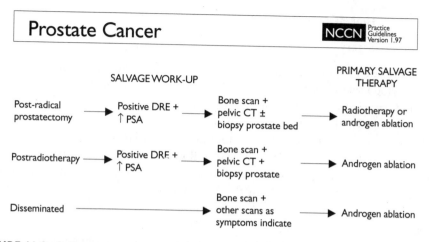

Prostate Cancer

NCCN Practice Guidelines Version 1.97

SALVAGE WORK-UP

PRIMARY SALVAGE THERAPY

Post-radical prostatectomy → Positive DRE + ↑ PSA → Bone scan + pelvic CT ± biopsy prostate bed → Radiotherapy or androgen ablation

Postradiotherapy → Positive DRE + ↑ PSA → Bone scan + pelvic CT + biopsy prostate → Androgen ablation

Disseminated → Bone scan + other scans as symptoms indicate → Androgen ablation

FIGURE 11-3. Salvage

PSA, prostate-specific antigen; DRE, digital rectal exam; CT, computed tomography.

The NCCN guidelines are a statement of consensus of its authors regarding their views of currently accepted approaches to treatment. Any clinician seeking to apply or consult any NCCN guideline is expected to use independent medical judgement in the context of individual clinical circumstances to determine any patient's care or treatment. The National Comprehensive Cancer Network makes no warranties of any kind whatsoever regarding their content, use, or application and disclaims any responsibility for their application or use in any way.

survival time for patients in the nilutamide group was 24.3 months compared with 18.9 months in the placebo group.

In an attempt to determine whether there is a difference in treatment outcomes between the antiandrogens used in TAB, the Casodex Combination Group[29] conducted a randomized, double-blind (for antiandrogen therapy), multicenter study. In this study, 813 men with Stage D2 prostate cancer were randomized in a ratio of 1:1 to bicalutamide or flutamide and 2:1 to goserelin or leuprolide. Although the patients receiving bicalutamide plus LHRH agonist had longer time to progression and disease-free survival, these endpoint results were not statistically significant.

The Casodex Combination Group further evaluated these data to assess the treatment outcomes among the LHRH agonists and among the four drug combination groups in the study.[30] The results indicated that goserelin plus antiandrogen and leuprolide plus antiandrogen were similarly well tolerated and had equivalent time to progression and survival. When the four groups were compared, leuprolide plus flutamide therapy appeared to be the least effective of the four TAB regimens. However, these results should be interpreted with caution, and further investigation is warranted.

Many patients with metastatic prostate cancer are being offered TAB as a treatment option, although its merits continue to be debated. The clinician must weigh the survival benefit of combined therapy with its additional costs. It has been estimated that the cost of 1 year of life extension using TAB is $20,000.[31]

NEOADJUVANT HORMONAL THERAPY

☐ Before Surgery

Androgen ablation has been used as neoadjuvant treatment to downstage (increase the likelihood that tumor is confined to prostate) patients before radical prostatectomy.[1] Fair and associates[32] reported on a Phase III study conducted to assess the effects of 3 months of neoadjuvant androgen ablation (NAA) with goserelin and flutamide on pathologic staging and PSA relapse rate. In this study, 114 men with clinically localized prostate cancer were randomized to NAA followed by surgery or surgery alone (control group). Organ-confined rates were 73% in the NAA group vs. 56% in the control group. Margin-positive rates were 17% in the NAA group vs. 36% in the control group. At a mean follow-up of 28.6 months, there was no statistically significant difference between the groups in terms of biochemical (serum PSA) failure.

NAA causes architectural changes in both benign and malignant prostatic epithelial cells. These changes may result in the reduced ability to identify capsular involvement and positive surgical margins.[33] Bazinet and colleagues[33] found that the use of cytokeratin immunohistochemistry revealed more tumor involvement and positive surgical margins than did conventional staining and suggested that the beneficial pathologic effects from NAA may be artifactual. Despite the apparent favorable pathologic findings, randomized trials have not demonstrated a benefit from NAA in reduced PSA progression rates. There is concern about the validity and biologic significance of the apparent downstaging and decreased rates of positive margins, and NAA has not been recommended outside of a clinical trial.[1, 34]

☐ Before Radiation Therapy

Because radiation and hormonally mediated apoptosis appear to be induced by different mechanisms, their interaction may be synergistic.[35] In a comparative trial of the Radiation Oncology Group,[36] patients with T2, T3, and T4 tumors (M0) were randomized to receive goserelin and flutamide for 2 months before and during external beam radiation therapy (EBRT) or EBRT alone. In this study, even patients with the more advanced stages of prostate cancer were treated with curative intent.

Results indicated a decrease in local progression rates in Arm I (NAA and EBRT) at 5 years (46%) compared with Arm II (EBRT alone)(71%). Progression-free survival rates were 36% in Arm I vs. 15% in Arm II (P < .001). A 4-month course of goserelin and flutamide before and during radiation therapy markedly reduced the incidence of treatment failures with no increase in major toxicity.[36]

Men who are at high risk for biochemical failure when treated with radiation therapy should probably receive a longer course of NAA, but the optimal duration and sequence of androgen ablation are not yet known.

Neoadjuvant therapy has also been shown to have a benefit in patients undergoing brachytherapy (radioactive seed implantation) for prostate cancer. In a study conducted by Stock and Stone,[37] 96 patients undergoing brachytherapy for prostate cancer were given 3 months of hormonal therapy (leuprolide and flutamide) before implantation. In 15 patients, NAA was used to downsize prostate glands larger than 50 cc. In 81 patients, it was used for high-risk features: PSA greater than 10 ng/mL, stage higher than T2a, or Gleason score greater than 6. The patients were separated into low- and high-risk groups for disease recurrence. At the 4-year follow-up point, the low-risk group had a significantly higher (P = .02) freedom from biochemical failure rate of 88% vs. 60% for the high-risk group. One way of potentially improving the outcome for high-risk patients is to combine EBRT with implantation.

There was a difference in negative biopsy rates (approaching significance); the NAA group had a rate of 94% compared with 77% for those treated with implant alone.[37] These results suggest that the benefits of neoadjuvant ablation before brachytherapy may be cytoreduction and improved local control.

ADJUVANT THERAPY

Many patients with asymptomatic early stages of disease are at high risk for disease recurrence and metastasis. These patients include those with positive nodes, those with locally advanced (T3) disease, and those with local disease with high-risk features.[1] With the goal of altering the natural history of high-risk patients, researchers have investigated the use of adjuvant therapy.

Van Aubel and colleagues[38] evaluated the results of immediate orchiectomy in patients with confirmed Stage D1 prostate cancer. Early hormonal therapy resulted in a 46% treatment failure rate after 45 months compared with shorter times to progression with delayed hormonal therapy, radical prostatectomy, and EBRT. In a retrospective study, Kramolowsky[39] analyzed 68 patients with Stage D1 disease, 30 of whom underwent immediate hormonal deprivation; the remainder received hormonal therapy when bone metastasis was diagnosed. At the 60-month follow-up, the median time interval to progression to bone metastasis was 100 months in the immediate hormonal deprivation group compared with 43 months in the delayed-treatment group. The immediate treatment group demonstrated a trend toward prolonged survival (150 months) compared with the delayed-treatment group (90 months).

These observations prompted clinicians to begin androgen ablation earlier in men with locally advanced disease but not necessarily metastatic prostate cancer. The anticipated benefits of early hormonal manipulation must be weighed against the potential risks of prolonged periods of androgen suppression.

SIDE EFFECT MANAGEMENT

Nursing plays a key role in patient education and side effect management. Patient education begins as the patient is contemplating treatment options (e.g., medical vs. surgical castration) and includes the patient's wife or significant other. The patient's understanding of these two options may be facilitated by using the analogy of a factory (testicles) supplied by electrical power (hormonal stimulation). The medical approach cuts off the

TABLE 11-5. Treatment Options for Relief of Hot Flashes

Drug	Dosage	Potential Side Effects
Megestrol acetate (Megace)	20 mg bid	Episodes of chills Appetite stimulation Weight gain Symptoms of carpal tunnel syndrome
Clonidine (Catapres)	Transdermal 0.1 mg weekly	Hypotension Allergic skin reaction to transdermal preparation
Medroxyprogesterone acetate (Depo-Provera)	400 mg IM	None reported when used every 6 mo or less

bid, twice a day; IM, intramuscularly; mo, month.

Data compiled from Loprinzi et al,[41] Quella et al,[42] and Parra and Gregory.[44]

electricity to the factory and the surgical approach removes the factory itself (John A. Heaney, MD, personal communication, June 1993). Side effects and potential interventions to minimize or treat them are reviewed (see Table 11-1). Patient education is ongoing as is assessment of side effects to ensure early intervention and management.

HOT FLASHES

Vasomotor hot flashes are a common symptom in men who undergo androgen suppression therapy for prostate cancer. In a study of 63 men treated with orchiectomy or LHRH agonist, Karling and others[40] noted that 68% reported hot flashes and 48% still had hot flashes 5 years after treatment. The degree of distress experienced is variable, but for some men hot flashes are significantly bothersome that they seek intervention. A summary of the current treatment options to alleviate hot flashes can be found in Table 11-5.

Mayo Clinic conducted a cross-over study that randomized participants to receive megestrol acetate (Megace), 20 mg twice daily for 4 weeks followed by placebo for 4 weeks, or vice versa in a double-blind manner.[41] Sixty-six men with prostate cancer who had undergone androgen deprivation therapy and experienced bothersome hot flashes enrolled in the study. After 4 weeks, hot flashes were reduced by 85% in the treatment group compared with 21% in the placebo group. A follow-up to this study was conducted to determine the long-term effectiveness of megestrol acetate in the management of hot flashes.[42] Forty-five percent of those contacted were continuing to take megestrol acetate for 3 years or longer with continued control of hot flashes. Potential toxicities related to megestrol acetate were identified and include episodes of chills, appetite stimulation and weight gain, and symptoms of carpal tunnel syndrome.

In a small, nonrandomized study, Bressler and colleagues[43] investigated the effects of 0.1 to 0.2 mg/day of transdermal or oral clonidine (Catapres), a centrally acting adrenergic agonist, in abating hot flashes in men receiving either leuprolide or goserelin for prostate cancer. All four participants reported symptomatic improvement. Although the study was small and did not control for the placebo effect, results suggest a potential benefit for the use of clonidine in alleviating hot flashes. Hypotension was found to be a limiting factor, and exclusion criteria included a diastolic blood pressure of 75 mm Hg or less. Parra and Gregory[44] also studied transdermal clonidine and found that a dose of 0.1 mg/week (delivers 0.1 mg/day and is changed every 7 days) decreased or abolished hot flashes after orchiectomy. However, there were some problems with allergic skin reactions to the transdermal preparation.

At the 19th Annual Meeting of the American Urological Association (April 1995), Brosman[45] presented the results of a study using medroxyprogesterone (Depo-Provera) as a treatment for hot flashes in men on androgen ablation therapy. Fifty-five men whose symptoms remained severe after an initial placebo injection were given an intramuscular injection of medroxyprogesterone, 400 mg. Significant improvement was reported by 51 (92.7%) participants monitored for a mean of 17.2 months. For 64% of men, the response lasted 4 to 12 months, and for 26.4% the benefit has lasted a year or longer; the typical patient received a dose every 6 months.

FATIGUE

Fatigue is a common symptom in patients with cancer and may be multifactorial. It can have a profound effect on quality of life. Potential causes of fatigue include anemia, pain, inadequate nutrition, medication, inadequate sleep or rest, endocrine abnormalities, depression, and anxiety.

In men taking androgen ablation therapy, fatigue seems to be a delayed rather than an immediate effect and variable in its severity. Although fatigue is likely related to testosterone suppression, the contributing factors just mentioned should be considered when assessing patients reporting this symptom. Interventions may include a program of regular physical exercise to increase stamina and endurance balanced with rest.[46] Exercise is important for men on androgen ablation therapy because of the potential for muscular atrophy.

It is important that patients experiencing fatigue understand the cause of the symptom as well as the treatment options and expected outcomes of intervention. Many patients may assume that their fatigue reflects progression of the prostate cancer. As part of the educational process, it may be helpful for patients to keep a diary of their fatigue. This information can help the clinician develop a management plan that modifies specific activities and allows for adequate rest periods.[46]

Persistent fatigue not only limits quality of life but can affect a patient's decision to continue treatment. Sometimes men on androgen ablation therapy will experience less fatigue with a change in LHRH agonist or a change in antiandrogen, although it is unclear why this is so. For those with intractable fatigue, intermittent hormonal therapy, although still under investigation, may be an option.

IMPOTENCE

Most treatments for prostate cancer affect sexual function, and for many men consideration of this potential side effect plays an important role in decision making. Testosterone suppression results in decreased libido and erectile dysfunction. This can have a signifi-

TABLE 11-6. Treatment Options for Men With Erectile Dysfunction

Treatment	Advantages	Disadvantages
External vacuum devices[47]	Inexpensive Can be used with other treatment options	Mechanical: requires preparation time Produces cool erection Side effects include bruising, discomfort
Sildenafil (Viagra)[48]	Oral tablet	Side effects include headache, flushing, dyspepsia, nasal congestion, abnormal vision Concurrent use of nitrates contraindicated
Alprostadil (Muse) urethral suppository*	Minimally invasive Produces rapid natural-appearing erection	Requires test dose Potential urethral burning, discomfort Potential for priapism Not effective with severe blood flow problem
Alprostadil penile injections[47] (Caverject, Edex)		Requires test dose Potential urethral burning, discomfort, priapism, fibrosis Not effective with severe blood flow problems
Implantable penile prosthesis[47]	Use as desired No preparation time Increases girth of penis	Expensive Requires surgical procedure Risk of infection, erosion of device, device failure

*Product information, Vivus, Inc., 1996.

cant impact on quality of life and the patient's self-perception of masculinity. Testicular and penile atrophy may result, further affecting body image.

For patients who wish intervention for sexual dysfunction, several options are available depending somewhat on the cause of the dysfunction and the level of function before initiation of hormonal therapy. Because erection is also affected by many medications and requires intact nerves and healthy blood vessels, dysfunction can be multifactorial, and patients should be referred as appropriate.

Current options to treat erectile dysfunction are summarized in Table 11-6.[47, 48]

OSTEOPOROSIS

Androgens play an important role in bone metabolism. With hormonal manipulation being initiated earlier and continued for prolonged periods, the potential for osteoporosis and subsequent risk for bone fractures need to be considered. Currently, there is a paucity of research addressing this issue in men, although numerous studies have documented the relationship between loss of estrogen and development of osteoporosis in women.

Stepan and associates,[49] in their long-term study of 12 men, reported on bone loss after surgical castration. A progressive decrease in lumbar bone density over time was noted at a rate of 7% per year for the first 2 years; this rate decreased to 1.5% per year 6 to 11 years after surgery.

The LHRH agonists are known to decrease bone mineral density. Townsend and others[50] conducted a study to determine the risk of bone fracture in men receiving LHRH agonists. They noted a 5% incidence of osteoporotic fractures, which was more than three times the incidence of hip fractures in age-matched controls.

Sisson de Castro[51] studied the effect of alendronate (Fosamax) on short-term bone mass response in 10 men with osteoporosis. Alendronate is a bisphosphonate that acts as a specific inhibitor of osteoclast-mediated bone resorption. Sisson de Castro demonstrated a mean increase in bone mass density of 3.8% at the L2-4 vertebral levels as well as a mean increase of 2.8% from baseline at the level of the femoral neck.

Daniell's[52] study of osteoporosis after castration provided evidence of an acceleration of osteoporosis in men treated with orchiectomy and suggested the need for bone mineral density determination at the beginning of hormonal manipulation and at periodic follow-up. In this study, cigarette smoking and an underweight body frame were also identified as risk factors for osteoporosis ($P < .10$). Among those men in this series who underwent orchiectomy, a habit of frequent exercise was most closely associated with a normal bone density. These findings suggest that lifestyle changes may be beneficial in reducing the risk for osteoporosis in this population.

Further research is necessary to determine the incidence of osteoporosis in men on androgen ablation therapy and the potential impact of drugs such as alendronate on minimizing its development and associated risk for fractures. In the meantime, osteoporosis is a factor to consider when deciding whether hormonal therapy or watchful waiting is more appropriate for the asymptomatic elderly patient with prostate carcinoma.[35]

Side effect management is an important factor as men adjust to living with prostate cancer and coping with the manifestations of the disease and its treatment. A prostate cancer support group provides additional psychosocial support and encouragement from those sharing similar experiences and is a vital component of a comprehensive program of cancer care. The mutual support inherent in these groups goes beyond what we as healthcare professionals can provide.

HORMONE-REFRACTORY DISEASE–ANDROGEN INDEPENDENCE

Hormone-refractory disease continues to be a treatment challenge. It was learned early on that the duration of response to androgen ablation was finite, lasting a median of 12 to 16 months.[24] Patients may have an additional response to secondary hormonal therapy or chemotherapy, but results have been variable and response rates low. Current research efforts are focused on developing successful treatment for those with progressive disease after initial hormonal manipulation.

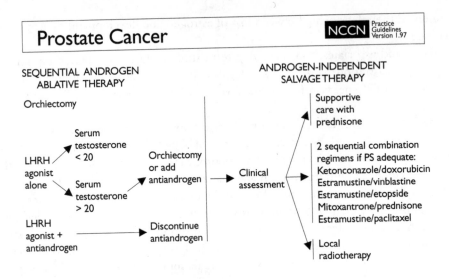

FIGURE 11-4. Androgen-independent salvage

LHRH, luteinizing hormone–releasing hormone; PS, performance status

The NCCN guidelines are a statement of consensus of its authors regarding their views of currently accepted approaches to treatment. Any clinician seeking to apply or consult any NCCN guideline is expected to use independent medical judgement in the context of individual clinical circumstances to determine any patient's care or treatment. The National Comprehensive Cancer Network makes no warranties of any kind whatsoever regarding their content, use, or application and disclaims any responsibility for their application or use in any way. From *Oncology,* November 1997, pp. 190, 192, and 193. Copyrighted by the National Comprehensive Cancer Network. All rights reserved. These guidelines and illustrations may not be reproduced in any form without the express written permission of the NCCN.

The cause of disease progression during hormonal manipulation is unclear but is potentially related to the heterogeneity of androgen responsiveness in the original tumor.[1] In animal testing, it has been demonstrated that the removal of androgens will promote the development of cell clones that are able to proliferate within an environment of minimal or no androgen support (androgen-independent clones).[53] Although androgen-independent cancers grow despite chemical or surgical castration, this does not necessarily mean they are resistant to further hormonal manipulations.[54]

ANTIANDROGEN WITHDRAWAL RESPONSE

Herrada and colleagues[55] evaluated the paradoxical decrease in PSA after flutamide withdrawal in 41 patients with progressive metastatic prostate cancer. Six weeks after discontinuing flutamide, 11 of 39 patients had a 50% decrease in PSA from baseline, and 3 of 11 continued to have suppressed PSA levels at 12+, 13+, and 20+ weeks. The serum PSA decrease was associated with improved clinical symptoms. Studies have shown that responders to withdrawal tend to have taken flutamide for longer periods of time than nonresponders.[55–57] Cells may become dependent on flutamide for their growth. Removal of flutamide support may result in their suppression. This hypothesis may help explain the observed flutamide withdrawal syndrome.[1]

TABLE 11-7. Biochemical Effects of Secondary Hormonal Manipulation

Biochemical Effect	DES	Ketoconazole	Aminoglutethimide	Progestins	Corticosteroids
Inhibits 5-α-reductase				Yes	
Inhibits LH secretion by pituitary	Yes				
Inhibits LHRH secretion by the hypothalamus	Yes			Yes	
Inhibits production of ACTH with resulting decrease in adrenal steroid production					Yes
Inhibits cytochrome P-450–mediated adrenal androgenesis		Yes	Yes	Yes	
Inhibits testicular androgenesis	Yes	Yes			
Blocks binding of DHT to androgen receptor				Yes	

DES, diethylstilbestrol; LH, luteinizing hormone; LHRH, LH-releasing hormone; ACTH, corticotropin; DHT, dihydrotestosterone. Data compiled from Brufsky and Kantoff,[1] Small and Srinivas,[57] and Small et al.[58]

Withdrawal responses have been observed for a number of agents known to act via the androgen receptor, including the antiandrogens, progestational agents (e.g., medroxy-progesterone), and estrogens.[54] In most instances, the patterns of response were similar. Among the antiandrogens, the response to withdrawal of flutamide occurred quickly, but PSA levels of patients taking bicalutamide continued to rise for up to 7 weeks before PSA decline was noted. This is likely due to the long half-life of bicalutamide (1 week) vs. that of flutamide (5.2 hours).[58]

Antiandrogen withdrawal is now considered the primary salvage therapy for patients who have demonstrated progressive disease despite androgen ablation (Figure 11-4). A trial of withdrawal therapy is warranted before initiation of more toxic therapies. Failure to control for this phenomenon in clinical trials may lead to the false attribution of response to the agent being studied.[54]

SECONDARY HORMONAL MANIPULATION

After antiandrogen withdrawal, other secondary hormonal therapies can be considered. It is recommended that testicular suppression of testosterone be continued for life because of the danger of an androgen-driven disease flare if LHRH agonists are withdrawn.[17]

Secondary hormonal therapies have been the subject of numerous studies, and their biochemical effects are summarized in Table 11-7. Corticosteroids suppress the pituitary production of corticotropin, which indirectly decreases production of adrenal androgens. Oral prednisone, dexamethasone, and hydrocortisone have been investigated as single agents in several small clinical trials.[59] Results indicated that corticosteroids produce response rates ranging from 20 to 25% in hormone-refractory disease.[59]

Ketoconazole is an imidazole antifungal agent that inhibits both testicular and adrenal androgenesis. Ketoconazole alone at doses of 200 to 400 mg three times per day has a response rate in the 20 to 30% range by National Prostate Cancer Project and European Organization for Research and Treatment of Cancer criteria.[57] Small and others[60] evaluated the response of 48 men with progressive disease after antiandrogen withdrawal to ketoconazole plus hydrocortisone. Whereas 30 men had a greater than 50% decrease in PSA, 23 had a decrease of greater than 80%. The median duration of response was 3.5 months. There was no difference in the ketoconazole response between those who had experienced an antiandrogen withdrawal response and those who did not. Potential side effects associated with ketoconazole include nausea, vomiting, skin rash, nail changes, edema, hepatotoxicity, and gynecomastia.

Like ketoconazole, aminoglutethimide suppresses adrenal androgenesis and is administered with hydrocortisone. In clinical trials, doses of aminoglutethimide have ranged from 1,000 to 1,750 mg/day, with response rates of 0 to 40%.[59] The majority of these response rates have represented stable disease. Aminoglutethimide commonly causes lethargy, nausea, and skin rash. Additional side effects include peripheral edema, hypothyroidism, and abnormal LFTs.

Estrogens have long been used in the treatment of prostate cancer. Estrogens suppress pituitary gonadotropins, thereby decreasing testosterone secretion. Diethylstilbestrol (DES) has been used extensively in the past. The dose administered ranges from 1 to 3 mg/day.[59] Response rates are in the range of 15 to 20%. Thromboembolic events have been associated with DES, and the introduction of LHRH agonists has significantly reduced the use of DES as primary therapy. Other potential side effects include nausea, vomiting, fluid retention, gynecomastia, mastodynia, and alterations in LFTs.[59]

Progestins have been shown to inhibit tumor growth, and in the United States, two agents have been used in the treatment of prostate cancer: medroxyprogesterone acetate and megestrol acetate. The primary benefit of medroxyprogesterone seems to be reduction in bone pain.[61–63] Dosages range from 500 to 1,200 mg/day. Peripheral edema and risk for cardiovascular events are potential side effects. Another progestin, megestrol acetate, has also been researched in hormone-refractory prostate cancer. In a study of 144 patients randomized to high-dose (840 mg/day) vs. standard dose (160 mg/day) megestrol, Dawson and colleagues[64] found one patient to have a partial response in each arm. Although further analysis is pending, megestrol appears to have minimal activity in hormone-refractory disease.

Secondary hormonal therapy produces minimal benefit in patients with hormone-refractory prostate cancer. The low response rate and short duration of response have led some to recommend that this population be considered for enrollment in clinical trials investigating new agents.[59]

CHEMOTHERAPY

For those patients with evidence of disease progression despite antiandrogen withdrawal or secondary hormonal therapy, chemotherapy may be an appropriate consideration. For several reasons, there has been renewed enthusiasm for the role of chemotherapy in hormone-refractory prostate cancer. Newer measurements of response, including PSA and quality of life measures, suggest activity with some older drugs that were previously thought to be inactive. New combinations of drugs appear to have synergistic activity, potentially enhancing clinical results. Improvements in the area of supportive care permit the safer administration of chemotherapy and reduced toxicity.[65]

Several systemic therapies are known to offer some palliative benefit in androgen-independent prostate cancer (see Figure 11-4) and, at present, it is impossible to guide choice among them.[17] Continued research efforts may provide guidance in the future. Ongoing clinical trials are examining combination therapies and such novel approaches as gene therapy.[65] A comprehensive discussion of chemotherapy for the treatment of advanced prostate cancer can be found in Chapter 12.

NOVEL APPROACHES TO HORMONAL MANIPULATION

To offer the potential benefit of early hormonal therapy while minimizing its side effects, several novel methods of androgen ablation are currently under investigation.

SEQUENTIAL ANDROGEN BLOCKADE

Sequential androgen blockade combines a 5 α-reductase inhibitor (finasteride [Proscar]) to reduce the conversion of testosterone to DHT and an antiandrogen to prevent residual androgen from reaching the androgen receptor. An example of such a regimen is finasteride, 5 mg twice daily, and flutamide, 250 mg every 8 hours.[66] Circulating testosterone is not reduced, thus minimizing the side effects usually associated with androgen suppression. Early results suggest that the time to progression is long, and the side effects are minimized compared with TAB.[67]

INTERMITTENT ANDROGEN SUPPRESSION

Intermittent androgen suppression (IAS) relies on the hypothesis that tumor cells that survive androgen suppression are forced into a normal pathway of differentiation by androgen replacement, resulting in restoration of apoptotic potential and possible delay of progression to androgen independence.[68] TAB is used to reduce serum testosterone rapidly and induce tumor regression. From time to time, treatment is stopped and testosterone levels rise.[67] This cycle of treatment and no treatment is repeated until evidence by PSA of androgen independence (successive increases in PSA despite androgen suppression therapy).

An IAS protocol[69] was developed for the treatment of Stage D2 prostate cancer with adaptations for the treatment of initially localized prostate cancer that has recurred after

TABLE 11-8. Potential Advantages of Intermittent Androgen Suppression

Preservation of androgen sensitivity of tumor

Possible prolongation of survival

Improved quality of life

   Recovery of libido and erectile dysfunction

   Greater sense of well-being

Reduction of treatment costs

Increased chemosensitivity of tumors

Application in treating all stages of prostate cancer

Reprinted from *Urology*, 52, G. Theyer and G. Hamilton, Current status of intermittent androgen suppression in the treatment of prostate cancer, p. 358, with permission from Elsevier Science.

either radiation therapy or radical prostatectomy. Treatment was initiated with TAB and continued until the PSA was less than 4 μg/L. TAB was administered for an average of 9 months. Afterward, the medication was interrupted and PSA levels were monitored monthly. When the PSA level increased to a value between 10 and 20 μg/L for patients with metastatic disease or more than 4 μg/L for patients with localized disease, the medication was restarted.[69] In clinical trials using this protocol, the off-treatment periods have lasted up to 50 months. During this time, patients regained potency and libido.[69]

Prostate cancer patients who seem to benefit from IAS include those with increasing PSA but without symptoms and those with a low tumor burden.[68] Because of their inherent genetic instability, large or aggressive tumors accumulate androgen-resistant clones quickly.[68] IAS may not be able to reestablish androgen responsiveness.[68]

The potential advantages of IAS are summarized in Table 11-8. IAS remains under investigation to understand better the factors that determine response and duration of the off-treatment periods. This additional knowledge is necessary to identify those patients most suitable for IAS, which, at this point in time, is not recommended outside of a clinical trial.[68]

MONOTHERAPY

The use of monotherapy with the pure antiandrogens is attractive because these drugs have the potential to preserve potency by maintaining serum testosterone levels. However, simultaneously, there is also the issue that maintained serum testosterone levels may reduce the effectiveness of prostate cancer treatment. This is related to the suppression of relatively androgen-insensitive clones in a heterogeneous prostate carcinoma, permitting androgen-sensitive clones to proliferate because of inadequate competition for the androgen receptor.[1]

Flutamide has been evaluated as monotherapy is several Phase II studies, and clinical trials have used bicalutamide as monotherapy. Bicalutamide at a dose of 150 mg was found to be nearly equivalent to castration in patients with locally advanced disease.[70]

Bicalutamide studies are ongoing with higher doses, 300 mg and above, to determine whether it is equivalent to castration in metastatic prostate cancer.[19]

Thus far, antiandrogen monotherapy has not been shown to be equivalent to standard hormonal therapy with orchiectomy or LHRH analogues or to TAB in advanced prostate cancer.[1] Patients contemplating the potential risks and benefits of monotherapy need to understand that these uncertainties still exist.

CONCLUSION

Over the last decade, we have seen advances that have led to the earlier detection of prostate cancer and, in some instances, earlier intervention with hormonal therapy. Research continues to evolve, attempting to clarify the appropriate timing of intervention and identify the optimal type of hormonal manipulation. With the new millenium, there is renewed optimism that the continued challenges of prostate cancer management will be met with success.

REFERENCES

1. Brufsky A, Kantoff PW. Hormonal therapy for prostate cancer. In: Ernstoff MS, Heaney JA, Peschel RE (eds). *Urologic Cancer.* Cambridge, MA: Blackwell Science, 1997:160–180.
2. McLeod DG, Crawford ED, DeAntoni EP. Combined androgen blockade: The gold standard for metastatic prostate cancer. *Eur Urol* 1997;32(Suppl 3):70–77.
3. Anderson KM, Laio S. Selective retention of dihydrotestosterone by prostatic cell nuclei. *Nature* 1968; 219:277–278.
4. Veldscholte J, Berrevoets CA, Zegers ND, et al. Hormone-induced dissociation of the androgen receptor–heat-shock protein complex: Use of a new monoclonal antibody to distinguish transformed from nontransformed receptors. *Biochemistry* 1992; 31:7422–7430.
5. Davies P, Rushmere NK. Association of glucocorticoid receptors with prostate nuclear sites for androgen receptors and with androgen response elements. *J Mol Endocrinol* 1990;5:117–127.
6. Labrie F. Intracrinology. *Mol Cell Endocrinol* 1991; 78:C113–C118.
7. Geller J. Basis for hormonal management of advanced prostatic cancer. *Cancer* 1993;71:1039–1045.
8. Baird DT, Uno A, Melbe JC. Adrenal secretion of androgens and estrogens. *J Endocrinol* 1969;45: 135–136.
9. Harper ME, Pike A, Peeling WB, et al. Steroids of adrenal origin metabolized by human prostatic tissue both in vivo and in vitro. *J Endocrinol* 1974;60: 117–125.
10. Labrie F, Belanger A, Simard J, et al. Combination therapy for prostate cancer: Endocrine and biologic basis of its choice as new standard first-line therapy. *Cancer* 1993;71:1059–1067.
11. Lachance Y, Luu-The V, Labrie C, et al. Characterization of human 3-beta hydroxysteroid dehydrogenase/delta-5 isomerase gene and its expression in mammalian cells. *J Biol Chem* 1990;265:20469–20475.
12. Briehl MM, Miesfeld RL. Isolation and characterization of transcripts induced by androgen withdrawal and apoptotic cell death in the rat ventral prostate. *Mol Endocrinol* 1991;5:1381–1388.
13. Kyprianou N, Martikainen P, Davis L, et al. Programmed cell death as a new target for prostate cancer therapy. *Cancer Surv* 1991;11:265–277.
14. Martikainen P, Kyprianou N, Tucker RW, et al. Programmed death of nonproliferating androgen-independent prostate cancer cells. *Cancer Res* 1991;51: 4693–4700.
15. Berges RR, Furuya Y, Remington L, et al. Cell proliferation, DNA repair, and p53 function are not required for programmed death of prostatic glan-

dular cells induced by androgen withdrawal. *Proc Natl Acad Sci.* U S A 1993;90:8910–8914.

16. Labrie F, Dupont A, Belanger A, Lachance R. Flutamide eliminates the risk of disease flare in prostatic cancer patients treated with luteinizing hormone-releasing hormone agonist. *J Urol* 1987;138:804–806.

17. Millikan R, Logothetis C. Update of the NCCN guidelines for treatment of prostate cancer. *Oncology* 1997;11:180–193.

18. Bennett CL. Quoted in: Crawford ED. The role of antiandrogens in hormonal therapy: Part 2. Recorded symposium of the Societe Internationale d'Urologie, September 1997. *Comtemp Urol* July 1998;38–57.

19. Boccon-Gibod L. Quoted in: Crawford ED. The role of antiandrogens in hormonal therapy: Part 1. Recorded symposium of the Societe Internationale d'Urologie, September 1997. *Comtemp Urol* June 1998;43–57.

20. Blackledge G. Clinical progress with a new antiandrogen, Casodex (bicalutamide). *Eur Urol* 1996;29 (Suppl 2):96–104.

21. Bennett CL. Quoted in: Crawford ED. The role of antiandrogens in hormonal therapy: Part 1. Recorded symposium of the Societe Internationale d'Urologie, September 1997. *Comtemp Urol* June 1998;43–57.

22. Harris MG, Coleman SG, Faulds D, Chrisp P. Nilutamide: A review of its pharmacodynamic and pharmacokinetic properties, and therapeutic efficacy in prostate cancer. *Drugs & Aging* 1993;3:9–25.

23. Fradet Y. Quoted in: Crawford ED. The role of antiandrogens in hormonal therapy: Part 1. Recorded symposium of the Societe Internationale d'Urologie, September 1997. *Comtemp Urol* June 1998;43–57.

24. Crawford ED, Eisenberger MA, McLeod DG, et al. A controlled trial of leuprolide with and without flutamide in prostatic carcinoma. *N Engl J Med* 1989;321:419–424.

25. Geller J, Albert JD, Nachtsheim OA, et al. Comparison of prostate cancer tissue dihydrotestosterone levels at the time of relapse following orchiectomy or estrogen therapy. *J Urol* 1984;132:693–696.

26. Goethuys H, Baert L, Van Poppel H, et al. Treatment of metastatic cancer of the prostate. *Am J Clin Oncol* 1997;20:40–45.

27. Resnick, MI. Hormonal therapy in prostatic cancer. *Urology* 1984;24:18–23.

28. Beland G, Elhilali M, Fradet Y, et al. A controlled trial of castration with and without nilutamide in metastatic prostatic carcinoma. *Cancer* 1990:66:1074–1079.

29. Schellhammer PF, Sharifi R, Block NL, et al. Clinical benefits of bicalutamide compared with flutamide in combined androgen blockade for patients with advanced prostatic carcinoma: Final report of a double-blind, randomized, multicenter trial. *Urology* 1997;50:330–336.

30. Sarosdy MF, Schellhammer PF, Roohollah S, et al. Comparison of goserelin and leuprolide in combined androgen blockade therapy. *Urology* 1998;52:82–88.

31. Bennett. Quoted in: Brufsky A, Kantoff PW. Hormonal therapy for prostate cancer. In: Ernstoff MS, Heaney JA, Peschel RE, eds. *Urologic Cancer.* Cambridge, MA: Blackwell Science 1997:160–179.

32. Fair WR, Cookson MS, Stroumbakis N, et al. The indications, rationale, and results of neoadjuvant androgen deprivation in the treatment of prostatic cancer: Memorial Sloan-Kettering Cancer Center results. *Urology* 1997;49 (3A Suppl):46–55.

33. Bazinet M, Zheng W, Begin LR, et al. Morphologic changes induced by neoadjuvant androgen ablation may result in underdetection of positive surgical margins and capsular involvement by prostatic adenocarcinoma. *Urology* 1997;49:721–725.

34. Abbas F, Scardino PT. Why neoadjuvant androgen deprivation prior to radical prostatectomy is unnecessary. *Urol Clin North Am* 1996;23:587–604.

35. Roach M. Neoadjuvant therapy prior to radiotherapy for clinically localized prostate cancer. *Eur Urol* 1997:32(Suppl 3):48–54.

36. Pilepich MV, Sause WT, Shipley WU, et al. Androgen deprivation with radiation therapy compared with radiation therapy alone for locally advanced prostate carcinoma: A randomized comparative trial of the Radiation Therapy Oncology Group. *Urology* 1995;45:616–623.

37. Stock RG, Stone NN. The effect of prognostic factors on therapeutic outcome following transperineal prostate brachytherapy. *Semin Surg Oncol* 1997;13;454–460.

38. Van Aubel OG, Hoekstra W, Schroder FH. Early orchiectomy for patients with stage D1 prostate cancer. *J Urol* 1985;134:292–294.

39. Kramolowsky E. The value of testosterone deprivation in stage D1 carcinoma of the prostate. *J Urol* 1988;139:1242–1244.

40. Karling P, Hammar M, Varenhorst E. Prevalence and duration of hot flushes after surgical or medical castration in men with prostatic carcinoma. *J Urol* 1994:152:1170–1173.

41. Loprinzi CL, Michalak JC, Quella SK, et al. Megestrol acetate for the prevention of hot flashes. *N Engl J Med* 1994;331:347–352.

42. Quella SK, Loprinzi CL, Sloan JA, et al. Long term use of megestrol acetate by cancer survivors for the treatment of hot flashes. *Cancer* 1998;82:1784–1788.

43. Bressler LR, Murphy CM, Shevrin DH, Warren RF. Use of clonidine to treat hot flashes secondary to leuprolide or goserelin. *Ann Pharmacother* 1993;27: 182–185.

44. Parra RO, Gregory JG. Treatment of post-orchiectomy hot flashes with transdermal administration of clonidine. *J Urol* 1990;143:753.

45. Brosman SA. Depo-Provera as a treatment for "hot flashes" in men on androgen ablation therapy. Proceedings of the 90th annual meeting of the American Urological Association. [Abstract 877] *J Urol* 1995;153(4):448A.

46. Portenoy RK, Miaskowski C. Assessment and management of cancer-related fatigue. In: Berger AM, Portenoy RK, Weissman DE (eds). *Principles and Practice of Supportive Oncology*. Philadelphia, PA: Lippincott-Raven, 1998:109–118.

47. Bryant R, Boarini J. Treatment options for men with sexual dysfunction. *J ET Nurs* 1992;19:131–142.

48. Goldstein I, Lue TF, Padma-Nathan H, et al. Oral sildenafil in the treatment of erectile dysfunction *N Engl J Med* 1998;338:1397–1404.

49. Stepan JJ, Lachman M, Zverina J, et al. Castrated men exhibit bone loss: Effect of calcitonin treatment on biochemical indices of bone remodeling. *J Clin Endocrinol Metab* 1989;69:523–527.

50. Townsend MF, Sanders WH, Northway RO, Graham SD Jr. Bone fractures associated with luteinizing hormone-releasing hormone agonists used in the treatment of prostate carcinoma. *Cancer* 1997;79: 545–550.

51. Sisson de Castro JA. Alendronate treatment of osteoporosis in men: Short term bone mass response. *J Bone Miner Res* 1995;11(Suppl 1):341.

52. Daniell HW. Osteoporosis after orchiectomy for prostate cancer. *J Urol* 1997;157:439–444.

53. Isaacs JT, Coffey DS. Adaptation vs. selection as the mechanism responsible for the relapse of prostate cancer to androgen ablation as studied in the Dunning R-3327-H adenocarcinoma. *Cancer Res* 1981; 41:5070–5075.

54. Scher HI, Zhang ZF, Nanus D, Kelly WK. Hormone and antihormone withdrawal: Implications for the management of androgen-independent prostate cancer. *Urology* 1996;47:61–69.

55. Herrada J, Dieringer P, Logothetis CJ. Characteristics of patients with androgen-independent prostatic carcinoma whose serum prostate specific antigen decreased following flutamide withdrawal. *J Urol* 1996:155:620–623.

56. Figg WD, Sartor O, Cooper MR, et al. Prostate specific antigen decline following the discontinuation of flutamide in patients with stage D2 prostate cancer. *Am J Med* 1995;98:412–414.

57. Small EJ, Srinivas S. The antiandrogen withdrawal syndrome. *Cancer* 1995;76:1428–1434.

58. Small EJ, Schellhammer P, Venner G, et al. A double-blind assessment of antiandrogen withdrawal from casodex or eulexin therapy while continuing luteinizing hormone releasing hormone analogue therapy for patients with stage D2 prostate cancer [Abstract]. *Proc Am Soc Clin Oncol* 1996;15:255.

59. Smith DC. Secondary hormonal therapy. *Semin Urol Oncol* 1997;15:3–12.

60. Small EJ, Baron AD, Fippin L, Apodaca D. Ketoconazole retains activity in advanced prostate cancer patients with progression despite flutamide withdrawal. *J Urol* 1997;157:1204–1207.

61. Johansson JE, Andersson SO, Holmberg L. High-dose medroxyprogesterone acetate vs. estramustine in therapy-resistant prostate cancer. *Br J Urol* 1991;68:67–73.

62. Sasagawa I, Satomi S. Effect of high-dose medroxyprogesterone acetate on plasma hormone levels and pain relief in patients with advanced prostate cancer. *Br J Urol* 1990;65:278–281.

63. Bezwoda WR. Treatment of stage D2 prostate cancer refractory to or relapsed following castration plus estrogens. *Br J Urol* 190;66:196–201.

64. Dawson NA, Conway M, Winer EP, et al. A randomized study comparing standard vs. moderately high dose megestrol acetate in advanced prostate cancer: A Cancer and Leukemia Group B study [Abstract 618]. *Proc Am Soc Clin Oncol* 1995; 14:236.

65. Oh WK, Kantoff PW. Management of hormone refractory prostate cancer: Current standards and future prospects. *J Urol* 1998;160:1220–1229.

66. Ornstein DK, Rao GS, Johnson B, Charlton ET, and Andriole GL. Combined finasteride and flutamide therapy in men with advanced prostate cancer. *Urology* 1996;48:901–905.

67. Trachtenberg J. Innovative approaches to the hormonal treatment of advanced prostate cancer. *Eur Urol* 1997;32(Suppl 3):78–80.

68. Theyer G, Hamilton G. Current status of intermittent androgen suppression in the treatment of prostate cancer. *Urology* 1998;52:353–359.

69. Goldenberg SL, Bruchronsky N, Gleave ME, et al. Intermittent androgen suppression in the treatment of prostate cancer: A preliminary report. *Urology* 1995;47:956–961.

70. Boccon-Gibod L. Are non-steroidal anti-androgens appropriate as monotherapy in advanced prostate cancer? *Eur Urol* 1998;33:159–164.

Chapter 12

CHEMOTHERAPY FOR PROSTATE CANCER

JEANNE HELD-WARMKESSEL

OVERVIEW

INTRODUCTION
CHEMOTHERAPY
  Single-Agent Chemotherapy
    Mitoxantrone
    Estramustine
    Vinblastine
    Cyclophosphamide
    Doxorubicin
    Paclitaxel
    Docetaxel
    Etoposide
  Combination Chemotherapy
    Mitoxantrone

    Estramustine
    Suramin
    Cyclophosphamide
    Docetaxel
    Doxorubicin
TREATMENT OPTIONS AFTER
  CHEMOTHERAPY FAILURE
CHEMOTHERAPY CANDIDATES
PATIENT EDUCATION
NURSING MANAGEMENT
PSYCHOSOCIAL ISSUES
CONCLUSION

INTRODUCTION

Recurrent or progressive prostate cancer developing after local radiation therapy or hormonal manipulation is a treatment problem. Patients die of metastatic cancer, of cancer that is androgen independent, or of disease that is hormone refractory. The prognosis of hormone-resistant prostate cancer (HRPC) carries a median survival rate of 6 to 12 months. Historically, prostate cancer has been poorly responsive to single-agent chemotherapy. Extensive research has been done to develop treatment modalities for this patient population that will improve survival and quality of life. Recently, several drug regimens have been developed that may provide palliation. However, no current drug or combination of drugs has been shown to improve survival.[1] The majority of men with HRPC are elderly and have other health problems. Many have poor bone marrow reserve from prior radiation therapy to bone marrow or from bone marrow metastases. Thus, chemotherapy is poorly tolerated if it is attempted in the latest stages of disease after multiple fields of radiotherapy have been administered.[1]

Progressive prostate cancer is defined as worsening symptoms, increasing prostate-specific antigen (PSA), or increased disease on diagnostic studies. Pain is the predominant symptom requiring palliation in metastatic prostate cancer.[2] Patients may also develop urinary obstruction and anemia as a result of tumor involvement of the soft tissues, visceral organs, or bone.[2] Progressive disease is usually detected by increasing PSA level or worsening disease present on bone scan or other imaging studies, such as magnetic resonance imaging or computed tomography scan.[3] Increasing soft tissue masses and worsening symptoms such as increasing pain, weight loss, bladder outlet obstruction, or fatigue may also occur.[3]

HRPC research has been hampered by difficulty in evaluating patient response to treatment. One problem is that bone is the principal site of metastases in patients with prostate cancer. Measurement of tumor in bone has not been precise because of the lack of easily measurable lesions on radionucleotide bone scans and plain radiographs.[4] Monitoring the response of bone disease with bone scans and radiographs is difficult. Bone heals slowly, and long time frames elapse before improvement or deterioration can be identified with these diagnostic studies.[4] Therefore, surrogate endpoints may be used as an early measure of evaluating treatment outcome.[5] A surrogate endpoint is the use of something that is easy to measure in place of another endpoint that is less easy to measure. It may substitute for or predict the results of an intervention. PSA has been used as a surrogate endpoint to assess treatment effect in many clinical trials.[1] Drugs may impact PSA levels without impacting the patient's disease. Therefore, it is necessary to exercise caution when evaluating PSA results because they may not reflect changes in how the patient feels or in how the disease is responding to treatment.[1] For example, suramin may reduce PSA levels without impacting on tumor volume.[6] Other endpoints that are used to assess response to drug therapy include survival and tumor volume reduction.[7] Studies have also used palliative response as an objective endpoint of trial outcome. Pain assessment tools and quality of life instruments have been used to monitor the effect of treatment on patient symptoms.[8] Additional symptom palliation may include improved urinary symptoms, fatigue, and weight loss.

Another problem encountered in studying the past HRPC research is the use of old diagnostic tests to evaluate patient response to treatment. Before the discovery of PSA, prostatic acid phosphatase (PAP) levels were used to evaluate patient response. PAP has generally been abandoned as a test because it is less specific and less frequently abnormal compared with other available tests. PSA is now frequently used as a trial endpoint.[4] Therefore, making comparison between trials that used PAP and PSA as the endpoints is difficult.

Clinical studies need to describe clearly the hormonal status of the study group to assess therapeutic effectiveness.[4] Flutamide withdrawal syndrome can confound the results of any drug trial and needs to be controlled for in clinical trials. With flutamide withdrawal syndrome, the discontinuation of flutamide can result in reduced PSA levels, and produce symptom improvement and changes in tumor size.[9, 10] This phenomenon has subsequently been identified with other hormonal agents. Patients are now observed off antiandrogens before beginning a clinical trial to avoid this confounding variable from altering the outcome of the trial.[7] Otherwise, hormonal treatment may be continued. This information should be clearly described in the treatment section of the published report.

Prostate cancer may progress through four different phases of hormone responsiveness.[11] At first, prostate cancer responds to hormonal therapy. In the androgen-dependent phase, the removal of androgens and the administration of antiandrogens promote tumor regression. Androgen independence is demonstrated by progressive disease after orchiectomy or luteinizing hormone–releasing hormone (LHRH) agonist, combined androgen therapy, or second-line therapy with antiandrogens.[11] As time passes, the tumor becomes less sensitive to hormonal manipulation and usually becomes hormone resistant. Patients with hormone-refractory tumors have progressive disease that does not respond to antiandrogens, androgen elimination by orchiectomy or LHRH therapy, steroids to block adrenal production of androgens, total androgen blockage, or any combination of these.[11]

Patients being considered for palliative chemotherapy may have painful metastases or other symptoms compromising quality of life. Because hormonal therapies produce fewer toxic side effects and are often tolerated better, candidates for systemic chemotherapy should first be evaluated for true hormonal resistance with a determination of serum testosterone levels to ensure that castration levels have been achieved.[12] Additional hormonal manipulations may be tried before beginning chemotherapy.[12] First, the patient's current antiandrogen is discontinued. Then the patient is monitored, and, if there is no withdrawal response, a different hormonal manipulation trial may be administered[12] (see Chapter 11, Hormonal Therapy). The patient is again monitored for response to the second hormonal trial. On demonstration of disease progression and hormonal insensitivity, chemotherapy may be considered. In patients who have not undergone orchiectomy, hormonal manipulation with LHRH analogues to maintain testosterone castrate levels is usually continued throughout additional interventions because of the risk of increased PSA levels confounding treatment response.[12] This is a particularly important issue in clinical trials. However, continuing hormonal manipulation in patients who demonstrate insensitivity is a controversial issue because ineffective cancer treatments are usually discontinued.

Toxicity of chemotherapy has been a major concern, along with limited antitumor activity, in the use of this modality for symptom palliation of HRPC.[1] The decision to palliate distressing symptoms such as pain produced by HRPC needs to be balanced against the side effects resulting from chemotherapy administration. Therefore, the search for a safe, well-tolerated regimen that improves rather than worsens quality of life has been a major goal of clinical research. Until recently, this goal has not been realized. In the following section, current research studies used in the management and palliation of patients with HRPC are presented, including the use of the drugs as single agents followed by their use in combination chemotherapy. New directions and agents are briefly discussed.

TABLE 12-1. Single-Agent Chemotherapy Used in the Treatment of Prostate Cancer

Study	N	Major Endpoints	Treatment-Doses Administered
Raghavan et al[14]	50	Measurable disease Symptoms	Mitoxantrone, IV 12–14 mg/m^2 q21 days, no steroids
Iversen et al[16]	129	Clinical progression • Death Adverse events • PSA Subjective response	280 mg estramustine PO bid (daily total 560 mg) vs. placebo
Roth et al[26]	21 evaluable	Measurable disease	Paclitaxel, IV by continuous infusion 135–170 mg/m^2 q21 days
Hussain et al[29]	22	Measurable disease PSA	VP-16 PO 50 mg/m^2/day for 21 days, repeated q28 days
Rangel et al[24]	111 from two different studies; 54 patients received doxorubicin only and are reported here	Measurable disease PSA Subjective response	Doxorubicin, 20 mg/m^2 IV weekly
Schultz et al[28]	21 evaluable	PSA	Docetaxel, 75 mg/m^2 q21 days
Dexeus et al[21]	39	Subjective response Measurable disease	Vinblastine, 1.5 mg/m^2/day for 5 days by CI repeated q3–4 weeks
Raghaven et al[23]	30	Symptom reduction Survival	Cyclophosphamide, 100 mg/m^2/day for 14 days, repeated q28 days; dose reduced to 100 mg/day for patients with prior pelvic radiation therapy

CHEMOTHERAPY

SINGLE-AGENT CHEMOTHERAPY

Extensive research has been performed using single-agent chemotherapy with the goal of identifying drugs active in treating HRPC. Drugs currently being investigated are included in Table 12-1.

❏ Mitoxantrone

Structurally related to doxorubicin, mitoxantrone is an anthracenedione antineoplastic agent previously identified as having antiproliferative effects in a variety of

Major Findings	Major Toxicities
Disease stabilization, 52%; reduced pain, 38%; reduced symptoms, 46%; no CRs, no PRs; median survival, 10 months	Myelosuppression Nail thickening Subungual hematomas
Median survival: placebo, 6.1 months; estramustine, 9.4 months; $P = $ ns Subjective response: placebo, 7%; estramustine, 18%; $P = $ ns	Breast tenderness Gynecomastia Diarrhea
Median survival, 9 months; 1 PR; 4 stable disease with PSA reductions of 16–24%; 11 stable disease	Leukopenia • Granulocytopenic fever • Cardiovascular events, including two deaths • Rash
2 PRs; minimally active drug; median survival, 31 weeks	Anemia • Granulocytopenia • Thrombocytopenia
Clinical improvement, 69%	Leukopenia • Alopecia • Mucositis • Cardiotoxicity
PRs, 24%	Fatigue • Stomatitis • Small bowel obstruction • Gluteal abscess • Death from lung toxicity-pneumonia, pulmonary embolus in two patients • Neutropenia • Anemia • Mild edema • Anorexia • Myalgia • Alopecia • Steroid-induced hyperglycemia
21% objective response median duration of response 28 weeks	Cardiac arrhythmias • Myelosuppression
Median survival from onset of treatment, 12.7 months; symptom reduction, 60%	Nausea • Vomiting • Anemia • Myelosuppression

IV, intravenous; PSA, prostate-specific antigen; NS, not significant; CI, continuous infusion; bid, twice daily.

tumors, including prostate cancer.[1] The usual dose is 12 to 14 mg/m^2 intravenously (IV) once every 3 weeks. Myelosuppression is the dose-limiting toxicity (DLT). Other less common side effects are mild nausea and vomiting, mouth sores, fatigue, and alopecia.[13] Patients need to be aware that their urine may turn a blue-green color from the drug.

A Phase II trial of mitoxantrone in the dosing schedule just mentioned was conducted in Australia from 1985 to 1986[14] (see Table 12-1). The importance of this trial is the demonstration of reduced symptoms and improved quality of life. Additionally, 52% of the patients experienced stabilization of disease. The authors concluded that mitoxantrone has activity against HRPC because of its ability to improve quality of life related to cancer-induced symptoms.[14]

❏ Estramustine

Estramustine, a combination of nornitrogen mustard and estradiol, is an antimitotic agent that has been studied extensively alone and in combination with other drugs. Like other single agents, it has not been shown to improve survival in patients with HRPC.[15] In one double-blind, randomized multicenter trial, estramustine produced a response rate similar to that of placebo[16] (see Table 12-1). Nonstatistically significant improvements were noted in survival, and improved subjective response also was found in the group receiving estramustine. Patients receiving estramustine had longer survival (> 11.6 months) if the PSA level was reduced by more than 25% when measured at 1-month follow-up ($P = .001$).[16] This trial demonstrated the ability of estramustine to impact the survival of a group of patients. The patients who were long-term survivors could be identified by early reduction in PSA level.[16]

Estramustine binds to tubulin and microtubule-associated proteins, thereby inhibiting microtubule function and mitosis.[17, 18] Unlike other antimicrotubule drugs such as vinblastine, paclitaxel, and docetaxel, it is rarely myelosuppressive. Thus, it is appropriate to combine it with other microtubule agents.[19, 20]

❏ Vinblastine

Vinblastine, a plant alkaloid, has also been investigated as a single agent in the treatment of HRPC.[21] Vinblastine produced improvements in pain, measurable disease in bone and soft tissue, and performance status. Side effects include neutropenia and neurotoxicity.

❏ Cyclophosphamide

Cyclophosphamide is a commercially available alkylating agent that comes in both oral and intravenous formulations. Side effects include myelosuppression, nausea, vomiting, hemorrhagic cystitis, alopecia, and nail changes.[22] Oral tablets should be taken early in the day with large amounts of water to enhance excretion, promote voiding, and prevent bladder irritation. Oral antiemetics are useful for patients experiencing nausea, and parenteral antiemetics are needed to manage vomiting. Low-dose oral cyclophosphamide may produce hair thinning as opposed to IV dosing, which often causes greater hair loss. Caps and hats will help keep the head warm and prevent excess heat loss. Patient education includes being aware of the need to notify the physician of signs and symptoms indicative of neutropenia or thrombocytopenia such as fever, chills, or bleeding and hemorrhagic cystitis. Oral cyclophosphamide has been studied in patients with HRPC. An early study reported overall response rate of 59% with improvement in symptoms such as pain.[23]

❏ Doxorubicin

Doxorubicin is an anthracycline antitumor antibiotic. Common side effects include red urine, alopecia, bone marrow depression, dose-limiting cardiotoxicity, mucositis, nausea, vomiting, and tissue damage with drug extravasation.[22] Patients receiving doxorubicin experienced weight gain, less pain, and increased appetite.[24]

❏ Paclitaxel

Paclitaxel also interferes with mitotic spindle action. Side effects include neutropenia, peripheral neuropathy, myalgias, arthralgias, hypersensitivity reactions, and bradycardia.[25] The drug is administered using glass, polypropylene, or other nonplastic container with a 0.2 μm in-line filter through non-polyvinyl chloride tubing. Premedications consisting of dexamethasone, 20 mg; diphenhydramine, 50 mg intravenously; plus cimetidine, 300 mg IV; or another histamine-2 blocker are administered 30 minutes before paclitaxel to reduce the incidence and severity of hypersensitivity reactions. As a single agent, however, paclitaxel given every 3 weeks by 24-hour infusion had little activity in HRPC.[26]

❏ Docetaxel

Docetaxel is a second taxane that interferes with mitotic spindle function.[22] Side effects include neutropenia, which is the dose-limiting toxicity, hypersensitive reactions, rash, alopecia, peripheral edema, and pleural effusion.[27] Premedication with steroids is required before administration to reduce the incidence of fluid retention. Hypotension may occur in some patients, so blood pressure should be checked before and after the infusion and as needed if hypotension is suspected. The patient should be weighed before each infusion to monitor for fluid retention. Hepatic enzymes are monitored before treatment because abnormal results are reasons for dose modifications. Docetaxel has been used in a clinical trial of men with HRPC. Side effects are significant at this dose (see Table 12-1) when administered to this patient population.[28]

❏ Etoposide

Etoposide (VP-16) inhibits topoisomerase II, resulting in DNA single-strand breaks and failure of cells to enter mitosis.[22] Etoposide side effects include allergic reactions, bone marrow depression, anorexia, nausea, vomiting, alopecia, and peripheral neuropathy. As a single agent, oral etoposide produces minimal response in the treatment of HRPC.[29]

Review of these single-agent trials sheds light on some potential areas for combining agents with the goal of improving symptom management. This next section addresses combination therapy.

COMBINATION CHEMOTHERAPY

❏ Mitoxantrone

One agent that has generated encouraging results is mitoxantrone. Up to 46% of patients receiving single-agent mitoxantrone experienced a palliative response with reduced pain and a reduction in other symptoms.[14] To enhance this effect or to prolong

TABLE 12-2. Mitoxantrone-Based Studies

Study	N	Major Endpoints	Treatment-Doses Administered
Moore et al[31]	27	Palliative response: pain, quality of life	Mitoxantrone, 12 mg/m2 IV q21 days with dose escalation by 2 mg/m^2 if nadir ANC > 1.0 × 109/L and platelets > 50 × 109/L at nadir, plus Prednisone, 5 mg bid
Tannock et al[8]	161 Phase III	Pain relief, Reduced analgesic scores	Mitoxantrone, 12 mg/m^2 IV q21 days Prednisone, 5 mg bid vs. Prednisone, 5 mg bid alone
Kantoff et al[32]	242	Survival Quality of life	Hydrocortisone, 40 mg/day with or without mitoxantrone, 14 mg/m^2 q21 days
Cohn et al[33]	10 preliminary results at 10 mg/m^2 mitoxantrone	PSA	Strontium 89 4 mCi IV q12 weeks. Escalating dose of mitoxantrone 10, 12, 14, 16 mg/m^2 q21 days beginning Day 22; hydrocortisone, 40 mg PO daily
Levine et al[34]	28 15, Arm I 13, Arm II	Response rate Response durability Safety	Mitoxantrone, 21 mg/m^2 IV q21 days (Arm I). History of pelvic radiation therapy–mitoxantrone, 17 mg/m^2 IV q21 days (Arm II) plus hydrocortisone, 40 mg PO daily, plus GM-CSF beginning Day 3 and given until ANC ≥ 1,500/mm^3 after Day 12
DeConti, et al[35]	14 evaluable	PSA Measurable disease Pain Quality of life	Mitoxantrone, 12 mg/m^2, plus paclitaxel, 175 mg/m^2 q21 days GM-CSF until ANC 1,500/mL

survival, other agents have been added. Prednisone has been used to manage HRPC with approximately a 32% response rate.[30] These agents have been combined in several studies (Table 12-2).

A Phase II nonrandomized multicenter trial examined the effect of the addition of 10 mg prednisone (5 mg twice daily) to 12 mg/m^2 IV mitoxantrone given every 3 weeks to hormone-refractory patients with metastatic or locally advanced disease[31] (see Table 12-2). The purpose of the trial was to evaluate the ability of mitoxantrone and prednisone to palliate patient symptoms. Survival was not the major emphasis of this study, although it was reported. This trial demonstrated that the addition of low-dose prednisone to mitoxantrone is well tolerated, improves quality of life, and reduces symptoms in responding patients. It also demonstrated that palliative response criteria can be used as endpoints in HRPC clinical trials.[31] Treatment can still be beneficial even though survival is not extended.

Major Findings	Major Toxicities
Palliative CR, 16%; palliative PR, 20%; stable disease, 41%; median survival, 5.7 months	Nausea, Neutropenia, Alopecia, Anorexia, Constipation
Mitoxantrone-prednisone responses, 29%; Prednisone alone, 12% ($P = .01$). Response duration: Mitoxantrone-prednisone, 43 weeks; Prednisone, 18 weeks ($P < .0001$). Mitoxantrone-prednisone response, 38%; Prednisone response, 21%; no effect on survival in either group	Nausea, Vomiting, Hair loss, Neutropenic fever Cardiac toxicity with cumulative doses of 116–214 mg/m^2 mitoxantrone
Median survival not affected 10.9 months (Mitoxantrone-hydrocortisone) vs. 11.8 months (hydrocortisone); pain level improved	Myelotoxicity
3/8 evaluable patients had reduced PSA levels	Thrombocytopenia
PR, 2 0%, arm I; PR, 17%, arm II All PSA alone	Neutropenic infection Granulocytopenia Thrombocytopenia Anemia
Median survival > 11 months; responses, > 50% improvement in PSA, 64%; pain, 77%	Anaphylaxis Myelotoxicity Neutropenic fever Neurotoxicity

ANC, absolute neutrophil count; bid, twice daily; CR, complete response; PR, partial response; IV, intravenous; GM-CSF, granulocyte-macrophage colony-stimulating factor; PO, orally.

After the Phase II trial, a Phase III prospective, randomized multicenter trial was done to examine the palliative endpoints of prednisone with or without mitoxantrone.[8] All patients in the study had pain. To be defined as achieving a palliative complete response (CR), the patient needed to achieve and maintain a decrease in pain for two consecutive evaluations, with each evaluation 3 weeks apart. Pain was assessed using the McGill-Melzack Pain Questionnaire. Reduction in pain by 2 points on a 6-point scale was required. Androgen ablative treatment continued throughout the trial. The same doses of prednisone and mitoxantrone (initial dose of 12 mg/m^2) were administered as previously described. Of the 161 patients entered into the trial, 80 received mitoxantrone and prednisone (MP) and 81 received prednisone alone. Twenty-three of the 80 patients (29%) receiving MP and 10 of the 81 patients (12%) receiving prednisone alone responded to treatment ($P = .01$).[8] The patients receiving both drugs had a 43-week duration of response versus 18 weeks in responding patients receiving prednisone alone ($P < .0001$).[8]

A second palliative endpoint in this trial was defined as a 50% reduction in analgesic score and no increase in pain level. Seven patients in each group fit this secondary response. In total, 38% of patients in the MP group and 21% of patients in the prednisone group responded with a palliative outcome.[8] There was a trend toward improved quality of life in the MP group in terms of pain, mood, physical activity, and constipation.

This trial demonstrated that MP is better than prednisone alone in disease palliation. Response duration was also improved in the mitoxantrone group. The cross-over design of the trial may have interfered with the ability to detect an effect on survival. Side effects were greater in the mitoxantrone group. Prednisone produced few side effects except in one patient with diabetes who stopped the drug because of toxicity.

A larger prospective, randomized trial of 242 patients using hydrocortisone (40 mg/day) with or without mitoxantrone (14 mg/m^2 every 3 weeks) has been reported in abstract form.[32] Pain was not a requirement for eligibility. There was no cross-over included in the trial, and quality of life was the secondary endpoint; survival was the primary endpoint. There was no statistically significant difference in survival between the two arms, but the patients receiving mitoxantrone had better pain control (level of significance not reported).[32] Myelotoxicity was greater in the mitoxantrone group. To assess quality of life, five assessment tools were used: FLIC, Symptom Distress Scale, Sexual and Urologic Functioning, Problems of Daily Activities, and Impact of Pain on Daily Activities.

Together, the mitoxantrone-steroid trials establish a role for chemotherapy in the palliative treatment of patients with HRPC, although neither trial demonstrated improved survival. Median survival ranged from 5.7 to 11.8 months.[31, 32]

In an attempt to increase the effectiveness of mitoxantrone and hydrocortisone, modification of this drug combination has been studied. In one trial, strontium 89 (4 mCi every 12 weeks) was given before mitoxantrone. In a preliminary report, 10 patients have been accrued and are reported to have complete pain relief and no longer require narcotics.[33] Thrombocytopenia has been severe and may limit the usefulness of this combination therapy.

Increasing the dose of mitoxantrone has also been evaluated. A trial was initiated to investigate the ability to increase the response rate, improve response duration, and determine the safety of high-dose mitoxantrone in patients with HRPC. Granulocyte-macrophage colony-stimulating factor (GM-CSF) was added. All responses to date (4 in 28 patients) have been partial responses (PR) with only reductions in PSA (response defined as reduction of PSA $\geq$ 75%). Further patient accrual will be necessary before the results can be analyzed. Thrombocytopenia has caused 14% of patients to withdraw from the study.[34]

Paclitaxel has also been added to mitoxantrone with GM-CSF support given every 3 weeks to assess drug synergy in HRPC.[35] The addition of paclitaxel increased the severity of bone marrow depression and neurotoxicity. The authors concluded that the combination of paclitaxel and mitoxantrone is useful in HRPC, but reduced doses should be used or docetaxel should replace paclitaxel.[35] However, single-agent docetaxel may also produce significant toxicity in this patient population (see Table 12-1).

❑ Estramustine

Estramustine and paclitaxel, both antimicrotubule agents, have been investigated for synergy in the laboratory.[20] Cell cultures were exposed to both drugs for 10 days. To approximate these laboratory conditions in the clinical setting, a 96-hour continuous infusion of paclitaxel was used with daily oral estramustine.[36] A Phase I trial using oral estramustine (600 mg/m^2/day in two or three divided doses beginning 24 hours before the paclitaxel infusion) in combination with paclitaxel was initiated.[19] The maximum tolerated dose (MTD) of paclitaxel was determined to be 140 mg/m^2, and the dose selected for a Phase II trial was 120 mg/m^2.[19, 36] All patients received prepaclitaxel medications (dexamethasone, 20 mg IV; cimetidine, 300 mg IV; and diphenhydramine, 50 mg IV) 30 minutes before initiation of the paclitaxel infusion (Table 12-3).

The follow-up Phase II study of this combination was completed in 1996.[36] Estramustine was given daily at the prior dosage along with paclitaxel, 120 mg/m^2 IV over 96 hours every 3 weeks. The same premedications were administered except the dose of dexamethasone was reduced to 10 mg. Androgen suppression was continued in the form of LHRH agonists in nonorchiectomy patients. Of the 34 patients entered on the study, 33 were evaluated for response and side effects.[36] The overall response rate was 30.3% (9 PRs, 1 CR) lasting an average of 9 months. Side effects included mild to moderate nausea, fluid retention, and gynecomastia from estramustine, and leukopenia, diarrhea, and stomatitis from paclitaxel. Fatigue and abnormal liver function tests could be attributed to both drugs. The effectiveness of this regimen in HRPC cannot be evaluated further without a prospective, randomized trial; however, this was not recommended by the authors.[36] Rather, they suggested pursuing additional studies of estramustine and paclitaxel to improve the ability to deliver the regimen to outpatients. Replacement of the 96-hour infusion of paclitaxel by a 1- to 3-hour weekly infusion and the development of the IV formulation of estramustine, which may be less toxic than the oral formulation, were the suggested modifications.[36]

The first recommended follow-up study was to shorten the paclitaxel infusion and administer it weekly.[37] A Phase I trial was initiated, and preliminary results have been published in abstract form. The estramustine dose was 600 mg/m^2 daily for 6 weeks. The dose of paclitaxel started at 60 mg/m^2/week IV and increased to 118 mg/m^2/week. Each cycle lasted 6 weeks followed by a 2-week rest. The MTD was estimated to be approximately 92 mg/m^2 when given with estramustine, 600 mg/m^2 daily for 6 weeks. DLTs included hepatotoxicity and myocardial infarction at the 118 mg/m^2 dose.[37] A Phase II trial of a similar regimen has been initiated using paclitaxel, 90 mg/m^2 weekly, by 1-hour infusion with oral estramustine.*

Oral estramustine often produces dose-limiting nausea and cardiovascular side effects related to hepatic metabolism of the oral drug.[36] It was hypothesized that an IV formulation would have less toxicity because of reduced or eliminated first-pass metabolic effect by the liver on the drug. In a Phase I trial, estramustine was administered IV weekly over 30 minutes in doses starting at 500 mg/m^2 and increasing by 500 mg/m^2 to a maxi-

*Information obtained from Fox Chase Cancer Center, Philadelphia (www.fccc.edu).

TABLE 12-3. Estramustine-Based Studies

Study	N	Major Endpoints	Treatment-Doses Administered
Hudes et al[19]	18 evaluable, 2 patients with prostate cancer and 2 additional patients treated off study	Response Toxicity	Estramustine, 600 mg/m² PO daily, beginning 24 h before paclitaxel infusion. Dose of paclitaxel increased from 80 to 140 mg/m² IV repeated q21 days, dose infused over 96 h. Prepaclitaxel medications administered
Hudes et al[36]	33 evaluable	Measurable disease PSA	Estramustine, 600 mg/m² PO daily, beginning 24 h before paclitaxel infusion; paclitaxel, 120 mg/m² IV over 96 h q21 days. Prepaclitaxel medications given
Garay et al[37]	8 evaluable for response	Measurable disease PSA	Estramustine, 600 mg/m² PO for 6 weeks; paclitaxel, escalating dose 60 to 118 mg/m²/wk over 3 h
Haas et al[38]	9	PSA	Estramustine, IV at 500, 1,000, or 1,500 mg/m² weekly × 4 weeks
Kelly et al[39]	5 (androgen independent)	Measurable disease PSA	Estramustine, 10 mg/kg, plus carboplatin at 0 or 6 AUC plus paclitaxel, 60, 80, or 100 mg/m²
Petrylak et al[40]	34 evaluable for toxicity, 33 evaluable for response	PSA	Estramustine, 280 mg PO tid Days 1–5 Docetaxel given at 4 dose levels on Day 2; 40 mg/m²; 60 mg/m²; 70 mg/m²; 80 mg/m² Dexamethasone, 20 mg, given 6 and 12 h and 15 min before docetaxel repeated q21 days
Attivissimo et al[41]	15	Measurable disease PSA	Vinblastine, 4 mg/m² IV weekly × 6 weeks; estramustine, 10 mg/kg PO in three divided doses × 6 weeks; Repeated q8 weeks
Hudes et al[42]	36	Measurable disease PSA	Estramustine, 600 mg/m² PO in three divided doses × 42 days, plus vinblastine, 4 mg/m² IV weekly × 6 weeks; repeated q8 weeks

mum of 1,500 mg/m².[38] Nine of 11 men with metastatic HRPC completed a minimum of one 4-week cycle. Side effects included transient rectal burning during the first treatment, nausea, thrombocytopenia, and thrombophlebitis. There were no Grade 3 or 4 toxicities. The authors reported that IV estramustine is well tolerated at dosages of up to 1,500 mg/m² weekly, and the study is ongoing. Dosages of 1,500 to 2,000 mg/m² weekly will be needed to produce plasma levels similar to those obtained with an oral dose of 300 mg/m² twice daily (G. Hudes, personal communication, January 1999).[38]

Oral estramustine and IV paclitaxel (EP) have also been investigated with the addition of carboplatin to enhance their effectiveness. In a preliminary report of this three-drug combination, 60% of patients with androgen-independent disease had significant declines of PSA.[39] The authors concluded that this regimen was safe at the doses administered (see Table 12-3). A randomized trial is required to determine whether the addition of carboplatin to EP is superior to EP alone.

Major Findings	Major Toxicities
2 PR in 2 patients 1, normalization of PSA and improved functioning; 1, 20% decrease in PSA and complete pain relief	Granulocytopenia (DLT), Sepsis, Mucositis (DLT), Hepatic enzyme elevations, Nausea
Median overall survival, 69 weeks; overall response rate, 9 PR, 1 CR	Nausea, Fluid retention, Fatigue, Leukopenia, Thrombocytopenia, Anemia
Measurable disease 3 PR; 5/8 with ≥ 75% PSA decrease	Nausea, Hepatotoxicity, MI, Edema
1/7 patients with > 50% PSA reduction	Transient rectal burning, Thrombophlebitis, Nausea
3/5 patients with > 50% reduction in PSA	Neutropenia
Overall PSA response, 63%; reduced analgesic requirements, 53%; measurable disease, 28%, PR	Fluid retention, Transaminitis, Granulocytopenia, Neutropenic fever, Nausea, Vomiting, Hyperbilirubinemia, CVA, DVT, Extravasation
0 CRs, 5 PRs, 1 stable disease; overall response, 40%; less pain in PRs; median survival in responders, 11.7 mo and in nonresponders, 13.2 mo (P = ns)	Minor only
≥ 50% PSA reduction, 61.1%; ≥ 75% PSA reduction, 22.9%; PRs, 11/36; > 50% reduction in pain or analgesic use, 42.9%; overall response, 58.3%	Leukopenia, Nausea, Leg edema, MI, DVT, TIA. Ileus

PSA, prostate-specific antigen; PO, orally; IV, intravenous; AUC, area under the curve; tid, three times daily; DLT, dose-limiting toxicity; PR, partial response; CR,complete response; ns, not significant; MI, myocardial infarction; CVA, cerebrovascular accident; DVT, deep vein thrombosis; TIA, transient ischemic attack; h, hour; wk, week; mo, month..

Oral estramustine has also been combined with the other taxane, docetaxel.[40] Two groups of androgen-independent patients were included in this trial. One group consisted of patients who had undergone fewer than two prior chemotherapy treatments, no more than 2 radiation therapy treatments, no prior radioisotope therapy, and no prior whole pelvic RT. The second group consisted of patients who had more extensive treatment. The 1-year survival rate is 68%. Side effects were tolerable. This combination produced a reduction in PSA, pain, and measurable disease. This promising Phase I trial deserves further evaluation.

Vinblastine is another vinca alkaloid antimitotic agent that has been used in combination with estramustine. These drugs have been used together in patients with HRPC[41, 42] (see Table 12-3). This regimen reduces symptoms but does not impact on survival.

TABLE 12-4. Oral Estramustine and Oral Etoposide Studies

Study	N	Major Endpoints	Treatment-Doses Administered
Pienta et al[44]	42	Measurable disease PSA	Estramustine, PO 15 mg/kg/day in four divided doses, plus VP-16, PO 50 mg/m²/day in two divided doses on Days 1–21
Pienta et al[45]	62	Measurable disease PSA	Estramustine, PO 10 mg/kg/day in three divided doses, plus VP-16, PO 50 mg/m²/day in two divided doses on Days 1–21 repeated q28 days
Dimopoulos et al[47]	56	Measurable disease PSA	Estramustine, 140 mg PO tid Days 1–21, plus VP-16 PO 50 mg/m²/day; repeated q28 days
Pienta et al[50]	23	Measurable disease PSA	Estramustine, PO 10 mg/kg/day for 14 days, plus VP-16 PO 50 mg/m²/day for 14 days plus paclitaxel, 135 mg/m² IV over 1 h on Day 2 with premeds; repeated q21 days
Colleoni et al[49]	25	Objective response	Estramustine, PO 400 mg/m² in three divided doses for 6 weeks, plus VP–16, PO 50 mg/m² on Days 1–14 and 28–42, plus vinorelbine, 20 mg/m² on Days 1, 8, 28, 35

Estramustine has also been studied in combination with oral etoposide both in vitro and in vivo using animals.[43] To test the observation that the combination of oral estramustine and oral etoposide have synergy against HRPC, a Phase II clinical trial was performed[44] (Table 12-4). A CR was defined as absence of disease, and a PR was defined as a reduction in size of the largest tumor of at least 50% for two evaluations of disease status 8 weeks apart. There were 3 CRs and 6 PRs in 18 patients with measurable soft tissue lesions, and the drug combination produced an overall response in 15 patients (36%) with bone or soft tissue disease. Responses included improvements in soft tissue and bone scans and reduced PSA levels. Performance status at the time of study entry was a predictor of survival. Using the Zubrod performance status scale, patients with a PS of 0 to 1 (ambulatory) lived longer than those with a PS of 2 to 3 (minimally ambulatory to non-ambulatory) (40 weeks vs. 12 weeks) ($P = .0001$)].[44] It is important to recognize that this is a nonrandomized Phase II trial.

Nausea is a serious problem with doses of estramustine in the range of 15 mg/kg or 600 mg/m² daily taken continuously, causing some patients to discontinue the drug. It was hypothesized that a lower dosage of estramustine (10 mg/kg/day) divided into three doses would produce less nausea and yet not affect the outcome of the previous etoposide-estramustine trials.[45] Sixty-two patients with HRPC and rising PSA levels off flutamide therapy received the lower dose of oral estramustine and the same dose of oral etoposide (50 mg/m²/day) as noted previously.[45] Nausea occurred in 24% of patients, causing 3 to withdraw from trial. As in the previous trial, patients with a good PS (0–1) lived longer than those with a poor PS (2–3).[44, 45] A 50% or greater reduction in PSA levels from baseline pretreatment level at 8 weeks was also associated with longer survival.[46] Nausea persists in being a problem even at this lower dose. The actual dose and number of days of

Major Findings	Major Toxicities
38% overall response rate; measurable disease response rate, 50%; median survival, 44 weeks; responders had improved survival	Alopecia, Leukopenia, Neutropenic fever, Bone marrow failure, DVT, CHF, Nausea, Allergic reactions, Cardiac-related death
Overall response rate for measurable disease, 53%; > 50% decrease in PSA, 39%; median survival, 56 weeks; PS 0–1 survival, 64 week; PS 2–3 survival, 48 weeks (P=.042)	Alopecia, Leukopenia, Neutropenic fever, Thrombocytopenia, DVT, Lower extremity edema
Measurable disease, 5 CR and 10 PR, 45% response rate, 58% PSA response rate	Neutropenia, Anemia, Thrombocytopenia, Alopecia, Nausea, Vomiting
Soft tissue disease response, 1 CR/7, 3 PR/7; decrease in PSA by > 50%, 13/23	Alopecia, Neutropenia, Asthenia
32% response rate, 8 PRs, 6 stable disease; ≥ 50% PSA reduction in 14/25; median survival, 11.7 mo	Neutropenia, Leukopenia, DVT, Anemia, Thrombocytopenia

PSA, prostate-specific antigen; PO, orally; DVT, deep vein thrombosis; CHF, congestive heart failure; tid, three times daily; IV, intravenous; premeds, premedications; CR, complete response; PR, partial response.

estramustine required for HRPC may not be this high. Current research trials are investigating lower doses or fewer days of estramustine to reduce the incidence of nausea and vomiting and improve patient tolerance without reducing the response rate.

Research into the oral etoposide-oral estramustine combination in patients with HRPC produces response rates in approximately 39 to 45% of patients.[45, 47] This combination may be an alternate treatment to the mitoxantrone-steroid combination for men with HRPC.[48] Other active combinations that may be useful include oral estramustine and paclitaxel or oral estramustine, oral etoposide, and paclitaxel.

Additional chemotherapeutic drugs have been added to the oral estramustine-oral etoposide duo, including vinorelbine and paclitaxel. Vinorelbine, 20 mg/m[2], and oral etoposide, 50 mg/m[2], were added to weekly estramustine, 400 mg/m[2], for 6 weeks to produce an overall response rate of 32%.[49] A higher response (57%) rate was seen with the addition of paclitaxel, 135 mg/m[2], on Day 2 to estramustine, 10 mg/kg/day for 14 days, and oral etoposide, 50 mg/m[2]/day for 14 days, although the results are preliminary.[50] Phase III trials are needed to determine the place of the estramustine-based combinations compared with mitoxantrone-steroid combinations.

Nausea is a problem for many patients taking oral estramustine. Patient education should include instruction to avoid taking the drug with food and dairy products because both interfere with drug absorption.[36] Antiemetics such as prochlorperazine, 10 mg, may be useful when given before meals.[45] It may be necessary to reduce the number of days of treatment or reduce drug dosage to improve tolerance.[47] When used in combination with paclitaxel and etoposide, signs and symptoms of neutropenia and neutropenic fever require prompt physician notification. Patients need to be aware of self-care management for fatigue and nausea. Drug-related leg edema is different from a deep vein thrombosis that requires anticoagulation therapy. Patients must be aware that they are not qualified to determine the difference between the two problems and need to seek medical intervention even if leg edema is bilateral. Diuretics may be useful in the management of leg edema.[45]

☐ Suramin

Suramin, an investigational agent, is a polysulfonated naphthylurea, which inhibits cellular growth factors and may, therefore, interfere with the growth of cancer cells.[51] Side effects include skin rash, edema, glucocorticoid insufficiency requiring hydrocortisone replacement, paresthesias, fatigue, malaise, anorexia, and renal impairment.[51, 52] Less common toxicities include mineralocorticoid insufficiency,[53] suramin keratosis,[54] and reversible acute renal failure.[55, 56] The development of severe sensorimotor polyneuropathy appears to be related to drug plasma concentrations. Limiting suramin drug dose to ≤157 mg/kg over 8 weeks, limiting the period of time plasma is exposed to more than 200 µg/mL of drug, and keeping the drug area under the curve to less than 200 µg/mL have been identified as useful steps in reducing toxicity.[57] Bleeding related to drug-induced coagulopathies can be managed with vitamin K supplements.[58]

Many suramin toxicities have been related to its long half-life of 55 days. This, along with the development of serious side effects when the plasma drug concentration exceeds 300 µg/mL, has made dosing and scheduling of drug administration complicated and time consuming.[59, 60] Numerous trials have been completed to identify the least toxic, most effective, easiest, and least complicated method of suramin administration. Many regimens have used intermittent piggyback administration of a test dose, a loading dose, and then infusions on several subsequent days or weeks.[61–64] A common drug schedule is a 200-mg test dose over 30 minutes followed by 1,000 mg/m^2 over 2 hours.[60, 61] With some regimens, on the following Days 2 to 5, lower doses are administered (400, 300, 250, 200 mg/m^2).[62]

A Phase III trial completed enrollment of patients to identify a fixed dose of suramin that would be appropriate in the treatment of HRPC.[65] Patients receive one of three fixed-dose regimens, which deliver lower doses of drug on the subsequent days of the 28-day cycle. This multiinstitution prospective, randomized trial should answer many questions about the safety, efficacy, dosing schedule, and toxicity of suramin.

In spite of the controversy regarding the best dose and scheduling sequence, multiple trials have been done to assess the effect of suramin on HRPC. Only one Phase III trial involving 458 patients has been completed and reported in abstract form. Men with HRPC, progressive disease, and bone pain requiring narcotics received either suramin and hydrocortisone or hydrocortisone alone. Patients receiving suramin and hydrocortisone had a better pain response ($P = .001$), longer pain relief (240 days vs. 69 days, $P = .0027$), and better PSA response (32% vs. 16%, $P = .001$).[66] Grades 3 and 4 side effects included peripheral edema, weakness, fatigue, anemia, dyspnea, neuropathy, coagulopathy, renal impairment, neutropenia, and thrombocytopenia. The authors concluded that

TABLE 12-5. Cyclophosphamide-Based Studies

Study	N	Major Endpoints	Treatment-Doses Administered	Major Findings	Major Toxicities
Maulard-Durdux et al[69]	20	Measurable disease, PSA	Cyclophosphamide, PO 100 mg/day, plus VP-16, PO 50 mg/day for 14 days; repeated q28 days	PSA, overall response 35%; bone pain, overall response rate 71%; median survival, 11 mo	No major
Small et al[68]	35	Measurable disease, PSA	Doxorubicin, 40 mg/m^2, plus cyclophosphamide, 800–2,000 mg/m^2, dependent on cohort (determined by prior radiation therapy) plus G-CSF, 5 μg/kg on Days 2–10 and ANC > 10,000/μL	Measurable disease response, 33%; median survival, 11 mo; PSA response, 46%; PSA >50% reduction, 23-mo survival; no PSA response, 7-mo survival (P=.02)	Neutropenia, Anemia, Thrombocytopenia

PSA, prostate-specific antigen; G-CSF, granulocyte colony-stimulating factor; ANC, absolute neutrophil count; mo, month.

suramin and hydrocortisone provide palliation and delay the disease progression. The relative risk of disease progression was 1.0 for the group receiving suramin compared with the hydrocortisone alone group (1.5 relative risk, P = .0003).[66] Survival was not affected. Results of the trial are awaited in a peer-reviewed journal. It is important to remember that suramin prevents the release of PSA, and patients receiving suramin have had PSA levels reduced by 50% or more in the presence of advancing disease.[67] In this setting, monitoring of PSA may not be a reliable indicator of patient response to therapy.

❏ Cyclophosphamide

In a 1996 study, cyclophosphamide was administered to 35 patients in escalating doses with doxorubicin and granulocyte colony-stimulating factor support (Table 12-5). Responses included 16 patients (46%) who had PSA levels decrease by more than 50%; 10 of these men experienced a decrease in PSA of more than 75%.[68] Toxicities included a 33.3 % incidence of Grade 4 neutropenia and a 7.8 % incidence of febrile neutropenia. Anemia and thrombocytopenia were also severe. Patients with a decline in PSA of greater than 50% lived longer than those who failed to obtain this level of PSA reduction (23 months vs. 7 months, P = .02).[68]

Oral cyclophosphamide and oral etoposide have also been studied in combination.[69] The majority of patients had previously failed two or more hormonal manipulations (75%) and had mild to moderate bone pain (70%). Only one patient required narcotics. Cyclophosphamide and oral etoposide were administered for 2 weeks followed by 2 weeks off treatment. Of the 14 patients with bone pain, 71% had symptomatic improvement. The regimen was well tolerated. Additional trials need to be done with oral cyclophosphamide, because these trials indicate the drug has some activity in HRPC.

❏ Docetaxel

Docetaxel has been added to estramustine to enhance drug activity.[70–72] Oral estramustine was given with docetaxel administered in escalating doses. The MTD of doc-

TABLE 12-6. Docetaxel-Based Studies

Study	N	Major Endpoints	Treatment/Doses Given	Major Findings	Major Toxicities
Shelton et al[71]	8 evaluable	PSA	Dexamethasone, 20 mg PO q6H × 3 doses on Day 2, plus docetaxel, 70 mg/m2 on Day 2, plus estramustine, 280 mg PO tid Days 1–5, repeated q21 days	≥ 50% PSA reduction in 7/8, ≥ 75% PSA reduction in 5/8	Granulocytopenia, Neutropenic fever, Elevated bilirubin
Kreis et al[70]	17	PSA	Estramustine, PO 14 mg/kg daily × 21 days, plus docetaxel, 40, 60, or 80 mg/m² q21 days, plus dexamethasone, 8 mg PO bid × 5 days to prevent fluid retention	5/6 patients with 94% reduction in PSA	Leukopenia, Fatigue, Diarrhea, Anemia, Increased LFTs, Anorexia, Stomatitis, Epigastric pain, Hyponatremia, Hypocalemia, Hypophosphatemia
Natale, et al[72]	13	PSA	Estramustine, 420 mg PO TID × 4 days reduced to 420 mg for first 4 doses followed by 280 mg for 5 more doses (total of 3 days), plus docetaxel, 35–40 mg/m² on Day 2 for 2 weeks; plus dexamethasone, 4 mg bid × 3 days, repeated q3 weeks	10/13 patients with ≥ 50% PSA reduction • 75% PSA reduction in 6/13 • 50% reduction in measurable disease 3/5	Neutropenia, Thrombocytopenia, Malaise, GI toxicity, Edema

PSA, prostate-specific antigen; tid, three times daily; bid, twice daily; LFTs, liver function tests; GI, gastrointestinal.

etaxel was determined to be 70 mg/m^2 when administered with oral estramustine at 14 mg/kg/day for 21 days.[70] At the MTD of 70 mg/m^2, five of six treated patients had a 94% PSA level reduction. The addition of dexamethasone did not appear to add to the observed response rate with docetaxel and estramustine[71] (Table 12-6).

❏ Doxorubicin

Another potentially useful drug combination is doxorubicin and ketoconazole[73] (Table 12-7). Ketoconazole is an oral antifungal agent used in the management of oral candidiasis but also has been identified as having an antitumor effect against prostate cancer cells.[74] Side effects include hepatotoxicity, fatigue, rash, and nausea.

Patients were treated with oral ketoconazole daily plus doxorubicin (20 mg/m^2) IV by continuous infusion over 24 hours once a week.[73] Vitamin C (250 mg) was administered with the ketoconazole to improve absorption, and 63% of the patients received 50 mg of hydrocortisone to manage adrenal insufficiency produced by the ketoconazole.[73] Median survival of all patients was 15.5 months.[73] Side effects included an unusual sticky-skin syndrome (where paper stuck to the skin), which occurred in 39% of patients.[73] Because patients were not stratified by whether or not hydrocortisone was given, the impact of the steroid cannot be assessed. The authors recommended additional study of this active but cardiotoxic combination.[73] Doxorubicin (adriamycin) may also be administered in an IV bolus weekly at the same dose.[75]

In conclusion, several drug combinations are active in HRPC, including mitoxantrone plus steroids, estramustine plus vinblastine, etoposide, and taxanes and weekly doxorubicin and ketoconazole. When discussing chemotherapy regimens, nurses need to be aware of the palliative endpoints for chemotherapy. Patients need to understand the benefits of reduced pain and analgesic requirements versus the risk of side effects and toxicities. Although these combinations may offer some patients palliative benefit, the overall impact on survival and quality of life remains uncertain. Until it is proven that combination therapy improves survival, nurses should focus on the palliative aspects of chemotherapy and its potential contribution to quality of life.

Certain genetic changes have been identified in HRPC. Increased expression of the *bcl*-2 protooncogene is found in hormone-independent cancers, resulting in reduced apoptosis (or programmed cell death).[76,77] It is also associated with the development of hormone independence.[76] The progression of prostate cancer from hormone dependence to hormone independence is also accompanied by changes in cell growth factors. These altered cellular growth factors include the secretion of PSA without androgen stimulation and the production of substances that promote the development of osteoblastic lesions such as transforming growth factor-β.[78–82]

Research continues into new and unique methods of managing patients with HRPC. Areas of investigation include matrix metalloproteinase inhibitors, which play a role in the metastatic spread of cancer.[83] Interfering with growth factor receptors may also be useful in managing HRPC. Several growth factors contribute to the growth of the cancer cells, and drugs that interfere with the binding sites may thus inhibit cancer cell growth.[84]

TABLE 12-7. Doxorubicin (Adriamycin)-Based Studies

Study	N	Major Endpoints	Treatment/Doses Given	Major Findings	Major Toxicities
Sella et al[73]	38 evaluable	Measurable disease PSA	Doxorubicin, 20 mg/m^2 as a 24-h continuous infusion weekly, plus PO ketoconazole, 1,200 mg/day in 3 divided doses beginning 1 week before IV doxorubicin	Median survival 15.5 months 55% response rate 50% reduction in PSA, 16% 50% PSA reduction and bone scan improvement, 18% 50% PSA reduction and reduced tumor size in soft-tissue, 13%	Neutropenia, Acral erythema, Stomatitis, Anal and urethral mucositis, "Sticky-skin syndrome," Infection, Nausea/vomiting, Central catheter thrombosis, CHF, Cardiac arrest, Hypokalemia
Culine et al[75]	31	Measurable disease PSA	Estramustine, 600 mg PO daily in 2 divided doses, plus weekly doxorubicin, 20 mg/m^2	58% with ≥ 50% reduction in PSA 6/18 with PSA normalization 5/11 with measurable disease PR median survival 12 months	Neutropenia, Vomiting, Increased LFTs, Septic shock, Death, Acral erythema, Alopecia, DVT

PSA, prostate-specific antigen; PO, oral; PR, partial response; CHF, congestive heart failure; LFTs, liver function tests; DVT, deep vein thrombosis.

Other potential modalities such as gene therapy, differentiation therapy, and antiangiogenesis therapy, with or without conventional antineoplastic drugs, hold promise for future management of HRPC.[85–87] Continuing research into these novel methods may unlock the door to improved palliation or improved survival in HRPC.

TREATMENT OPTIONS AFTER CHEMOTHERAPY FAILURE

Failure of chemotherapy to provide palliation may be a crisis point for patients and their family members. Nurses play a vital role in encouraging verbalization, providing support, and helping patients adapt and adjust to the situation. Referrals appropriate at this time include social service, hospice, and home care. For the patient with a good performance status, another chemotherapy regimen could be considered. Palliative care should be instituted for patients who are no longer chemotherapy candidates. Pain management needs to include adequate doses of short-acting and long-acting narcotics in addition to adjuvant analgesics such as corticosteroids and nonsteroidal antiinflammatory drugs for bone pain. A bowel regimen consisting of a laxative and stool softener promotes easier elimination. Nurses need to monitor urine output so that signs of bladder outlet obstruction are promptly recognized. An indwelling urinary catheter needs to be inserted to relieve this uncomfortable symptom.

CHEMOTHERAPY CANDIDATES

The goal of chemotherapy is palliation.[88] Chemotherapy has not been shown to prolong survival in HRPC. Therefore, it may be prudent to monitor patients who are potential chemotherapy candidates until symptoms develop. PSA levels should be monitored regularly. Increased PSA levels may signify recurrent or new sites of disease.[88] Although symptoms such as bone pain and decreasing performance status usually follow PSA elevations, some patients may develop signs and symptoms of progressive tumor without significant change or elevation in PSA.[89] Diagnostic tests, such as bone scan, then demonstrate abnormalities. The decision to institute chemotherapy depends on several factors, including extent of tumor, rate of tumor growth, presence and severity of symptoms, general medical condition, including comorbidities that may limit tolerance to chemotherapy, and patient's willingness to tolerate side effects with potential but uncertain benefit. Patients being considered for a clinical research trial must first meet the eligibility criteria for the study. Response to therapy can be monitored by PSA values, reports of how the patient feels (subjective response), symptom response (pain, measurable tumor response), performance status response, and assessments by the nurse and physician.[13, 90]

PATIENT EDUCATION

Patient education is important during the initial phase of treatment planning so that the patient understands the goal of treatment. The family and spouse or significant other should be included in the teaching. Education should be provided when the topic of chemotherapy is first initiated by the physician. Initial information provided by the physician includes the plan and palliative goal of treatment, risks and benefits of treatment, other treatment options, and prognosis.[91] General chemotherapy information may also be provided. Information is often useful when a patient is making a decision about pursuing treatment.[92] Once the decision is made to pursue chemotherapy, information should be provided regarding the specific drugs, administration route, frequency of drug administration, expected and potential drug side effects, and specific self-care measures. Nurses should supplement oral teaching with written materials and frequent reviews and reinforcement of previously taught material. Appropriate patient education materials include drug information sheets, chemotherapy booklets, and techniques to manage side effects and promote self-care. The patient also needs to be aware of signs and symptoms that cannot be managed at home. Nausea and vomiting that interfere with fluid and food consumption, decreased urine output, leg-calf swelling, mouth sores, diarrhea, fever, chills, and hematuria all require the notification of the nurse and physician. The best plan is for patient education to start before treatment and continue with each treatment. One must not assume that the patient will remember everything he has been taught. Ongoing reinforcement is necessary. The nurse must teach the patient what he needs to know to undergo treatment. Rare or unusual side effects may be presented in the form of written information and discussed when needed. [91] The nurse should encourage the patient and family to ask questions. This gives the nurse an opportunity to clarify information, correct misconceptions, and assess what the patient understands. When teaching is complete, the nurse should document the verbal and written information provided and the patient's understanding of the information.

NURSING MANAGEMENT

Nursing management of the patient receiving chemotherapy for HRPC usually occurs in the outpatient clinic, in the physician's office, or at home. Patient education is a critical aspect of self-care management and allows patients and families to manage mild symptoms at home with previously provided information. It also makes the patient and family aware of symptoms that require nursing or medical intervention.

It is helpful to follow up on office or clinic visits for chemotherapy administration with a telephone call.[13] The nurse making follow-up telephone calls needs to be aware of the patient's history, treatment, and disease symptomatology.[93] After adequate information has been obtained regarding chemotherapy-related side effects, the nurse can identify problems that may be developing and actively intervene to solve the problem. The physician may need to be contacted based on the nurse's assessment of the situation. The problem may be solved over the telephone, or the patient may need to be seen by the physician. At the time of follow-up telephone calls, questions can be answered and the nurse has the opportunity to provide more teaching, as appropriate. At the end of the telephone call, the patient should be encouraged to call with any problems or concerns.

Nursing care is critical to the management of the patient with HRPC. The nurse provides education related to chemotherapy and side effect self care but may also need to educate the patient about supportive therapies such as administration of growth factors at home. Visiting nurse follow-up should be arranged to expedite administration of growth factors at home, when appropriate. The patient needs to be questioned about the impact of treatment on pain, activities of daily living, and quality of life.[13] The nurse should emphasize the improvement of quality of life and symptom improvement from treatment. If these goals have not been achieved, the physician may need to reevaluate treatment.

The nurse actively intervenes to assess, plan, intervene, and evaluate the nursing care of the patient (Table 12-8).[94–98] Problems requiring nursing intervention include knowledge deficit, alopecia, fatigue, altered nutrition, and mucositis. The nurse consults and collaborates with the physician in the management of other patient problems to enhance the quality of life and provide quality care to the patient with HRPC. Areas of consultation and collaboration include pain management.

PSYCHOSOCIAL ISSUES

Men with HRPC are usually middle-aged or older adults. They may have older children or have already raised children to adulthood. Often the patient's career is established, or the patient may be retired.[99] The patient may have experienced the loss of other family members, such as his parents or spouse. In addition to these real losses, the patient could now be facing the loss of his own life within approximately 1 year. This is a time of significant stress and crisis.[100] The addition of pain or other symptoms can reduce the patient's quality of life.

The nurse plays an important role in helping the patient to adapt and adjust to this difficult time. Education related to drug side effects and self-care management will help the patient manage some symptoms at home and be aware of when to notify the physician of symptoms such as bleeding or fever. Symptoms, such as pain, are assessed, monitored, and managed by the nurse in collaboration with the physician. When chemotherapy is no longer an option, hospice care should be recommended and the family involved as much as possible in the patient's decision and care. The patient and family should be encouraged to express their thoughts and feelings regarding end-of-life care. Improving the quality of life is a major component of hospice care.[101]

CONCLUSION

In the past several years, progress has been made in the treatment of HRPC. Commercially available drugs are being used in new ways and combinations. Useful regimens include mitoxantrone plus steroids or one of the oral estramustine combinations. Phase III trials are needed to determine the best antineoplastic treatment for patients with HRPC. Patient education and nursing care are critical components of patient care.

I thank Gary R. Hudes, MD, for his helpful comments and critique of the final drafts of this chapter.

TABLE 12-8. Standard of Care: Chemotherapy for the Management of Hormone-Resistant Prostate Cancer

NURSING DIAGNOSIS: *Knowledge deficit related to palliative nature of chemotherapy, side effects, and self-care activities*
OUTCOME: Pt will verbalize understanding of purpose of chemotherapy, side effects, and how to manage side effects at home.
NURSING INTERVENTIONS:
1. Assess pt/SO understanding of the purpose of chemotherapy, side effects, and self-care.
2. Educate pt/SO as to drug action, expected side effects, and management (appropriate for regimen): Myelo-suppression; Anorexia, nausea, vomiting; Diarrhea; Changes in urine color; Alopecia; Mucositis; Peripheral edema; Neuropathy; Altered LFTs; Allergic reactions; Fatigue; Cardiac-cardiovascular; Hemorrhagic cystitis; Myalgia; Steroid-induced hyperglycemia.
3. Educate pt as to s-s requiring nurse-physician notification: fever (T $\geq$ 101°F), chills, bleeding, vomiting, dehydration, profound fatigue, mucositis, leg swelling.
4. Encourage pt/SO to verbalize questions, concerns about treatment, side effects and self-care.
5. Provide pt/SO with printed education materials to use as reference at home.

NURSING DIAGNOSIS: *Body image disturbance related to alopecia*
OUTCOME: Pt will verbalize methods of managing hair loss.
NURSING INTERVENTIONS:
1. Assess pt/SO understanding of hair loss induced by antineoplastic regimen.
2. Teach pt about why hair loss occurs and what body hair will be affected (scalp, body, face).
3. Teach pt to wear hat or cap to retain body heat and cover head.
4. Pt should consider preparing for hair loss by having hair cut short before loss or thinning or purchase a wig or head coverings before hair loss.
5. Encourage pt/SO to verbalize effect of hair loss on body image.
6. If hair thinning is expected as opposed to total hair loss, teach pt to use a gentle shampoo and avoid tugging or pulling hair

NURSING DIAGNOSIS: *Fatigue related to chemotherapy*
OUTCOME: Pt will use methods to promote adaptation to fatigue.
NURSING INTERVENTIONS:
1. Assess pt/SO understanding of cause of fatigue and methods of fatigue management.
2. Encourage pt/SO to verbalize impact of fatigue on usual lifestyle.
3. Encourage periods of rest and activity, midday naps, and routine times of arising and retiring, mild exercise routine, such as walking.
4. Remind pt to ask for assistance when required. Assess need for help at home (e.g., home health aide, homemaker).
5. Monitor H/H results and report low counts to physician. Treat as per hospital standard.
6. Teach pt to report incidence and severity of fatigue.
7. Teach pt to administer prescribed erythropoietin injections.

NURSING DIAGNOSIS: *Risk of infection or bleeding from myelosuppression-steroids*
OUTCOME: Pt will promptly notify nurse-physician of s-s of bleeding or infection. Pt will verbalize under-standing of serious potentially life-threatening nature of infection and that hospitalization may be required for IV antibiotics.
NURSING INTERVENTIONS:
1. Assess pt/SO understanding of s-s of bleeding or infection.
2. Educate pt to notify nurse-physician of bleeding, fever, sore throat, cough, episodes of chills or diaphoresis, dysuria. Emphasize need to notify the physician promptly of s-s of infection.
3. Have pt monitor temperature each afternoon and whether he feels warm or has the chills. Have pt keep a record of temperatures.
4. Have pt avoid infection sources such as children and adults who are sick, large crowds, pet stool, plants and flowers.
5. Pt should avoid aspirin, NSAIDs, other over-the-counter meds that contain aspirin or NSAIDs.
6. Pt should shave with electric razor and avoid other activities that may cause bleeding.

7. Obtain cultures (blood, urine, central lines), chest radiograph as ordered.
8. Administer IV antibiotics as prescribed.
9. Administer platelets as prescribed.
10. Monitor CBC-differential. Calculate ANC. Notify physician when ANC < 1.0.
11. Educate pt on correct method of taking antibiotics at home.
12. Monitor pt for change in vital signs, increased temperature, RR and HR, decreasing blood pressure. Report changes to physician.
13. Arrange for home care for infusion therapy of antibiotics when pt ready for discharge.
14. Administer acetaminophen to manage fever.
15. Avoid rectal suppositories, enemas, IM injections, other procedures that violate the integrity of skin or mucous membranes.
16. Institute platelet-bleeding or neutropenic precautions when appropriate.
17. Promote good hygiene with daily bath.
18. Promote good hand-washing technique by all health care providers.
19. No fresh fruits or vegetables in diet; cooked foods should be consumed.
20. Monitor skin and mucous membranes for infection, bleeding.
21. Send stool for Hematest as ordered. Monitor urine for blood.
22. Apply pressure to venipuncture sites until bleeding stops.
23. Monitor neurologic signs for change in mental status.
24. No straining on bowel movement. Administer laxatives and stool softeners to maintain regular soft formed stools.

NURSING DIAGNOSIS: *Altered comfort related to edema*
OUTCOME: Pt will manage leg edema at home.
NURSING INTERVENTIONS:
1. Assess weight and edema before each treatment.
2. Educate pt to elevate legs while sitting and avoid prolonged standing.
3. Diuretics may be useful in managing leg edema.
4. Ascertain that appropriate premedications have been taken.
5. Compression stockings may be useful.
6. Educate pt to notify physician at onset of leg edema because cause may be related to DVT.
7. Drug dose may need to be modified.

NURSING DIAGNOSIS: *Risk for altered nutrition related to nausea, vomiting, diarrhea. Risk for altered fluid and electrolyte balance related to vomiting, diarrhea*
OUTCOME: Pt will verbalize understanding of how to manage nausea, vomiting, or diarrhea. Pt will recognize s-s of dehydration and notify physician.
NURSING INTERVENTIONS:
1. Assess pt understanding of methods to manage nausea, vomiting, and diarrhea.
2. Administer antiemetic before treatment and have pt take antiemetics on a routine basis if oral antineoplastics cause nausea at home.
3. Have pt notify physician if s-s of dehydration develop: dry mouth, reduced urine output, concentrated urine, weakness; or causes of dehydration: vomiting, diarrhea.
4. Have foods prepared in room different from where foods are consumed because odors may cause nausea.
5. Educate pt as to low-residue diet and to consume large amounts of fluids and electrolytes if diarrhea occurs.
6. Administer antidiarrheal medication as prescribed.
7. Administer IV fluids and electrolytes as prescribed.
8. Monitor BUN and creatinine values.
9. Measure I&O; include volume of liquid stool in output.
10. Weigh twice each week.
11. Consult dietitian.
12. Keep emesis basin and commode clean and odor free.
13. Encourage resting in a quiet place.
14. Use distraction such as deep breathing, music therapy, guided imagery.
15. Keep pt NPO during vomiting episodes and slowly restart clear liquids when vomiting stops. Have pt try tea, crackers, toast, bland foods.

(Continued on next page)

TABLE 12-8. Continued

16. Avoid foods containing lactose, fat, and sweet or spicy foods.
17. Perform frequent mouth care and frequent perianal care after diarrhea.

NURSING DIAGNOSIS: *Altered oral mucous membrane integrity*
OUTCOME: Pt will be able to perform good oral care to keep mucous membranes clean and moist.
NURSING INTERVENTIONS:
1. Teach pt about good oral care: Brush teeth after meals with soft toothbrush and fluoride toothpaste and floss if it does not cause pain or bleeding. Pt should rinse mouth well with warm tap water or saline, and rinse mouth several times each day to keep mouth moist and clean.
2. Pt should consume bland low-acid diet high in protein and calories.
3. Topical analgesics or anesthetics are useful for mouth sores such as a mixture of viscous lidocaine (xylocaine), antacid, and liquid pediatric diphenhydramine mixed in a 1:1:1 solution. Use 5 mL as needed by mouth.
4. Encourage large fluid intake (≥ 2 L/day).
5. Monitor oral cavity for pain, difficulty swallowing, sore throat, white patches, and other signs of oral infection, and notify physician. Obtain cultures as ordered.

NURSING DIAGNOSIS: *Risk for altered neurovascular dysfunction related to peripheral neuropathy*
OUTCOME: Pt will use safety measures to reduce risk of injury.
NURSING INTERVENTIONS:
1. Assess pt for altered sensation, altered gait.
2. Educate pt as to safety issues, concerns related to neuropathies.
3. Have pt wear shoes at all times to avoid foot injury.
4. Pt should use care with sharp and hot items because sensation is reduced.
5. Altered sensation will slowly improve over time.
6. Pt should notify nurse of altered sensation.
7. Pt may need assistance with tasks requiring fine motor function such as buttoning shirts.
8. Drug doses may need to be modified because of neuropathies.
9. Assess level of pain resulting from neuropathies and consider use of medications to reduce pain.
10. Monitor pt for injuries.
11. Consult PT/OT, home care as needed.

NURSING DIAGNOSIS: *Risk for altered nutrition related to anorexia, taste changes*
OUTCOME: Pt will verbalize understanding of how to alter foods to enhance food intake.
NURSING INTERVENTIONS:
1. Consult with dietitian. Perform calorie counts for 3 days to assess caloric intake.
2. Encourage pt to experiment with different flavorings, herbs, spices to promote food intake.
3. Encourage pt to eat favorite foods.
4. Provide high-calorie nutrient-concentrated foods that are easy to prepare and consume.
5. Consider use of appetite-stimulating medication.
6. Provide recipes and written information on methods of increasing calorie intake without needing to eat more food.
7. Assess ability to obtain and prepare foods.
8. Weigh weekly.
9. Encourage mild exercise such as walking after consulting with physician.
10. Encourage use of liquid diet supplements.
11. Experiment with different foods, different culturally appropriate foods; cold, cool, or room temperature foods; and those without odor. Have family provide foods from home.

NURSING DIAGNOSIS: *Risk for altered tissue perfusion*
OUTCOME: Pt will have prompt recognition of s-s of anemia.
NURSING INTERVENTIONS:
1. Educate pt as to s-s of anemia (↑HR, ↑RR, ↑fatigue, pallor, dizziness, palpitations) and need to notify nurse should these develop.
2. Monitor H/H, and report >1g reduction in Hgb or Hgb < 8.0.
3. Transfuse blood products as ordered.

4. Teach pt to change positions slowly to avoid dizziness.
5. Monitor pulse oximetry.
6. Educate pt to self-administer erythropoietin.
7. Teach pt about foods high in iron.
8. Assess need for supplemental oxygen.

NURSING DIAGNOSIS: *Potential for constipation as a result of reduced mobility, decreased dietary fiber intake*
OUTCOME: Pt will have an easily formed bowel movement at least every other day.
NURSING INTERVENTIONS:

1. Educate pt about need to have soft but formed easy-to-pass stools.
2. Teach pt to take stool softeners and laxatives daily.
3. Teach pt how to titrate laxatives and stool softeners to manage bowels (increase dose with hard stools, decrease dose with diarrhea).
4. Increase amount of fiber and fluid in diet if tolerated.
5. Encourage mild exercise such as walking after discussion with physician.

NURSING DIAGNOSIS: *Risk for cardiac toxicity*
OUTCOME: Pt will have prompt recognition of s-s of cardiac toxicity.
NURSING INTERVENTIONS:

1. Assess pt for s-s of preexisting heart disease: chest pain, poor exercise tolerance, edema, shortness of breath, abnormal ECG, low ejection fraction, cough, JVD, ↑HR, extra heart sounds.
2. Monitor cumulative dose of cardiotoxic agents.
3. Educate pt to notify nurse or physician if any of these symptoms develop.

NURSING DIAGNOSIS: *Risk for arthralgia, myalgia related to chemotherapy*
OUTCOME: Pt will verbalize an understanding of how to manage arthralgia, myalgia.
NURSING INTERVENTIONS:

1. Educate pt as to cause of myalgia and arthralgia and its time-limited course.
2. Acetaminophen, two regular-strength tablets q4h PRN, may be useful in managing discomfort. Pt needs to follow package directions.
3. Pt should notify nurse if analgesic not effective.

NURSING DIAGNOSIS: *Risk for hypersensitivity reaction related to taxane chemotherapy*
OUTCOME: Pt will not experience a hypersensitivity reaction.
NURSING INTERVENTIONS:

1. Monitor vital signs before, q15min during, and at end of infusion.
2. Administer prescribed steroids, antihistamine and histamine-$_2$ blocker before infusion.
3. Monitor for hypotension, bronchospasm, facial flushing, dyspnea, abdominal and leg pain. Most reactions occur in the first 10 min of the infusion.
4. Immediately terminate infusion with development of s-s of reaction and notify physician.
5. Maintain pt IV site.
6. Have emergency drugs available.

NURSING DIAGNOSIS: *Risk of hemorrhagic cystitis related to cyclophosphamide therapy*
OUTCOME: Pt will not experience hemorrhagic cystitis.
NURSING INTERVENTIONS:

1. Educate pt as to need to take oral drug in morning.
2. Pt needs to consume 2–3 L of fluid each day.
3. Pt needs to void hs to avoid having drug lay in bladder during night. Pt should void promptly at initial urge to void.
4. Pt needs to notify nurse or physician of hematuria promptly

NURSING DIAGNOSIS: *Risk of hepatotoxicity related to chemotherapy*
OUTCOME: Pt will have prompt recognition of s-s of hepatotoxicity.
NURSING INTERVENTIONS:

1. Assess pt for abnormal LFTs before initiation of therapy. Assess pt for history of alcohol abuse, which may promote liver toxicity.
2. Educate pt as to s-s of liver toxicity: dark urine, light-colored stool, yellow skin or sclera, itching.
3. Monitor LFT results and notify physician of abnormal results.

(Continued on next page)

TABLE 12-8. Continued

4. Have pt notify nurse or physician promptly if s-s of hepatotoxicity develop.
5. Drug doses may be modified in presence of altered LFT results.
6. Pt is to avoid alcohol and other drugs that may increase risk of hepatotoxicity.

NURSING DIAGNOSIS: *Risk for hyperglycemia from steroid therapy*
OUTCOME: The pt will have prompt recognition of s-s of hyperglycemia.
NURSING INTERVENTIONS:

1. Educate pt as to s-s of hyperglycemia: thirst, hunger, increased urination.
2. Monitor blood glucose results.
3. Notify physician of increased glucose levels.
4. Consult with dietitian regarding diabetic diet.
5. Institute diabetic education.
6. Set up home visits by visiting nurse.

PT, patient; SO, significant other; LFTs, liver function tests; H/H, hematocrit and hemoglobin; IV, intravenous; NSAIDs, nonsteroidal antiinflammatory drugs; meds, medications; CBC, complete blood cell count; ANC, absolute neutrophil count; IM, intramuscular; DVT, deep vein thrombosis; BUN, blood urea nitrogen; I&O, intake and output; NPO, nothing by mouth; RR, respiration rate; HR, heart rate; Hgb, hemoglobin; ECG, Electrocardiogram; JVD, jugular venous distention; T, temperature; hs, at bedtime; s-s, signs-symptoms.
Data compiled from Doenges and Moorhouse,[94] Wilkes et al,[95] Wilkes,[96] Anderson et al,[97] and Tortoria.[98]

REFERENCES

1. Moore MJ, Tannock IF. Overview of Canadian trials in hormonally resistant prostate cancer. *Semin Oncol* 1996;23(6, Suppl 14):15–19.
2. Esper PS, Pienta KJ. Supportive care in the patient with hormone refractory prostate cancer. *Semin Urol Oncol* 1997;15:56–64.
3. Scher HI, Steineck G, Kelly WK. Hormone-refractory (D3) prostate cancer: Refining the concept. *Urology* 1995;46:142–148.
4. Kelly WK, Slovin S, Scher HI. Clincial use of posttherapy prostate-specific antigen changes in advanced prostate cancer. *Semin Oncol* 1996;23(6, Suppl 14):8–14.
5. Schatzkin A, Freedman LS, Dorgan J, et al. Surrogate endpoints in cancer research: A critique. *Cancer Epidemiol Biomarkers Prev* 1996;5:947–953.
6. Thalmann GN, Sikes RA, Change SM, et al. Suramin-induced decrease in prostate-specific antigen with no effect on tumor growth in the LNCaP model of human prostate cancer. *J Natl Cancer Inst* 1996;88:794–801.
7. Dreicer R. Metastatic prostate cancer: Assessment of response to systemic therapy. *Semin Urol Oncol* 1997;15:28–32.
8. Tannock IF, Osoba D, Stockler MR, et al. Chemotherapy with mitoxantrone plus prednisone or prednisone alone for symptomatic hormone-resistant prostate cancer: A Canadian randomized trial with palliative end points. *J Clin Oncol* 1996;14:1756–1764.
9. Kelly WK, Scher HI. Prostate specific antigen decline after antiandrogen withdrawal: The flutamide withdrawal syndrome. *J Urol* 1993;149:607–609.
10. Scher HI, Kelly WK. Flutamide withdrawal syndrome: Its impact on clinical trials in hormone-refractory prostate cancer. *J Clin Oncol* 1993;11:1566–1572.
11. Newling D, Fossa SD, Andersson L, et al. Assessment of hormone refractory prostate cancer. *Urology* 1997;49(Suppl 4A):46–53.
12. Oesterling J, Fuks Z, Lee CT, Scher HI. Cancer of the prostate. In: DeVita, VT, Hellman, S, Rosenberg, SA (eds). *Cancer: Principles and Practice of Oncology,* 5th ed. Philadelphia: Lippincott-Raven, 1997:1322–1386
13. Moore MJ, MacLeod M, Brittain M-A, et al (eds). *Mitoxantrone to Control Pain in Patients with Hormone Refractory Prostate Cancer.* Pittsburgh: Oncology Education Services, 1997:1–26.
14. Raghavan D, Coorey G, Rosen M, et al. Management of hormone-resistant prostate cancer: An Australian trial. *Semin Oncol* 1996;23(6, Suppl 14):20–23.
15. Hudes G. Estramustine-based chemotherapy. *Semin Urol Oncol* 1997;15:13–19.

16. Iversen P, Rasmussen F, Asmussen C, et al. Estramustine phosphate versus placebo as a second line treatment after orchiectomy in patients with metastatic prostate cancer: DAPROCA study 9002. *J Urol* 1997;157:929–934.

17. Dahllof B, Billstrom A, Cabral F, Hartley-Asp B. Estramustine depolymerizes microtubules by binding to tubulin. *Cancer Res* 1993;53:4573–4581.

18. Rowinsky EK, Donehower RC. Antimicrotubule agents. In: DeVita VT, Hellman S, Rosenberg SA (eds). *Cancer: Principles and Practice of Oncology,* 5th ed. Philadelphia: Lippincott-Raven, 1997:467–483.

19. Hudes GR, Obasaju C, Chapman A, et al. Phase I study of paclitaxel and estramustine: Preliminary activity in hormone-refractory prostate cancer. *Semin Oncol* 1995;22 (3, Suppl 6):6–11.

20. Speicher LA, Barone L, Tew KD. Combined antimicrotubule activity of estramustine and taxol in human prostatic carcinoma cell lines. *Cancer Res* 1992;52:4433–4440.

21. Dexeus F, Logothetis CJ, Samuels ML, et al. Continuous infusion of vinblastine for advanced hormone-refractory prostate cancer. *Cancer Treat Rep* 1985;69:885–886.

22. Burke MB, Wilkes GM, Ingwersen KC, et al. *Cancer Chemotherapy: A Nursing Process Approach,* 2nd ed. Sudbury, MA: Jones and Bartlett, 1996:243–247, 284–289, 427–430.

23. Raghavan D, Cox K, Pearson BS, et al. Oral cyclophosphamide for the management of hormone-refractory prostate cancer. *Br J Urol* 1993;72:625–628.

24. Rangel C, Matzkin H, Soloway MS. Experience with weekly doxorubicin (Adriamycin) in hormone-refractory stage D2 prostate cancer. *Urology* 1992;39:577–582.

25. Fischer DS, Knobf MT, Durivage HJ. *The Cancer Chemotherapy Handbook,* 5th ed. St. Louis, MO: Mosby-Year Book, 1997:170–172.

26. Roth BJ, Yeap BY, Wilding G, et al. Taxol in hormone-refractory carcinoma of the prostate. *Cancer* 1993;72:2457–2460.

27. Cook GA, Troutner K. *Taxotere: An Important Advance in the Treatment of Metastatic Breast Cancer.* Collegeville, PA: Rhone-Poulenc Rorer Pharmaceuticals, 1996:15–16, 20–24.

28. Schultz M, Wei J, Picus J. A phase II trial of docetaxel in patients with hormone refractory prostate cancer (HRPC) [abstract 1320]. *Proc Am Soc Clin Oncol* 1998;17:342a.

29. Hussain MH, Pienta KJ, Redman BG, et al. Oral etoposide in the treatment of hormone-refractory prostate cancer. *Cancer* 1994;74:100–103.

30. Tannock I, Gospodarowicz M, Meakin W, et al. Treatment of metastatic prostatic cancer with low-dose prednisone: Evaluation of pain and quality of life as pragmatic indices of response. *J Clin Oncol* 1989;7:590–597.

31. Moore MJ, Osoba D, Murphy K, et al. Use of palliative endpoints to evaluate the effects of mitoxantrone and low-dose prednisone in patients with hormonally resistant prostate cancer. *J Clin Oncol* 1994;12:689–694.

32. Kantoff PW, Conaway M, Winer E, et al. Hydrocortisone (HC) with or without mitoxantrone (M) in patients (pts) with hormone refractory prostate cancer (HRPC): Preliminary results from a prospective randomized Cancer and Leukemia Group B study (9182) comparing chemotherapy to best supportive care [abstract 2013]. *Proc Am Soc Clin Oncol* 1996;14:1748.

33. Cohn H, Pincus J, Vogelzang NJ. Strontium-89 (SR-89), mitoxantrone (M), and hydrocortisone (H) in hormone refractory prostate cancer (HRPC): A phase I-II study with intriguing PSA kinetics [abstract 1265]. *Proc Am Soc Clin Oncol* 1998;17:328a.

34. Levine EG, Halabi S, Hars V, et al. Preliminary results of CALGB9680: A phase II trial of high dose mitoxantrone/GM-CSF and low dose steroids in hormone refractory prostate cancer (HRPC) [abstract 1297]. *Proc Am Soc Clin Oncol* 1998;17:336a.

35. DeConti R, Balducci L, Einstein A, et al. A phase II trial of mitoxantrone/paclitaxel in hormone-refractory prostate cancer [abstract 1270]. *Pr Am Soc Clin Oncol* 1998;17:329a.

36. Hudes GR, Nathan F, Khater C, et al. Phase II trial of 96-hour paclitaxel plus oral estramustine phosphate in metastatic hormone-refractory prostate cancer. *J Clin Oncol* 1997;15:3156–3163.

37. Garay C, Roth B, Hudes G, et al. Phase I trial of weekly paclitaxel by 3-hour infusion plus oral estramustine (EMP) in metastatic hormone refractory prostate cancer (HRPC) [abstract 1278]. *J Clin Oncol* 1998;17:331a.

38. Haas NB, Hartley-Asp B, Kopreski M, et al. Phase I pharmacokinetic trial of intravenous (IV) estramustine phosphate (EMP) in patients with hormone refractory prostate cancer (HRPC) [abstract 1250]. *Proc Am Soc Clin Oncol* 1998;17:324a.

39. Kelly WK, Slovin S, Curley TC, et al. Weekly 1 hour paclitaxel (P) in combination with estramustine (E) and carboplatin (C) in patients with advanced prostate cancer (PC) [abstract 1249]. *Proc Am Soc Clin Oncol* 1998;17:324a.

40. Petrylak DP, Macarthur RB, O'Connor J, et al. Phase I trial of docetaxel with estramustine in androgen-dependent prostate cancer. *J Clin Oncol* 1999;17:958–967.

41. Attivissimo LA, Fetten JV, Kreis W. Symptomatic improvement associated with combined estramustine and vinblastine chemotherapy for metastatic prostate cancer. *Am J Clin Oncol* 1996;19:581–583.

42. Hudes GR, Greenberg R, Krigel RL, et al. Phase II study of estramustine and vinblastine, two microtubule inhibitors, in hormone-refractory prostate cancer. *J Clin Oncol* 1992;10:1754–1761.

43. Pienta KJ, Lehr JE. Inhibition of prostate cancer growth by estramustine and etoposide: Evidence for interaction at the nuclear matrix. *J Urol* 1993;149:1622–1625.

44. Pienta KJ, Redman B, Hussain M, et al. Phase II evaluation of oral estramustine and oral etoposide in hormone-refractory adenocarcinoma of the prostate. *J Clin Oncol* 1994;12:2005–2012.

45. Pienta KJ, Redman BG, Bandekar R, et al. A phase II trial of oral estramustine and oral etoposide in hormone refractory prostate cancer. *Urology* 1997;50:401–407.

46. Smith DC, Dunn RL, Strawdermann MS, Pienta KJ. Change in serum prostate-specific antigen as a marker of response to cytotoxic therapy for hormone refractory prostate cancer. *J Clin Oncol* 1998;16:1835–1843.

47. Dimopoulos MA, Panopoulos C, Bamia C, et al. Oral estramustine and oral etoposide for hormone-refractory prostate cancer. *Urology* 1997;50:754–758.

48. Vogelzang N. Editorial comment to Pienta KJ, Redman BG, Bandekar R, et al. *Urology* 1997;50:406–407.

49. Colleoni M, Graiff C, Vicario G, et al. Phase II study of estramustine, oral etoposide, and vinorelbine in hormone-refractory prostate cancer. *Am J Clin Oncol* 1997;20:383–386.

50. Pienta K, Smith DC. Paclitaxel, estramustine, and etoposide in the treatment of hormone-refractory prostate cancer. *Semin Oncol* 1997;24(5, Suppl 1S):S15-72–S15-77.

51. Fischer DS, Knobf MT, Durivage HJ. *The Cancer Chemotherapy Handbook*, 5th ed. St. Louis, MO: CV Mosby, 1997.

52. Eisenberger MA, Sinibaldi V, Reyno L. Suramin. *Cancer Pract* 1995;3:187–189.

53. Kobayashi K, Weiss RE, Vogelzang NJ, et al. Mineralocorticoid insufficiency due to suramin therapy. *Cancer* 1996;78:2411–2420.

54. Kenner JR, Sperling LC, Waselenko J, et al. Suramin keratosis: A unique skin eruption in a patient receiving suramin for metastatic prostate cancer. *J Urol* 1997;158:2245–2246.

55. Figg WD, Cooper MR, Thibault A, et al. Acute renal toxicity associated with suramin in the treatment of prostate cancer. *Cancer* 1994;74:1612–1614.

56. Smith A, Harbour D, Liebmann J. Acute renal failure in a patient receiving treatment with suramin. *Am J Clin Oncol* 1997;20:433–434.

57. Bitton RJ, Figg WD, Venzon DJ, et al. Pharmacologic variables associated with the development of neurologic toxicity in patients treated with suramin. *J Clin Oncol* 1995;13:2223–2229.

58. Konety BR, Getzenberg RH. Novel therapies for advanced prostate cancer. *Semin Urol Oncol* 1997;15:33–42.

59. Clark JW, Chabner BA. Suramin and prostate cancer: Where do we go from here? *J Clin Oncol* 1995;13:2155–2157.

60. Jodrell DI, Reyno LM, Sridhara R, et al. Suramin: Development of a population pharmacokinetic model and its use with intermittent short infusions to control plasma drug concentrations in patients with prostate cancer. *J Clin Oncol* 1994;12:166–175.

61. Eisenberger MA, Sinibaldi VJ, Reyno LM, et al. Phase I and clinical evaluation of a pharmacologically guided regimen of suramin in patients with hormone-refractory prostate cancer. *J Clin Oncol* 1995;13:2174–2186.

62. Reyno LM, Egorin MJ, Eisenberger MA, et al. Development and validation of a pharmacokinetically based fixed dosing scheme for suramin. *J Clin Oncol* 1995;13:2187–2195.

63. Kobayashi K, Vokes EE, Vogelzang NJ, et al. Phase I study of suramin given by intermittent infusion

without adaptive control in patients with advanced cancer. *J Clin Oncol* 1995;13:2196–2207.

64. Hussain M, Fisher E, Wood D, et al. Androgen deprivation (AD) + 4 – courses of fixed-schedule suramin in D2 prostate cancer (PCA) patients (PTS): A Southwest Oncology Group phase II study [abstract 1211]. *Proc Am Soc Clin Oncol* 1998; 17:314a.

65. Vogelzang NJ, Small EJ, Halabi S, et al. A phase III trial of 3 different doses of suramin (SUR) in metastatic hormone refractory prostate cancer (HPRC): Safety profile in CALGB 9480 [abstract 1339]. *Proc Am Soc Clin Oncol* 1998;17:347a.

66. Small EJ, Marshall ME, Reyno L, et al. Superiority of suramin + hydrocortisone (S+H) over placebo + hydrocortisone (P+H): Results of a multi-center double-blind phase III study in patients with hormone refractory prostate cancer (HRPC) [abstract 1187]. *Proc Am Soc Clin Oncol* 1998;17:308a.

67. Siu LL, Moore MJ. Other chemotherapy regimens including mitoxantrone and suramin. *Semin Urol Oncol* 1997;15:20–27.

68. Small EJ, Srinivas S, Egan B, et al. Doxorubicin and dose-escalated cyclophosphamide with granulocyte colony-stimulating factor for the treatment of hormone-resistant prostate cancer. *J Clin Oncol* 1996;14:1617–1625.

69. Maulard-Durdux C, Dufour B, Hennequin C, et al. Phase II study of the oral cyclophosphamide and oral etoposide combination in hormone-refractory prostate carcinoma patients. *Cancer* 1996;77:1144–1148.

70. Kreis W, Budman DR, Fetten J, et al. Phase I trial of the combination of daily estramustine phosphate and intermittent docetaxel in patients with metastatic hormone refractory prostate cancer. *Ann Oncol* 1999;10:33–35.

71. Shelton G, Gerson H, Zuech N, et al. Activity of docetaxel (D) + estramustine (E) after dexamethasone (DEX) treatment in patients (PTS) with androgen insensitive prostate cancer (AIP) [abstract 1324]. *Proc Am Soc Clin Oncol* 1998;17:343a.

72. Natale RB, Zaretsky S. Phase I/II trial of estramustine (E) with taxotere (T) or vinorelbine (V) in patients (PTS) with metastatic hormone-refractory prostate cancer (HRPC) [abstract 1302]. *Proc Am Soc Clin Oncol* 1998;17:338a.

73. Sella A, Kilbourn R, Amato R, et al. Phase II study of ketoconazole combined with weekly doxorubicin

in patients with androgen-independent prostate cancer. *J Clin Oncol* 1994;12:683–688.

74. Eichenberger T, Trachenberg J, Toor P, et al. Ketoconazole: A possible direct cytotoxic effect on prostate carcinoma cells. *J Urol* 1989;141:190–191.

75. Culine S, Kattan J, Zanetta S, et al. Evaluation of estramustine phosphate combined with weekly doxorubicin in patients with androgen-independent prostate cancer. *Am J Clin Oncol* 1998;21: 470–474.

76. McDonnell TJ, Troncoso P, Brisbay S, et al. Expression of the protooncogene bcl-2 in the prostate and its association with emergence of androgen-independent prostate cancer. *Cancer Res* 1992;52:6940–6944.

77. Colombel M, Symmans F, Gil S, et al. Detection of the apoptosis-suppressing oncoprotein bcl-2 in hormone refractory human prostate cancers. *Am J Pathol* 1993;143:390–400.

78. Gleave ME, Hsieh JT, Wu HC, et al. Serum prostate specific antigen levels in mice bearing human prostate LNCaP tumors are determined by tumor volume and endocrine growth factors. *Cancer Res* 1992;52:1598–1603.

79. Wu HC, Hsieh JT, Gleave ME, et al. Derivation of androgen-independent human LNCaP prostate cancer cell sublines: Role of bone stromal cells. *Int J Cancer* 1994;57:406–412.

80. Hsieh JT, Wu HC, Gleave ME, et al. Autocrine regulation of prostate specific antigen expression in human prostatic cancer (LNCaP) subline. *Cancer Res* 1993;53:2852–2857.

81. Mundy GR. Mechanisms of bone metastases. *Cancer* 1997;80:1546–1556.

82. Goltzman D. Mechanisms of the development of osteoblastic metastases. *Cancer* 1997;80:1581–1587.

83. Roth BJ. New therapeutic agents for hormone-refractory prostate cancer. *Semin Oncol* 1996;23 (6, Suppl 14):49–55.

84. Slovin SF, Livingston PO, Rosen N, et al. Targeted therapy for prostate cancer: The Memorial Sloan-Kettering Cancer Center approach. *Semin Oncol* 1996;23(6, Suppl 14):41–48.

85. Sanda MG. Biologic principles and clinical development of prostate cancer gene therapy. *Semin Urol Oncol* 1997;15:43–55.

86. Carducci MA, DeWeese TL, Nelson WG, et al. Prostate cancer treatment strategies based on

tumor-specific biologic principles: Future directions. *Semin Oncol* 1996;23(6, Suppl 14): 56–62.

87. Campbell SC. Advances in angiogenesis research: Relevance to urologic oncology. *J Urol* 1997;158: 1663–1674.

88. Baker LH, Hanks G, Gershenson D, et al. NCCN prostate cancer practice guidelines. *Oncology*, 1996, 10(11, Suppl):265–288.

89. Newling DWW, Denis L, Vermeylen K. Orchiectomy plus goserelin and flutamide in the treatment of newly diagnosed metastatic prostate cancer. *Cancer* 1993;72:3793–3798.

90. Kelly WK, Scher HI, Mazumdar M, et al. Prostate-specific antigen as a measure of disease outcome in metastatic hormone-refractory prostate cancer. *J Clin Oncol*, 1993;11:607–615.

91. Goodman M, Riley MB. Chemotherapy: Principles of administration. In: Groenwald SL, Frogge MH, Goodman M, Yarbro CH (eds). *Cancer Nursing: Principles and Practice,* 4th ed. Sudbury, MA: Jones and Bartlett, 1997:283–316.

92. Padberg RM, Padberg, LF. Patient education and support. In: Groenwald SL, Frogge MH, Goodman M, Yarbro CH (eds). *Cancer Nursing: Principles and Practice,* 4th ed. Sudbury, MA: Jones and Bartlett, 1997:1642–1677.

93. Camp-Sorrell D. Chemotherapy: Toxicity management. In: Groenwald SL, Frogge MH, Goodman M, Yarbro CH (eds). *Cancer Nursing: Principles and Practice,* 4th ed. Sudbury, MA: Jones and Bartlett, 1997:385–425.

94. Doenges ME, Moorhouse MF. *Nurse's Pocket Guide: Diagnosis, Interventions and Rationales,* 6th ed. Philadelphia: FA Davis, 1998.

95. Wilkes GM, Ingwersen K, Burke MB. *1997–1998 Oncology Nursing Drug Handbook.* Sudbury, MA: Jones and Bartlett, 1997.

96. Wilkes GM. Potential toxicities and nursing management. In: Burke MB, Wilkes GM, Ingwersen KC, et al (eds). *Cancer Chemotherapy: A Nursing Process Approach,* 2nd ed. Sudbury, MA: Jones and Bartlett, 1996:97–186.

97. Anderson L, Ward D. Nutrition. In: Otto SE (ed). *Oncology Nursing,* 3rd ed. St. Louis, MO: CV Mosby, 1997:728–745.

98. Tortoria PV. Chemotherapy: Principles of Therapy. In: Groenwald SL, Frogge MH, Goodman M, Yarbro CH (eds). *Cancer Nursing: Principles and Practice,* 4th ed. Sudbury, MA: Jones and Bartlett, 1997:283–316.

99. Anastasia PJ, Carroll-Johnson RM. Gender and age differences in the psychological response to cancer. In: Carroll-Johnson RM, Gorman LM, Bush NJ (eds). *Psychosocial Nursing Care Along the Cancer Continuum.* Pittsburgh: Oncology Nursing Press, 1998:53–60.

100. Northouse LL, Peters-Golem H. Cancer and the family: Strategies to assist spouses. *Semin Oncol Nurs* 1993;9:74–82.

101. Gorman, LM. Hospice care. In: Carroll-Johnson RM, Gorman LM, Bush NJ (eds). *Psychosocial Nursing Care Along the Cancer Continuum.* Pittsburgh: Oncology Nursing Press, 1998:341–348.

QUALITY OF LIFE AFTER TREATMENT FOR PROSTATE CANCER

13

ESTHER MUSCARI LIN
MARIA D. KELLY

OVERVIEW

QUALITY OF LIFE DEFINITION

REASONS FOR QOL RESEARCH IN PROSTATE CANCER

Questionable Prostate Disease Course

Decision Making

Credibility in Prostate Cancer QOL Studies

Predictor Ability

CHALLENGES TO QOL RESEARCH IN PROSTATE CANCER

HRQOL INSTRUMENTS

HRQOL IN LOCALIZED PROSTATE CANCER

TREATMENT OPTIONS FOR LOCALIZED PROSTATE CANCER

URINARY INCONTINENCE

Types of Incontinence

Incontinence Assessment

Nursing Interventions

SEXUAL DYSFUNCTION

Management of Erectile Dysfunction

BOWEL DISTURBANCES

HRQOL IN ADVANCED PROSTATE CANCER

CONCLUSION

QUALITY OF LIFE DEFINITION

Quality of life (QOL) research has gained increased attention as more patients are surviving cancer and its therapies. Increased activity in QOL research is reflected in contributions by multidisciplinary healthcare team members. The contributions include a proliferation of measurement tools, conceptual frameworks, definitions, and ongoing recommendations for enriching future studies and results.[1-4] QOL is complex, often related to who is doing the defining, what the researcher is intending to measure, to whom the QOL pertains, and the situation at the time of the definition.[1, 4-6] The history of health-related QOL (HRQOL) research reflects how the definition has evolved and how researchers have struggled to capture all the domains that contribute to a comprehensive QOL definition.[1, 3, 7]

Overall, QOL encompasses HRQOL and many nonmedical phenomena the patient may be experiencing.[8] The purpose of QOL research is to quantify and describe the short-term and long-term sequelae from therapies. QOL research is intended to capture the impact of cancer, side effects from cancer and treatment, and consequences of patients' decisions regarding treatment options. Identifying aspects of a man's experience with prostate cancer that are significant to him yet that may lie outside the usual focus of clinical studies is a benefit of QOL research.[9] The impact of disease and treatment on QOL needs to be quantified in a manner that is understood by all involved: the patient, significant other, and all healthcare providers.

A starting point in the early prostate QOL studies was the three domains of health identified by the World Health Organization (WHO) of physical, mental, and social well-being.[10] Functional scales such as the Karnofsky or Eastern Cooperative Oncology Group (ECOG) scales require the care provider to evaluate and assign a quantitative measure of a patient's functional status.[11, 12] Although the scales continue to be used, they have shown a weak correlation with overall HRQOL.[9, 13, 14] The care provider's judgment of a person's QOL is just that: a third's person's estimation and not the survivor's subjective perspective.[1, 2]

As QOL has gained increasing respect for the importance it plays in everyone's life, its definition has evolved and taken on numerous dimensions. Researchers and clinicians have included physical functioning, emotional status, occupational functioning, sexuality, spirituality, social functioning, cognitive functioning, general health perceptions, pain, emotional well-being, vitality, political and cultural dimensions, activity limitation, and bed disability as dimensions of QOL.[1, 3, 13, 15–17] Altwein and others[13] defined HRQOL research as "assessing the effects of disease and the therapy on psychological and social functions, which may be expressed as anxiety, depression, satisfaction with life, and relationship to family and friends" (p. 67). Sharp[18] expanded the description of QOL to include families' and caregivers' perspectives, which contribute to the complexity of the definition and what is subsequently measured.

REASONS FOR QOL RESEARCH IN PROSTATE CANCER

The information gained from QOL research is consistent with the goals of oncology nursing care, which are to provide holistic and supportive interventions and to assist patients and their families throughout the illness continuum.[1] It is recognized that supportive nursing care during the diagnostic and the acute periods is necessary for symptom control and successful coping. Yet the impact of the diagnosis, the disease, and treatment side effects on psychological, social, physical, and spiritual well-being can continue through the remainder of a patient's life. A description of survivor experiences and perspectives can provide the nurse with valuable information of what the newly diagnosed or previously treated prostate patient encounters, how to prepare him, and how to support him in the future.[7]

QUESTIONABLE PROSTATE DISEASE COURSE

Rossetti and Terrone[19] argued that, because of the slow-growing nature of the disease, combined with the age at diagnosis, how a person's prostate cancer will progress tends to be a statistical prediction because the natural history and disease outcomes from different treatment options are not yet clear. Disease symptoms or therapy side effects can result in physical, social, spiritual, and psychological impairment.[7, 20] The extent of prostate cancer disease at the time of diagnosis and the treatment decisions will, at some point, affect a person's QOL. Long-term cancer survivors' views of side effects of treatment may be very different from those of side effects experienced during the initial time after diagnosis and treatment, because day-to-day functioning and coping may be altered over time.[7] The natural progression of prostate cancer warrants the need to capture the experience and the impact of that experience at various points along the disease, treatment, and observation continuum.[2, 21, 22] Schellhammer and colleagues[23] expressed the concern that, because an adequate time interval for detection of a decrease in mortality has yet to elapse in men with localized disease treated aggressively, early and aggressive therapy may not be appropriate in this group. Therefore, a lack of answers regarding benefit, morbidity, and mortality leads to QOL research for insight and information surrounding treatment choices.

Traditionally, outcomes for medical interventions in the management of prostate cancer have been overall survival time, disease-free survival, tumor response, and symptom management. Because uncertainty has arisen regarding the best course of management at different disease stages in men with prostate cancer, new endpoints for evaluation have been needed. QOL research broadens the dimension of cancer therapy outcomes. Comprehensive cancer care not only means disease and side effect management but also implies attention to the impact of disease and treatment modalities on a person's QOL. The treatment and disease impact information gained from QOL research may help patients, families, and care providers make informed decisions among alternative treatment strategies.

DECISION MAKING

With the knowledge that prostate cancer is the most common non-skin cancer in men older than 60,[24] there is a strong impetus to include QOL information when describing potential treatments and providing informed consent. QOL research provides patients with other patients' perceptions regarding the impact of their therapies on QOL. It is credible information because it originates from other patients and reflects what is important to them. This information may help patients decide among different therapies. Although patients and physicians have been found to agree on the preference for aggressive therapy, they differ in their definition of efficacy.[25] More than 90% of surveyed physicians equated treatment efficacy with survival extension, whereas 45% of patients defined treatment efficacy as preservation of QOL, 29% of patients as extension of expected QOL, and 13% of patients as delaying disease progression.[25] QOL information is most credible when shared with men and their partners if it is obtained from studies that reflect men's perspectives with same-stage disease and treatment courses.

CREDIBILITY IN PROSTATE CANCER QOL STUDIES

Studies have shown that physicians and patients prioritize QOL domains differently and have different overall health perceptions and evaluations of subjective morbidity.[20, 25–27] Fossa and associates[28] noted significant underestimation by physicians of subjective morbidity in 30 to 50% of patients with progressive hormone-resistant prostate cancer. Watkins-Bruner and colleagues[29] noted significant differences between medical professionals' and patients' severity ratings of problems with dysuria and diarrhea during curative radiotherapy.

Previously used instruments measuring QOL in the prostate cancer population were primarily functional scales and were completed by physician observation, resulting in low complication rates with localized treatment options. Questions arise regarding the validity of these low rates because the research captured the physicians' perceptions of the patients' side effects rather than the patients' perceptions.[30–32] Ferrell[2] emphasized the importance of patient perspective in QOL research by pointing out that the patients are the "experts" from whom the research or healthcare team is learning. Results may also be inaccurate if physicians or patients minimize symptoms and side effects.[33–35] For reasons of coping or in attempts to ward off hospitalization or further intervention, patients may minimize or deny the occurrence or severity of their experiences.[7] Because of this possibility, Ferrell and associates[7] suggested that how questions are asked of patients can greatly enrich the results.

Conducting QOL research in men with prostate cancer requires comparison with an age-matched group in the general population. This is important because this population tends to be elderly, and with advancing age, comorbidities increase, as do problems with sexual, urinary, and bowel function.[34]

PREDICTOR ABILITY

There is some suggestion that baseline measurements of QOL domains serve as predictors of overall health perceptions.[15] Assessment of social, physical functioning, and emotional aspects of HRQOL tend to be the strongest predictors of general overall health perceptions in prostate cancer patients.[5, 15, 36] This information can be used by care providers to recommend services and resources for patients' treatment plans.

CHALLENGES TO QOL RESEARCH IN PROSTATE CANCER

With the need for a comprehensive and yet globally accepted definition of QOL comes the added challenge of being able to standardize measurement tools.[18] The broad definition and lack of specific, universally accepted domains that comprise QOL are the

TABLE 13-1. Necessary Characteristics for Prostate Cancer Health-Related Quality of Life Research

- Not lengthy
- Reliable and valid
- Sensitive to changes in a patient's health status
- Multidimensional
- Nonburdensome
- Capable of international and cross-cultural standardization
- Contains global questions regarding the cancer experience
- Captures prostate cancer-specific morbidity
- Captures prostate cancer treatment-specific morbidity
- Self-administration capabilities
- Paper based
- Distress measurement in addition to frequency and degree
- Prospective design
- Captures baseline status and is able to be administered longitudinally

result of the vast number of ideas, definitions, studies, tools, and data published on QOL.[1, 3, 4, 37, 38] The numerous definitions of QOL, combined with the need to choose a tool that accurately captures family, socioeconomic, and cultural aspects, raise the issue of whether or not it is possible and credible for one tool to accommodate all patient populations. Ferrell and colleagues[3] described QOL of long-term cancer survivors using a comprehensive QOL model, and yet the majority of respondents were breast cancer survivors. Identifying an instrument that might be applicable for QOL measurement across many different cancer trials is challenging.[39] Ferrell[2] suggested a professional goal of identifying relevant core issues across cancer populations while refining population specific aspects. This goal is consistent with the 1996 development of the prostate cancer-specific module of the European Oncology Research and Treatment Cooperative Quality of Life Questionnaire (EORTC-QLQ-C30).[40]

Physician skepticism regarding the value of QOL research combined with a lack of familiarity with instruments contributed to the slow process of incorporating QOL tools into existing and evolving prostate cancer clinical trials.[5, 17, 28, 34] Finally, compliance has been poor in some prostate cancer studies because of lack of research support, patients' low motivation, lack of time in patients' schedule, and decline in health.[14]

Although the oncology nursing literature reflects QOL research in other patient populations,[41–43] the prostate cancer group has only recently received increased attention. Until very recently, prostate cancer QOL research has been designed and conducted as an adjunct to therapeutic clinical trials.

HRQOL INSTRUMENTS

Questionnaires measuring symptoms, problems, and experiences need to be written in a manner that can be easily and quickly completed by patients. Ideally, questionnaires should not take more than 40 minutes to complete.[13] Table 13-1 lists characteristics of

HRQOL instruments that are necessary for comprehensive measurement of symptoms, functional status, and QOL.

Because HRQOL is a subjective measure, instruments are often designed for self-report.[44] A number of QOL instruments that have been used in prostate clinical trials are now discussed.

The Medical Outcomes Short-Form General Health Survey (RAND SF-36) is a global health status–QOL questionnaire. Not limited to use in the oncology population, this tool is applied to the study of a variety of chronic disease patient populations.[45–47] It captures eight domains of health: physical functioning, role-physical (limitations in performing one's daily role because of physical health), role-emotional (limitations in performing one's daily role because of mental health), bodily pain, general health, vitality, social functioning, and mental health. Scores range from 0 to 100; higher scores represent better levels of functioning. Scales of this instrument differentiate between patient sample and the general population. The psychometric properties of this instrument have been studied and supported.[39]

The EORTC Quality of Life Questionnaire (EORTC-QLQ-C30, Version 2) is specially designed to study QOL in patients with cancer. The domains include physical function, role function, urologic symptoms, fatigue, sexual function, emotional function, social function, and pain.[14] Composed of 30 questions, it has an overall health-related QOL scale and is divided into five functioning scales (physical, role, cognitive, emotional, and social) and three symptom scales (fatigue, pain, and nausea and vomiting). For functional scales and overall QOL, higher scores reflect a higher level of functioning. Higher scores within the symptom scales indicate higher levels of symptomatology.[48] This questionnaire has been validated in lung, head, and neck cancer patients; is able to detect baseline differences between subgroups of patients with different clinical status; and has excellent psychometric properties.[44, 49] A prostate cancer–specific questionnaire, using the same response format and shown to be psychometrically sound, was developed to cover areas not adequately evaluated in the EORTC QLQ-C30.[40] The combination provides a comprehensive and accurate picture of the patient's experience.

The Cancer Rehabilitation Evaluation System—Short Form (CARES-SF) is a rehabilitation and QOL instrument that measures information about the day-to-day problems of cancer patients. The five overall domains are physical, psychosocial, medical interaction, marital, and sexual. Psychometric properties and sensitivity to changes in health status over time are excellent.[50]

The Functional Assessment of Cancer Therapy—General (FACT-G) is a 33-item general cancer QOL questionnaire. Five subscales covered are as follows: physical, functional, social, emotional, and relationship with doctor.[51] The scale is sensitive enough to differentiate patients on the basis of disease stage, performance status, and hospitalization status. Psychometric properties of this instrument are high. FACT-P is a 12-item prostate cancer subscale reported in the literature in 1997. Initial psychometric testing has been conducted, but further study is still required.

HRQOL IN LOCALIZED PROSTATE CANCER

Although radical prostatectomy and radiation therapy demonstrate similar survival patterns in men with localized disease, the risk of side effects that significantly influence health perceptions and HRQOL accompany both treatment modalities.[21] Studies that measure side effects from curative radiotherapy or prostatectomy and their impact on HRQOL, both short term and long term, are necessary. Also required is QOL research in men who choose watchful waiting and monitor the natural course of the disease. If the side effect impact on HRQOL was well established, this information could be shared with men at the time of diagnosis and assist in treatment decision making.

TREATMENT OPTIONS FOR LOCALIZED PROSTATE CANCER

Localized prostate cancer is usually treated with radical prostatectomy, external beam radiotherapy, or watchful waiting. Variables that enter into treatment decision making include age, accompanying comorbidities, and the preferences of the patient and significant other. Prostatectomy and radiation therapy can result in serious side effects, which can affect a person's QOL. Thus, treatments that seem equal based on disease response and survival may not be "equal" if QOL is considered.[52] Because two thirds of men diagnosed with prostate cancer have localized disease, will be older than 70, and have a cancer that is slow growing, it is very likely that patients will die from other medical problems before prostate cancer.[33] Therefore, the majority of newly diagnosed prostate patients make decisions about treatment options that will have significant side effects for the rest of their lives to prevent metastatic disease that will lead to death in only a minority of these patients.[33]

In an analysis of 260 men with newly diagnosed, localized disease, Talcott and colleagues[33] found that the men who chose prostatectomy over external beam radiotherapy were, on average, 6 years younger. Increased screening for prostate cancer has resulted in younger men being diagnosed and increasing numbers of radical prostatectomies being performed. Among patients who have undergone a radical prostatectomy, the most common reports of side effects tend to be urinary incontinence and impotence. Among postradiotherapy patients, bowel disturbances have been most often reported.

A number of QOL studies have begun to capture the incidence and distress (how bothersome) of sexual, urinary, and bowel dysfunction.[33, 34, 53] Litwin and colleagues,[34] in their study of side effect outcomes, reported no significant difference in overall HRQOL between groups of men who underwent radical prostatectomy and those who received external beam radiotherapy for localized prostate cancer despite physical symptoms and sexual dysfunction. Maintenance of sexual activity may be less important to patients when they compare it with the attempt to cure the disease; thus, radical prostatectomy may be viewed as having a minimal effect on overall QOL.[19, 35, 54]

URINARY INCONTINENCE

Although continence has been reported as being regained in as many as 94% of men 18 months after prostatectomy, there are also reports of a high prevalence of incontinence (2–87%) lasting years after a radical prostatectomy.[55] A factor in the vast difference in prevalence is that the definition of incontinence is not standardized across studies.[56] In some studies, incontinence is defined as any amount or frequency or urine leakage. Such a strict definition would result in more people being categorized as incontinent.[57]

Significantly more urinary dysfunction is reported in men after prostatectomy than in men who receive radiotherapy.[30, 34, 58, 59] In Talcott and associates'[33] study, pretreatment incontinence was uncommon in both treatment groups (surgery and radiotherapy), occurring in 3% or less. After treatment, there was a significantly higher incidence of urinary incontinence in the prostatectomy group; 58% at 3 months and 35% at 12 months. At 12 months, 5% of patients who reported leaking or dribbling had used a penile clamp within the previous week. Litwin and colleagues[34] reported a 40% incidence of urine leakage; 10% of men used more than two pads a day for leakage 2 years after surgery. Fowler and associates[53] reported that at 5 to 6 years after surgery, 31% of men used pads, adult diapers, or penile clamps to manage urinary incontinence.

The increasing number of prostatectomies being performed correlates with the increasing number of men dealing with incontinence.[60–64] Because men undergoing prostatectomy are, on average, 10 to 15 years younger than their radiotherapy counterparts, incontinence is going to be a problem for a greater number of years.

Urinary problems include greater frequency and amounts of urine leakage, increased leaking with coughing or sneezing, more interference in sexual function as a result of leakage, and greater use of devices such as disposable absorbent products, clamps, and external catheters.[65] Although the level of urinary dysfunction has been shown to be significantly higher in the surgery group than in the radiotherapy group, the level of distress with incontinence (how bothered) is reported as equal between the two groups. Patients report being moderately or extremely upset because of their incontinence regardless of treatment modality.[66] Patients may experience anxiety, hopelessness, loss of control, and low self-esteem because of their bladder problems.[56] Increased depression and anger has been noted in men with incontinence 12 months after prostatectomy.[35] Incontinence can result in feelings of shame and sensitivity to the attitudes and reactions of others.[67] Hesitancy to be away from home for fear of leakage can limit social activities and lead to feelings of isolation. Fear of urine leakage can also cause a man to withdraw from his partner and avoid sexual relations, often adding to the stress of the prostate experience.[62]

TYPES OF INCONTINENCE

The four common types of urinary incontinence (the involuntary loss of urine per the urethra) are stress, urge, overflow, and functional incontinence. The causes of postprostatectomy incontinence are complex, not clearly understood, and most likely multifactorial.[61, 68, 69] Stress incontinence occurs with an increase in intraabdominal pressure such as coughing, straining, sneezing, and laughing. Stress incontinence after prostatectomy is due to sphincteric insufficiency. The proximal sphincter located in the prostate gland is removed during surgery, leaving only the distal urethral sphincter to control postoperative continence. If the distal urethral sphincter is unable to resist bladder-filling pressures or increased pressures resulting from, for example, coughing and sneezing, incontinence results. Ficazzola and Nitti[60] found postprostatectomy incontinence to be due to intrinsic sphincter deficiency in 90% of incontinent men. Symptoms of stress incontinence after prostatectomy are 95% accurate for predicting intrinsic sphincter deficiency.[60]

Urge incontinence is accompanied by a feeling or urgency to void. It is primarily because of bladder dysfunction; the bladder is unable to store urine. The bladder may be unable to store urine for a number of reasons, including involuntary detrusor contractions (bladder spasms), low bladder compliance, sensory urgency, or a fistula.[56] Detrusor instability can be manifested by urgency, frequency, and urge incontinence.[57] Bladder dysfunction, although a contributor to postprostatectomy incontinence, has been shown to be the sole cause of postprostatectomy incontinence in only 3% of patients. In fact, bladder dysfunction can be present without actually causing incontinence.[60] Urge incontinence and bladder dysfunction usually occur in combination with stress incontinence and sphincter deficiency. Additionally, before prostatectomy, it is thought that men have bladder contractions to overcome the tumor obstruction, but after surgery or radiotherapy, the bladder contractions persist, with resultant incontinence.[62]

Overflow incontinence is the loss of urine resulting from the inability to empty the bladder completely because of the bladder itself or outlet obstruction.[56] Overflow incontinence is characterized by reports of frequent voiding and the feeling that there is still the need to void. Functional incontinence is associated with altered mental status or physical disability that interferes with getting to the bathroom or removing clothes. Although these may occur in men with prostate cancer, they are not common types of prostate cancer–associated incontinence.

INCONTINENCE ASSESSMENT

The first step in attempting to help patients manage their incontinence is assessment to identify characteristics and contributing factors of urinary incontinence. A bladder diary or record of intake, number and amount of continent and incontinent episodes, precipitating events, urgency and leakage, and number of pads used provides a patient profile. Analysis of the profile leads to identification of causes and serves as an evaluation by which to measure the success of interventions.[56, 61, 70, 71] This type of in-depth and specialized assessment and physical examination of the patient with urinary incontinence can be performed by an advanced practice nurse or urologist. Physical examination of the abdominal and rectal muscles is important for determining strength and the potential for successful execution of pelvic muscle exercises. Postvoid residuals and cystograms can be done in the office, are inexpensive, and provide information about uninhibited detrusor contractions, bladder dysfunction, obstructive incontinence, and stress incontinence.

Before any interventions, patients should first be educated about fluid and dietary intake, limiting fluids to 48 to 64 ounces/day. This fluid intake is sufficient to stimulate bladder stretch receptors while also diluting the urine. Avoidance of caffeine and alcohol is recommended to minimize bladder irritants.

Goals of interventions are to gain as much continence as possible through interventions that are not invasive and are, therefore, low risk. The Clinical Practice Guidelines for Urinary Continence in Adults by the Agency for Health Care Policy and Research (AHCPR)[72] are standards that promote using behavioral interventions first before progressing to pharmacologic and surgical options. Because postprostatectomy urinary incontinence is probably due to a combination of stress and urge incontinence, behavioral interventions stand a good chance of being successful.

The majority of urinary incontinence studies have involved women; thus, research regarding behavioral interventions for postprostatectomy incontinence is limited. Behavioral techniques have been associated with significant improvements in reducing incontinent episodes.[73–75] Improvements have been found with the use of pelvic muscle exercises (PMEs), voiding schedules, and urgency training.[76, 77]

NURSING INTERVENTIONS

Continence interventions are intended for avoidance of long-term use of indwelling catheters.[78] Nursing care begins with a knowledge of the different options available to patients. A comprehensive assessment of the patient and social situation assists the nurse in identifying educational needs, dexterity abilities, support system, and, most importantly, the patient's wishes and goals. Regardless of the interventions chosen, patients require in-depth and repeated education, informal as well as formal demonstration sessions. Repeated encounters with the patient and partner, whether in person or via the telephone, allow for repeated explanations and reinforcement based on the patient's needs.

PMEs, or Kegel exercises, are intended to contract the pubococcygeal muscle and, by increasing the muscle strength, increase urethral resistance.[61] PMEs support, lengthen, and compress the urethra.[79] PMEs are useful in treating stress incontinence and possibly urge incontinence.[71] The most important challenge in teaching PMEs is helping the patient correctly identify his pelvic muscle. If the patient is unable to identify and contract the muscle correctly, intraabdominal pressure can increase, thereby worsening the incontinence. PMEs can be taught verbally, with patients correctly contracting the muscle during a rectal examination, or through biofeedback.[56, 61, 70, 72] Biofeedback is a teaching mechanism that lets patients know how they are performing the exercises through visual or auditory feedback. Biofeedback is particularly helpful when patients are having difficulty contracting the appropriate muscle or have no awareness of function. The goal of biofeedback in the patient with urinary incontinence is to "alter physiologic responses of the detrusor and pelvic muscles that mediate urine loss" by providing information back to the patient which assists in learning the new skill (p. 130).[73] The combination of biofeedback and PMEs has reportedly resulted in a 95% reduction in urinary incontinent episodes.[80]

A biofeedback program instituted postoperatively by the fourth week involves two to three office visits per week for approximately 15 to 40 minutes. This program can include a home biofeedback component. Patients progress at their own pace, and instructional programs can last an average of 3 to 6 weeks for 4 to 20 sessions. A personal home monitor and a specific protocol are designed for each patient. Surface electrodes, placed on external pelvic floor sites, measure, record, and amplify muscle exercise activity.[81] Patients are instructed to practice these exercises a set number of times per day. Information is given to the patient about their pelvic muscle activity as they exercise from auditory and visual information on the home monitor. The monitor also stores information so that the certified biofeedback clinician can review the patient's home activity and evaluate whether the protocol is being carried out as prescribed.[80] Before becoming incontinent, patients are most likely unaware of the physiologic functions associated with bladder control. Biofeedback brings these visceral functions to a conscious level so that the patient can then begin to modify them.[82]

Bladder training can be used for both stress and urge incontinence. A bladder training program is aimed at teaching patients to void on a schedule rather than in response to sensations. The program consists of a mandatory voiding schedule that gradually extends to voiding every 3 to 4 hours. A bladder training program is intended to decrease voiding frequency, increase bladder capacity, and suppress the bladder urgency.[74] Patients are encouraged to note and control their fluid consumption, because average intake volumes are incorporated into their training plan. In addition to an established schedule, patients are taught distraction and relaxation techniques for use during episodes of urgency.

Electrical stimulation may be helpful for stress and urge incontinence. It is used to strengthen and tone pelvic muscles by innervating the pelvic viscera, pelvic muscle, or nerve supply; increasing urethral resistance; or inhibiting bladder contractility.[70] Bladder instability is inhibited, and sphincter contractility is improved. Electrical stimulation may also be helpful with pelvic muscle exercises by helping patients who have weak muscles or who do not know where the muscles are located.[71] Patients can be trained in their own home with a home electrical stimulation unit.

Pharmacologic interventions include anticholinergics or tricyclic antidepressants for reducing involuntary detrusor contractions (bladder contractions) and increasing bladder capacity. These are indicated in the patient with urge incontinence.[72] Side effects of dry mouth, visual disturbances, constipation, and dry skin are often intolerable for patients, resulting in drug cessation. Alpha-adrenergic agents used to increase smooth muscle tone are indicated for stress incontinence because urethral resistance can be improved.[72] Side effects of anxiety, insomnia, agitation, respiratory difficulty, sweating, cardioarrhythmia, and hypertension can lead to drug discontinuation (Table 13-2).[83–85] Caution is warranted when prescribing or caring for patients taking different agents for urinary incontinence because adverse reactions are likely, particularly in the elderly. The elderly are also at greater risk for confusion, tachycardia, urinary retention, postural hypotension, hallucinations, and nightmares. Side effects are often dose dependent and

TABLE 13-2. Pharmacologic Therapy for Stress-Urge Incontinence

Drug	Dose	Indications	Side Effects
ANTICHOLINERGICS AND ANTIMUSCARINICS*			
Oxybutynin	2.5–5 mg tid-qid	Direct relaxant effect on detrusor muscle. AHCPR-recommended anticholinergic drug of choice for treatment of detrusor instability	Dry mouth*[†] Blurred vision[†] Constipation[†]
Propantheline (synthetic analogue of atropine with pure anticholinergic properties)	7.5–30 mg 3–5 times/day up to 60 mg qid	Recommended second-line agent for urge incontinence secondary to detrusor instability in patients who can tolerate full dosage	Headache, Xerostomia[†] Blurred vision[†] Drowsiness, Constipation, Tachycardia, Inhibition of gut motility, Dizziness[†]
Dicyclomine (synthetic antimuscarinic with direct smooth muscle relaxant effect)	10–20 mg bid	May be used as alternative agent to propantheline for urge incontinence	
Emepronium bromide		Only available in Europe for detrusor instability	
TRICYCLIC ANTIDEPRESSANTS‡			
Imipramine	10–25 mg 1–3 times/day, increased to a maximum of 150 mg/day; less frequent administration often possible because of long half-life.	Urine storage facilitated by decreasing bladder contractility and increasing outlet resistance	Dry mouth[†], Blurred vision, Constipation
Doxepin	Used interchangeably with imipramine; 50 mg qhs with or without 25 mg in the AM		Gut motility inhibition, Arrhythmias, Drowsiness and confusion at higher doses, Weakness, Fatigue, Orthostatic hypotension may be marked in elderly, Anxiety, Anorexia
ADRENERGIC AGENTS§			
Phenylpropanolamine	50–100 mg bid	Stress incontinence	Anxiety, Insomnia, Agitation, Dyspnea, Headache, Sweating, Hypertension, Arrhythmias, Dry mouth[†], Tachycardia

[†]Most common. *Anticholinergics are AHCPR recommended first-line therapy for patients with detrusor instability. These drugs act on muscarinic and acetylcholine receptors throughout the bladder, suppressing involuntary as well as normal contractions, which result in urge incontinence. ‡Widely used in the treatment of urge incontinence, especially nocturnal incontinence. §These drugs act at α-adrenoceptors in the bladder neck, base, and proximal urethra, treating the urethral sphincter insufficiency that causes stress incontinence. tid, three times a day; qid, four times a day; AHCPR, Agency for Health Care Policy and Research; bid, twice daily; qhs, every bedtime.

can limit optimal dosing.[65] At each health visit, repeated assessments of medications the patient might be taking and any side effects can assist in identifying potential problems or risk for complications.

Artificial sphincters are used when behavioral or pharmacologic interventions have failed to control urinary incontinence. Surgical placement is required, and artificial sphincters are usually not placed until bladder pressures are controlled, because high bladder pressure dysfunction will lead to sphincter failure.[62] Surgery is usually not conducted until all other therapies are proven unsuccessful and the incontinence is debilitating to the patient.[68] An artificial sphincter cuff, available in a variety of sizes, is surgically placed into the bladder neck or bulbar urethra.[86] Side effects of an artificial sphincter include infection, persistent incontinence, and erosion of the device through the tissue.[86]

The condom catheter and external collecting pouch are external continence devices. A penile shaft of sufficient length is necessary for the device to fit, and large collection bags should be avoided so that the urine collection does not pull the device off the penis. Manual dexterity is required because the device needs to be changed every 24 to 48 hours. Patients are taught to start with a clean, dry surface and apply the device carefully to avoid ulceration and pressure to the delicate skin.

Penile clamps prevent leakage by closing off the urethra externally. Care in application is taught so that not too much pressure is applied, resulting in ulceration and necrosis. Patients should be taught to release the clamp every 2 hours to urinate or immediately if they experience discomfort. To avoid pressure problems, clamps should not be worn at night. Clamps can be recommended to patients during high-stress activities, which, in the past, have resulted in leakage, such as sports, dancing, and yard work. Men will often discontinue their use because they find them uncomfortable.

Pads and continence garments can be either disposable or reusable. Disposable garments, although convenient, can become costly over time. Costs vary depending on the patient and the number of incontinent episodes. Urinary containment products in the United States are a multimillion dollar industry.[87] Although reusable products are cost effective, they are costly and time consuming to wash and maintain. Regardless of the type of product, all pads and continence garments can result in dependence and inhibit patients from seeking options for other interventions. These types of easy but costly products lead men to learn to live with the incontinence rather than intervene. Patients should be encouraged to use them for the short term: in the postoperative period, during high-stress activities, or while they are learning other means of management. Because of the high risk of skin breakdown from constant urine contact, meticulous skin care with barrier creams, ointments, and films should be included in patient education.

SEXUAL DYSFUNCTION

Sexual dysfunction, as referred to in the research literature, includes decreased frequency and quality of erections, decreased morning erections, decreased intercourse, and decreased ability to achieve sexual climax; changes in sexual desire; and change in orgasm.[34, 88] Erectile dysfunction can include the inability to obtain an erection with arousal regularly, the permanent inability to obtain an erection (complete impotence), and the inability to obtain an erection firm enough for penetration. In addition, sexual dysfunction can include decreased libido, deficiency in arousal, and inability to achieve an orgasm. Although sexual function may decline with age, it has not been validated that its importance to men declines as well. Many people continue sexual relations well into their 70s, and men older than 65 are just as likely as those younger than 65 to regard impotency as a major issue.[35]

Litwin and others[34] noted no distinguishable statistically significant differences in sexual function and how "bothered" or how much distress existed among the active treatment groups for localized prostate cancer (surgery, radiotherapy, watchful waiting). All three treatment option groups scored significantly worse than the age-matched nonprostate comparison group. Reports of worsening sexual function in men having undergone radiotherapy or prostatectomy do not necessarily translate into overall decreased QOL.[15, 54] Despite an overall impact on QOL, sexual dysfunction may still be a major issue for patients but may be viewed as separate from QOL.[35] Despite sexual dysfunction, patients report that they would repeat their treatment again.

After adjusting for age, postprostatectomy men have significantly worse sexual dysfunction than radiotherapy patients.[34, 59] Talcott and others[33] noted an 85% complete impotence rate at 3 months and 75% at 12 months after radical prostatectomy. Incomplete erections were reported by 96% at 3 months and 93% at 12 months. These rates are significantly higher than pretreatment impotency rates of 11% experiencing complete dysfunction and 32% experiencing erections inadequate for sexual intercourse. When analyzing only those men who had erections before treatment, the surgery group had significantly higher rates of erectile dysfunction after treatment than the radiotherapy group. Impotency rates within the radiotherapy groups are higher with larger pelvic fields, as opposed to three-dimensional conformal therapy.

Although men who underwent radiotherapy retain a higher level of some type of sexual functioning than men who had prostatectomy, there are consistent reports of a general decline in the quality and frequency of sexual function.[32, 40, 88–90] Helgason and colleagues[88] reported that 1½ to 2 years after radiotherapy, a majority of men believed their QOL was reduced because of alterations in sexual capacity. Posttreatment changes included sexual desire, erection capacity, and orgasm. Eighty-four percent of the men in the study[88] reported an overall decrease in frequency of sexual functioning, whereas 44% reported a decrease in the importance of sex. Beard and associates[91] noted prominent sexual dysfunction pretreatment, which is consistent with other studies, and worsening erectile dysfunction 12 months after treatment. Almost 40% of 337 men (average age, 69) reported markedly decreased sexual desire and overall sexual dissatisfaction before treatment. These dimensions did not change significantly after treatment despite the worsening erectile function. Risk factors for erectile dysfunction in men who underwent radiotherapy for localized prostate cancer are older age before treatment, size of field to be irradiated, and dose and fractionation of the radiotherapy.

Rosseti and Terrone[19] reported that 91% of 161 men, when informed of the possibility of conserving potency by using a nerve-sparing surgical intervention, wanted to have the surgery with the greater chance of cure as opposed to maintenance of sexual activity. Despite nerve-sparing procedures, which aim to leave the neurovascular bundles intact, thus allowing for erection, erectile dysfunction can still occur after prostatectomy.[92] Litwin and colleagues[34] noted no significant difference in men who had a nerve-sparing prostatectomy compared with men who underwent the standard procedure. Men older than 70 are unlikely to regain potency regardless of the type of surgical approach. Risk factors for erectile dysfunction in men after prostatectomy include age, preoperative erectile dysfunction, tumor extension, the surgical procedure itself, and circulatory problems.[93] Tumor extension into the seminal vesicles or outside the capsule is a risk factor for impotency. Patients with atherosclerosis or whose blood supply to the corpora cavernosa has been interrupted may experience dysfunction.

Fowler and colleagues'[53] assessment of sexual function 2 to 4 years after radical prostatectomy supports the significant incidence of erectile dysfunction. They reported that 61% of men had no erections after 2 to 4 years. In a review of results from a study completed more than 5 years after prostatectomy, 52% of men reported complete impotence and only 29% reported erections adequate for intercourse or foreplay.[34]

Spouses and partners of men with erectile dysfunction after treatment for prostate cancer need to be included in all education sessions so that they are aware of potential changes. Partners are active participants, accompanying the men to healthcare sessions for treatment of erectile dysfunction. Wives report similar needs for intimacy and physical contact; their levels of satisfaction measured similarly to those of men when they are involved and maintaining close communication and physical contact with their spouses. For some couples, intimacy without intercourse is just as satisfying, and, with good communication, they can work out their needs. Couples with past patterns of difficulty expressing their feelings or their needs to their spouses may benefit from referral to a psychosocial healthcare team member or sexual counselor.

MANAGEMENT OF ERECTILE DYSFUNCTION

Three options for erectile dysfunction exist: vacuum constriction devices (VCDs), penile implants, and pharmacologic therapy.

Sexual dysfunction needs to be understood in the context of the patient's history, disease status, and psychosocial situation. Determining options for the patient involves considering the least invasive intervention and the patient's and his partner's strengths and preferences. It is necessary to have an integrated approach to patients with input from the urologist, radiation oncologist, oncology nurses, psychosocial team, and others specializing in sexuality.

VCDs are considered the least invasive, least expensive, and safest option available.[93] VCDs, available by prescription, consist of a clear plastic cylinder, an attached vacuum pump with tubing, and constriction bands or rings (Figure 13-1). The VCD is effective in producing erections in approximately 89% of men, has a dropout rate of less than 20%,

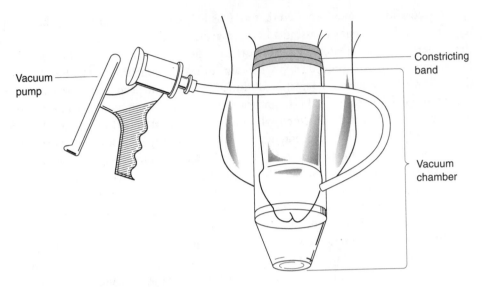

FIGURE 13-1. Vacuum chamber device
Illustration by Esther Muscari Lin. Used with permission.

and has been shown to improve psychological well-being and marital relationships.[94] Requirements for successful VCD use include manual dexterity and motivation of the patient and partner to understand the device and practice before regular use.

With the VCD, a vacuum is created around the penis with a battery-driven pump, creating a negative pressure so that the penis becomes passively engorged with blood and tumescence results. The erection-like state can be maintained for 30 minutes with a ring or band that is slid off the vacuum chamber onto the penis base.

Side effects from a VCD are usually limited to the time the band is on the penis base. Decreased penile skin temperature, penile numbness, penile cyanosis, and increased penile girth result from decreased blood flow and extracorporal tissue and superficial vein congestion.[93, 95] Pain can occur if the device is pumped too quickly, scrotal tissue is pulled into the cylinder, or the constriction band is too tight. Excessive pressure during pumping is avoided with current devices equipped with safety valves. Petechiae or hematomas may result if pressures approach 180 mm Hg during pumping.[96] A pressure of 100 mm Hg is usually sufficient to achieve tumescence. Blocked ejaculation can occur in a large percentage of men if the band is so tight that the urethra is obstructed.

Patient education begins with emphasizing the amount of preparation time necessary before regular use. Patients need to practice applying the device and pumping the vacuum chamber up a number of times before they apply a band. Some devices come in a variety of sizes, which decreases the chance of catching scrotal tissue in the chamber. Instruct patients that foreplay with achievement of a partial erection can be helpful before applying the VCD. VCD application after a partial erection may also decrease the chance of blocked ejaculation, because the constriction band does not need to be as tight.[94]

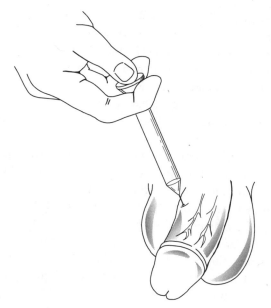

FIGURE 13-2. Intracavernosal injections (hand is above the penis)
Illustration by Esther Muscari Lin. Used with permission.

Patients should be informed that if the band is too tight, discomfort and numbness can result. If the constriction band is not tight enough, the erection will slowly lose rigidity and they may need to use two or more bands.[94] Because of the constriction and resultant penile coolness, partners need to be forewarned about the cold temperature and the liberal use of lubricant.[97]

Instruct patients to avoid salicylate preparations and nonsteroidal anti-inflammatories. Caution is warranted with VCD use if patients are taking anticoagulants or are thrombocytopenic. As patients pump the device, they should be instructed not to pump too rapidly and to hold the scrotum down so that the tissue is not pulled into the chamber. Refraining from lubrication during pumping can help avoid scrotal tissue being pulled into the chamber. Lubrication should be applied after a band has been applied and may help raise the penile temperature.

Patient and partner support is necessary, particularly during the first few weeks of learning to use the VCD. Dissatisfaction resulting in device discontinuation is usually because of premature loss of penile tumescence and pain or discomfort.[98] Contacting patients after their initial attempts with the device in their home can be very helpful. It allows patients and partners to validate the procedure, ask questions, and receive encouragement to try again. Psychosocial support groups with other men and their partners contribute practical tips and help decrease some of the isolation that patients and their partners feel. Groups also assist in validating the gamut of emotions couples experience in their attempts to achieve satisfying sexual relations.

Intracavernosal, or penile, injections involve inserting a small (1-mL) syringe with a 27- or 30-gauge needle into the side of the penis (the corpora cavernosa) and injecting a vasoactive medication to produce an erection (Figure 13-2). Intracavernosal injections are capable of initiating a rapid-onset erection in approximately 90% of patients.[99] Vasoactive agents used alone or in combination include prostaglandin E (alprostadil [Muse]), papaverine, and phentolamine.[99–102] Combination use allows for smaller doses of each drug and injection volume. Sexual stimulation also lowers the drug dose necessary for erection.[93]

Minor potential side effects of intracavernosal injections include pain, ecchymosis at the injection site, local infections, prolonged erections, and mild liver enzyme elevations.[103] Pain, when it occurs, tends to be at the time of injection and is less of a problem when drugs are mixed in lower alcohol concentrations.[100] Elevated liver enzymes that have been reported have been associated with alcohol.[103] Although infections at the site of injection can occur, they are extremely rare. Prolonged erections usually occur during the period of dose determination in the clinic setting. During the dose titration phase, approximately 10% of patients experience a prolonged erection.[93] This percentage drops drastically once injections begin in the home.

Major complications are fibrotic changes in the corporeal tissue (focal or diffuse) and vasovagal responses.[93, 99, 103] Fibrosis in the corpora occurs in the form of nodules or plaques.[93] Fibrosis is associated with papaverine injection alone or in combination with prostaglandin E.[103] Lakin and others[103] reported fibrotic complications in 31% (N = 100) of patients at 12 months, correlating significantly with the number of injections and number of months injections have been administered. When prostaglandin E is used alone, the risk of fibrosis is lower. The typical presentation is one of asymmetric curvature, sometimes associated with an area of induration.[94] Patients with significant cardiovascular or cerebrovascular disease, in whom hypotension could be harmful, should be carefully screened by their primary care physician because of the risk of a vasovagal response. Although unusual, during the dose titration phase, hypotension or hypertension can occur.[93]

Ascertaining patients' comfort level with intracavernosal injection therapy is important because it may be unappealing to some patients. Once patients have expressed a desire to learn about the therapy, patient education begins, teaching patients and their partners about candidacy for intracavernosal injections. A good candidate has adequate visual acuity, manual dexterity, and no morbid obesity or significant cardiovascular-cerebrovascular disease. Intracavernosal injection therapy should be avoided in men with a history of priapism or corpora fibrosis, elevated liver enzymes, or the sickle cell trait or disease.[93] The patient is educated about the risks; the necessary titration period, with patients remaining in the clinic until detumescence has occurred; and potential complications (minor and major). Patients need to be instructed to contact their healthcare provider in the case of a prolonged erection lasting more than 3 to 4 hours, because detumescence usually occurs 1 hour after injection. Intracavernosal therapy erections can be reversed with intracorporal injections of phenylephrine and epinephrine at 5-minute intervals until detumescence occurs.

Transurethral prostaglandin E (alprostadil) is self-administered via an applicator 3 cm into the distal urethra. Doses begin at 125 to 250 μg and are titrated to a total dose of 500 to 1000 μg for an erection sufficient for intercourse.[99] The majority of alprostadil is absorbed through the urethral mucosa within 10 minutes, and erections should last 30 to 60 minutes.[104] Use of alprostadil has been shown to be effective in 70% of men with post-prostatectomy erectile dysfunction.[105]

Side effects of transurethral administration consist primarily of local burning or pain associated with the drug metabolism.[99, 105] Other less common side effects include hematuria from urethral bleeding, dizziness, hypotension, and priapism.[99]

Patient education includes instructing patients to pull the penis upright before suppository insertion. After insertion, rubbing the penis for 30 seconds helps with drug absorption. If pain or stinging occurs, they should continue rubbing the penis between their hands until the discomfort dissipates.

The U.S. Food and Drug Administration has approved oral pharmacologic therapy in the form of sildenafil (Viagra) for erectile dysfunction. It enhances the normal sexual response by potentiating penile tumescence. Sildenafil stimulates the relaxation of smooth muscles in the corpora cavernosa so that blood flow to the penis increases, filling the spongy tissue within the corpora cavernosa and leading to penile tumescence. Full rigidity is maintained when veins exiting the corpora are compressed, limiting outward blood flow. Sexual stimulation is required for onset of action because sildenafil does not result in a rapid-onset erection, as with pharmacologic injections, and does not cause an erection in the absence of sexual stimulation.[106–108] The recommended dose is 25 to 100 mg 1 hour before anticipated sexual activity. Goldstein and colleagues[106] reported that 69% of all sexual intercourse attempts were successful in a group of 329 men with varying underlying causes of erectile dysfunction in a sildenafil dose-escalating study. The mean number of successful monthly attempts was significantly greater than in the group of men taking placebo. To date, studies of sildenafil in men after prostatectomy and stratified by procedure (nerve sparing or nonnerve sparing) are limited.[109] Although patient numbers are small, Zippe and colleagues[109] suggested that the success of sildenafil in men after prostatectomy depends on the presence of bilateral neurovascular bundles.

Sildenafil is generally well tolerated; because its half-life is 3 to 5 hours, all side effects are mild and transient.[106, 110] The more common side effects include headaches, facial flushing, and dyspepsia.[106] Nasal congestion and visual disturbances (described as blue-tinged vision, sensitivity to bright light, and blurred vision) are less common and are associated with increasing doses.[99, 106, 108, 110]

Patient education includes instruction regarding usage (only one dose daily), expected side effects, and symptoms to report to their healthcare provider. Sildenafil is strictly contraindicated in patients using oral or transdermal nitrates.[107] Patients with a history of hypotension are also warned of potential hypotensive side effects.

Penile prostheses are usually not considered an option in men who underwent prostatectomy until 1 year after the procedure to be sure that no sexual function has returned. Although penile prostheses have the highest rate of patient satisfaction, they also are accompanied with the most significant complications. Implants are usually reserved for men who have considered vacuum devices and pharmacologic therapy first. Devices can be broadly categorized as semirigid, malleable, or hydraulic inflatable and multicomponent or one-piece instruments. Prostheses require surgery, and a number of different devices are available; the urologist can select the most appropriate device for the patient based on his general health and age, patient's and partner's degree of manual dexterity, penile size, and patient preference.[93]

Potential side effects of penile implants include component failure, infection, and erosion.[69, 93, 99] Infection usually occurs within the first 3 months but can occur later. Prophylactic antibiotics should be considered in the patient who undergoes a procedure in which there is the possibility of a bacteremia.[111] Because of the way the prosthesis is made, the penis is unable to be in a completely flaccid state, which can sometimes be embarrassing or lead to discomfort.

Patient education is vital before surgery because unrealistic expectations can result in dissatisfaction. Patients need to understand that potential complications requiring reoperation do exist and that device removal is always a possibility. In addition, it should be emphasized that, once they have undergone penile prosthetic surgery, other alternatives cannot be offered subsequently.[99] Preoperatively, patients should understand that the penis is, on average, 1/2 to 1 inch shorter, with even more marked shortening in those who have corporal scarring from a previous injection program.

BOWEL DISTURBANCES

Patients who received radiotherapy for prostate cancer report more problems of bowel dysfunction than those who underwent prostatectomy.[13, 34, 59, 91, 112] Diarrhea, rectal urgency, crampy abdominal pain, and bleeding associated with bowel movements are the problems patients report as bothersome.[34, 59, 69, 90] Although bowel dysfunction is reported as bothersome, its impact on overall HRQOL has been reported as minor.[13]

Radiotherapy side effects can be acute or short term, associated with the treatment period, and often resolve within 1 year after treatment completion. Common acute side effects associated with prostate cancer treatment are diarrhea, rectal urgency, and pain with bowel movements. Sixty percent of patients on treatment experience one or more of these symptoms during the third week of treatment, requiring pharmacologic intervention.[113] Pharmacologic management is directed at reducing gastric motility and water content of stool. Commonly used drug classifications are opiates, anticholinergics, and bulk-forming drugs.[114] Commonly used agents are pectin, atropine sulfate with diphenoxylate hydrochloride, loperamide hydrochloride, tincture of opium, psyllium, methylcellulose, and octreotide acetate.[115] Johnson and colleagues[116] showed that weekly education on expected side effects and self-care suggestions resulted in a 31 to 60% decrease in disruption of patients' usual life activities. This study is an example of interventions that may influence overall HRQOL during the treatment phase.

Long-term or chronic complications can occur years after treatment completion. Long-term treatment sequelae from radiation therapy for prostate cancer are more often gastrointestinal complications.[117] Beard and others [91]reported that the incidence of these symptoms increases 3 months after treatment and then, although still elevated above baseline, declines substantially by 1 year. Radiation proctopathy, often referred to as radiation proctitis, is an outcome of radiation therapy directed at the pelvis. Features associated with radiation proctopathy include diarrhea, fecal incontinence, rectal pain, rectal urgency (tenesmus), rectal bleeding (with potential drops in hemoglobin), anal stricture, and fistula.[117–123] The prevalence of any of these symptoms in the radiation-treated prostate group ranges from 5 to 19%.[119, 120, 122] Chronic radiation proctopathy is defined as existing if rectal mucosa changes (cell loss, inflammation, edema, and ulceration), connective tissue fibrosis, and endarteritis of the arterioles occur, and clinical symptoms appear or persist 3 months after treatment completion.[118, 120] Endoscopic findings include mucosal pallor, friability, spontaneous oozing, and angiectasis usually confined to the distal 18 cm of the rectum.[118, 119] Fibrosis is cumulative and progressive and can continue for years before a patient experiences symptoms.

The bleeding that occurs usually develops 6 months to 2 years after treatment is completed, results from friable mucosal angiectasis, and is the most difficult problem to manage successfully. The chronic bleeding can be daily or episodic, can accompany bowel movements, or can occur in isolation as frank blood or clots. Topical agents administered via enemas consist of steroid, sucralfate, or formulin preparation; reported results suggest short-term relief, although formulin instillations can result in decreased angioectatic lesions and decreased friability. There have been reports of recurrent bleeding after laser therapy aimed at coagulating the angioectatic lesions.[119, 120] The effectiveness of laser therapy has not been adequately assessed.

Surgery, consisting of either a diverting colostomy or resection with coloanal pull-through anastomosis, is reserved for patients unresponsive to other treatment attempts or who are also experiencing an obstruction, perforation, or fistula.[118, 122] Surgery is a last resort because morbidity is significant and has been reported to be as high as 79%.[118]

Hyperbaric oxygen treatment (HBO), a relatively new treatment modality for chronic proctopathy, has had some successful reports.[121, 122] HBO, having an angiogenic effect, supposedly helps heal irradiated tissue that is hypovascular, hypocellular, and hypoxic. The therapeutic effect of HBO for patients with progressive microvascular ischemia characterizing radiation-induced proctopathy requires further investigation.

HRQOL IN ADVANCED PROSTATE CANCER

Although the definition of HRQOL does not change with cancer stage, endpoints for evaluation may be different depending on the extent and responsiveness of disease.[124] For patients faced with metastatic prostate cancer, anxieties are real concerning the risk of adverse effects of the disease and can transform someone from a nonsymptomatic status to symptomatic.[13] Compounding the risk of disease side effects are the risk of side effects from treatment and comorbidities.[36] Schag and others[36] noted that QOL did not improve with longer survival times in men with prostate cancer and may be due to the fact that the incidence occurs later in life with the concomitant problems of aging.

In the palliative care population, prolonging life is not the primary aim of treatment.[16, 21, 125] Health perceptions and priorities may be different for the man with advanced disease as opposed to the man with localized disease because differences of health perceptions have been noted among men within metastatic disease. Although extending survival time is hoped for in advanced prostate cancer, it should not occur in isolation of trying to improve QOL. Preserving function and maintaining a satisfying QOL become priorities and endpoints of evaluation for the man with metastatic prostate cancer.[126] According to Altwein and others,[13] the goal of palliation is to relieve distress, prevent distress, and maintain a good HRQOL as long as possible. Ferrell,[2] in a review of methodologic issues in QOL, noted the importance of assessing the QOL of terminally ill patients.

Identifying the side effects of metastatic treatments influencing HRQOL is vital because, by controlling distressing symptoms, a person's HRQOL is improved. Herr and others[66] found that asymptomatic men with newly diagnosed metastatic prostate cancer who deferred hormonal therapy had fewer sexual problems, more physical energy, and less psychological distress than those with comparable disease status who chose to initiate hormonal therapy. This study underscores the value of QOL research and suggests that active treatment does not necessarily translate into improved QOL.

Another factor to consider within the metastatic group is sensitivity of disease to intervention. Albertsen and colleagues[48] found that men with metastatic disease in remission who responded to hormonal therapy had a QOL similar to that of someone without end-stage cancer and significantly better than that of men who were hormone resistant. Even with separate analyses of men stratified by extent of disease (minimal vs. extensive), a significant difference persisted in those whose disease responded compared with those whose disease was resistant. Because therapy in the metastatic prostate cancer population has questionable efficacy in extending life span and may negatively influence QOL, clinical trials in this population would be more holistic and comprehensive if accompanied by QOL assessment.

Symptoms and problems that have been identified through HRQOL research in the advanced prostate cancer population include pain, vitality, impaired performance status, altered sex life, social function, altered body image, altered perceptions of the effectiveness of treatment, satisfaction with treatment decisions, and fatigue.[9, 20, 48] Kornblith's group[127] found that patients experiencing problems adapting to prostate cancer were more likely to have advanced disease or were experiencing side effects related to the disease or treatment modality. There are also greater reports of pain, fatigue, and urinary problems that correlate with deteriorating physical functioning. Additionally, hormonal therapy, commonly used in end-stage disease, can cause loss of libido, erectile dysfunction, gynecomastia, hot flashes, and nausea, influencing QOL.[128]

CONCLUSION

As patients listen to treatment options, they need to hear that, although overall HRQOL may not be affected by their treatment choice, they will still most likely experience significant changes in bowel, urinary, and sexual function. It is unclear as to why HRQOL is not impacted by physical problems in some patients. Patients may compartmentalize physical problems resulting from disease or treatment, separating them from their definition of QOL. Patients may very well be consciously weighing their symptoms against the possibility of death without treatment. Regardless of these types of conscious decisions, satisfaction with overall HRQOL suggests adaptation and adjustment to the changes that prostate cancer brings to patients' lives.

REFERENCES

1. King CR, Haberman M, Berry DL, et al. Quality of life and the cancer experience: The state-of-the-knowledge. *Oncol Nurs Forum* 1997;24:27–41.
2. Ferrell BR. The quality of lives: 1,525 voices of cancer. *Oncol Nurs Forum* 1996;23:909–916.
3. Ferrell BR, Dow KH, Leigh S, et al. Quality of life in long-term cancer survivors. *Oncol Nurs Forum* 1995;22:915–922.
4. Mast ME. Definition and measurement of quality of life in oncology nursing research: Review and theoretical implications. *Oncol Nurs Forum* 1995;2:957–964.
5. Cleary PD, Greenfield S, McNeil BJ. Assessing quality of life after surgery. *Control Clin Trials* 1991;12:189s-203s.
6. Pannek J, Hallner D, Kugler J, et al. Quality of life of patients with renal cell carcinoma or prostate cancer after radical surgery. *Int J Urol Nephrol* 1997;29:637–643.
7. Ferrell BR, Dow KH, Grant M. Measurement of the quality of life in cancer survivors. *Qual Life Res* 1995;4:523–531.
8. Gill T, Feinstein A. A critical appraisal of the quality of quality-of-life measurements. *JAMA* 1994;272:619–626.
9. Clark JA, Wray N, Brody B, et al. Dimensions of quality of life expressed by men treated for metastatic prostate cancer. *Soc Sci Med* 1997;45:1299–1309.
10. World Health Organization. *The First Ten Years of the World Health Organization.* Geneva: Author, 1958.
11. Karnofsky PA, Bunchenal JH. The clinical evaluation of chemotherapeutic agents in cancer. In: MacCleod CM (ed). Evaluation of Chemotherapeutic Agents. New York: Columbia Press, 1949:119–205.
12. Ganz PA, Haskell CM, Figlin RA, et al. Estimating the quality of life in a clinical trial of patients with metastatic lung cancer using the Karnofsky performance and the Functional Living Index-Cancer. *Cancer* 1988;61:849–856.
13. Altwein J, Ekman P, Barry M, et al. How is quality of life in prostate cancer patients influenced by modern treatment? The Wallengberg symposium. *Urology* 1997;49(4A):66–76.
14. da Silva FC, Fossa SD, Aaronson NK, et al. The quality of life of patients with newly diagnosed M1 prostate cancer: Experience with EORTC clinical trial 30853. *Eur J Cancer* 1996;32A:72–77.
15. Cleary PD, Morrissey G, Oster G. Health-related quality of life in patients with advanced prostate cancer: A multinational perspective. *Qual Life Res* 1995;4:207–220.
16. Fossa SD. Quality of life in advanced prostate cancer. *Semin Oncol* 1996;23:32–34.
17. Lubeck DP, Litwin MS, Henning JM, Carrol PR. Measurement of health-related quality of life in men with prostate cancer: The CaPSURE database. *Qual Life* 1997;6:385–392.
18. Sharp JW. Expanding the definition of quality of life for prostate cancer. *Cancer* 1993;71(Suppl):1078–1082.

19. Rossetti SR, Terrone C. Quality of life in prostate cancer patients. Eur J Urol 1996;30(Suppl 1): 44–48.

20. da Silva FC, Reis E, Costa T, et al. A feasibility study. Quality of life in patients with prostate cancer. *Cancer* 1993;71:1138–1142.

21. Esper P, Mo F, Chodak G, et al. Measuring quality of life in men with prostate cancer using the functional assessment of cancer therapy-prostate instrument. *Urology* 1997;50:920–927.

22. Talcott JA. Quality of life in early prostate cancer: Do we know enough to treat? *Hematol Oncol Clin North Am* 1996;10:691–701.

23. Schellhammer P, Cockett A, Boccon-Gibod L, et al. Assessment of endpoints for clinical trials for localized prostate cancer. *Urology* 1997;49(Suppl 4A): 27–38.

24. Haas G, Sakr W. Epidemiology of prostate cancer. CA: *A Cancer J Clin* 1997;47:273–287.

25. Crawford ED, Bennett CL, Stone NN, et al. Comparison of perspectives on prostate cancer: Analyses of survey data. *Urology* 1997;50:366–372.

26. Fossa, SD, Waehre H, Kurth KH, et al. Influence of urological morbidity on quality of life in patients with prostate cancer. *Eur Urol* 1997;3(Suppl 3):3–8.

27. Bennett CL, Chapman G, Elstein AS, et al. A comparison of perspectives on prostate cancer: Analysis of utility assessments of patients and physicians. *Eur J Urol* 1997;32(Suppl 3):86–88.

28. Fossa SD, Aaronson NK, Newling D, et al. Quality of life and treatment of hormone resistant metastatic prostatic cancer. *Eur J Cancer* 1990;26:1133–1136.

29. Watkins-Bruner D, Scott C, Lawton C, et al. RTOG's first quality of life study—RTOG 90-20: A Phase II trial of external beam radiation with etanidazole for locally advanced prostate cancer. *Int J Radiat Oncol Biol Phys* 1995;33:901–906.

30. Catalona WJ, Basler JW. Return of erections and urinary continence following nerve sparing radical retropubic prostatectomy. *J Urol* 1993;150:905–907.

31. Steiner M, Morton R, Walsh P. Impact of anatomical radical prostatectomy on urinary continence. *J Urol* 1991;145:512–514.

32. Zinreich ES, Derogatis LR, Herpst J. Pre- and post-treatment evaluation of sexual function in patients with adenocarcinoma of the prostate. *Int J Radiat Oncol Biol Phys* 1990;19:729–732.

33. Talcott JA, Rieker P, Clark JA, et al. Patient-reported symptoms after primary therapy for early prostate cancer: Results of a prospective cohort study. *J Clin Oncol* 1998;16:275–283.

34. Litwin MS, Hays RO, Fink A, et al. Quality-of-life outcomes in men treated for localized prostate cancer. *JAMA* 1995;273:129–135.

35. Braslis KG, Santa-Cruz C, Brickman AL, Soloway MS. Quality of life 12 months after radical prostatectomy. *Br J Urol* 1995;75:48–53.

36. Schag CAC, Ganz PA, Wing DS, et al. Quality of life in adult survivors of lung, colon and prostate cancer. *Qual Life Res* 1994;3:127–141.

37. Cella D, Tulsky D. Measuring quality of life today: Methodological aspects. *Oncology* 1990;4:29–38.

38. Stenstrup E. Review of quality of life instrumentation in the oncology population. *Clin Nurs Spec* 1996;10:164–169.

39. Moinpour C, Feigl P, Metch B, et al. Quality of life endpoints in cancer clinical trials: Review and recommendations. *J Natl Cancer Inst* 1989;81:485–493.

40. Borghede G, Sullivan M. Measurement of quality of life in localized prostatic cancer patients treated with radiotherapy. Development of a prostate cancer-specific module supplementing the EORTC-C30. *Qual Life Res* 1996;5:212–222.

41. Bush N, Haberman M, Donaldson G, Sullivan K. Quality of life of 125 adults surviving 6-18 years after bone marrow transplantation. *Soc Sci Med* 1995; 40:479–490.

42. Dow KH, Ferrell BR, Leigh S, et al. An evaluation of the quality of life among long-term survivors of breast cancer. *Breast Cancer Res Treat* 1996;39:261–263.

43. Germino B. Quality of life for families with cancer. Research issues. *Qual Life Nurs Challenge* 1993;2: 39–45.

44. Kaasa S. Measurement of quality of life in clinical trials. *Oncology* 1992;49:288–294.

45. Stewart AL, Hays R, Ware JE. The MOS Short-form General Health Survey: Reliability and validity in a patient population. *Med Care* 1988;26:724–735.

46. Ware JE, Sherbourne CD. The MOS 36-item short form health survey (SF-36): I. Conceptual framework and item selection. *Med Care* 1992;30:473–483.

47. McHorney CA, Ware JE, Lu JF, Sherbourne CD. The MOS 36-item short form health survey (SF-36): II. Pyschometric and clinical tests of validity in measuring physical and mental health constructs. *Med Care* 1993;31:247–263.

48. Albertsen PC, Aaronson NK, Muller MJ, et al. Health-related quality of life among patients with metastatic prostate cancer. *Urology* 1997;49:207–217.

49. Curran D, Fossa S, Aaronson N, et al. Baseline quality of life of patients with advanced prostate cancer. *Eur J Cancer* 1997;33:1809–1814.

50. Schag CA, Ganz PA, Heinrich RL. Cancer rehabilitation evaluation system-short form (CARES-SF): A cancer specific rehabilitation and quality of life instrument. *Cancer* 1991;68:1406–1413.

51. Cella D, Tulsky D, Gray G, et al. The functional assessment of cancer therapy scale: Development and validation of the general measure. *J Clin Oncol* 1993;11:570–579.

52. Dawson NA, McLeod DG. The assessment of treatment outcomes in metastatic prostate cancer: Changing endpoints. *Eur J Cancer* 1997;33:560–565.

53. Fowler F, Barry J, Lu-Yao G, et al. Patient reported complications and follow-up treatment after radical prostatectomy. The National Medicare Experience: 1988–1990. *Urology* 1993;42:622–629.

54. Perez M, Meyerowitz B, Lieskovsky G, et al. Quality of life and sexuality following radical prostatectomy in patients with prostate cancer who use or do not use erectile aids. *Urology* 1997;50:740–746.

55. Chang M, Joseph A. Evolution of a bladder behavior clinic for patients after prostatectomy. *Urol Nurs* 1993;13:62–66.

56. Gallo M, Fallon P, Staskin D. Urinary incontinence: Steps to evaluation, diagnosis, and treatment. *Nurse Pract* 1997;22:21–41.

57. Foote J, Yun S, Leach G. Postprostatectomy incontinence: Pathophysiology, evaluation and management. *Urol Clin North Am* 1991;18:229–241.

58. Sall M, Madsen FA, Rhodes PR, et al. Pelvic pain following radical retropubic prostatectomy: A prospective study. *Urology* 1997;49:575–579.

59. Shrader-Bogen CL, Kjellberg JL, McPherson CP, Murray CL. Quality of life and treatment outcomes: Prostate carcinoma patients' perspectives after prostatectomy or radiation therapy. *Cancer* 1997;79:1977–1986.

60. Ficazola M, Nitti V. The etiology of post-radical prostatectomy incontinence and correlation of symptoms with urodynamic findings. *J Urol* 1998;160:1317–1320.

61. Harris J. Treatment of postprostatectomy urinary incontinence with behavioral methods. *Clin Nurs Spec* 1997;11:159–166.

62. Leach G, Trockman B, Wong A, et al. Post-prostatectomy incontinence: Urodynamic findings and treatment outcomes. *J Urol* 1996;155:1256–1259.

63. Klutke C, Nadler R, Tiemann D, Andriole G. Early results with antegrade collagen injection for post-radical prostatectomy stress urinary incontinence. *J Urol* 1996;156:1703–1706.

64. Diokno A. Post prostatectomy urinary incontinence. *Ostomy/Wound Management* 1998;44:54–60.

65. Nasr S, Ouslander J. Urinary incontinence in the elderly: Causes and treatment options. *Drug Aging* 1988;12:349–360.

66. Herr HW, Kornblith AB, Ofman U. Comparison of the quality of life of patients with metastatic prostate cancer who received or did not receive hormonal therapy. *Cancer* 1993;71:1143–1150.

67. Newman D, Burns P. Significance and impact of urinary incontinence. *Nurse Pract Forum* 1994;5:130–133.

68. Yalla S. Management of urinary incontinence—Progress and innovative strategies [editorial]. *J Urol* 1998;159:1520–1522.

69. Freedman A, Hahn G, Love N. Follow-up after therapy for prostate cancer. Treating problems and caring for the man. *Postgrad Med* 1996;100:125–136.

70. Beckman N. An overview of urinary incontinence in adults: Assessments and behavioral interventions *Clin Nurse Spec* 1995;9:241–248.

71. Wyman J. Level 3: Comprehensive assessment and management of urinary incontinence by continence nurse specialists. *Nurse Pract Forum* 1994; 5:177–185.

72. Agency for Health Care Policy and Research. Quick reference guide for clinicians: Managing acute and chronic urinary incontinence. *J Am Acad Nurse Pract* 1996;8:390–403.

73. Smith D, Newman D. Treatment strategies for urinary incontinence: Basic elements of biofeedback therapy for pelvic muscle rehabilitation. *Urol Nurs* 1994;14:130–135.

74. Wyman J, Fantl J. Bladder training in ambulatory care management of urinary incontinence. *Urol Nurs* 1991;11:11–17.

75. Sale P, Wyman J. Achievement of goals associated with bladder training by older incontinent women. *Nurse Pract Forum* 1994;5:93–96.

76. Meaglia JP, Joseph AC, Chang M, Schmidt JD. Post-prostatectomy urinary incontinence: Response to behavioral training. *J Urol* 1990;144:674–676.

77. Burgio KL, Stutzman RE, Engel BT. Behavioral training for post-prostatectomy urinary incontinence. *J Urol* 1989;141:303–306.

78. Smith D. Devices for continence. *Nurse Pract Forum* 1994;5:186–189.

79. Newman D, Smith D. Pelvic muscle reeducation as a nursing treatment for incontinence. *Urol Nurs* 1992;12:9–15.

80. Messick G, Powe C. Applying behavioral research to incontinence. *Ostomy/Wound Management* 1997; 43:40–48.

81. Bray D. Biofeedback. In: Rankin-Box (ed.) *The Nurses' Handbook of Complimentary Therapies.* Edinburg: Churchill Livingstone, 1995:65–73.

82. Denis P. Methodology of biofeedback. *Eur J Gastroenterol Hepatol* 1996;8:530–533.

83. Wein A. Pharmacologic options for the overactive bladder. *Urology* 1998;51(Suppl 2A):43–47.

84. Owens R, Karram M. Comparative tolerability of drug therapies used to treat incontinence and enuresis. *Drug Safety* 1998;19:123–139.

85. Moore K, Richardson V. Pharmacology: Impact on bladder function. *Ostomy/Wound Management* 1998; 44:30–45.

86. Kreder K, Webster G. Evaluation and management of incontinence after implantation of the artificial urinary sphincter. *Urol Clin North Am* 1991;18: 375–381.

87. Gallo M, Staskin D. Patient satisfaction with a reusable undergarment for urinary incontinence. *J Wound Ostomy Continence Nurse* 1997;24:226–236.

88. Helgason A, Fredrikson M, Adolfsson J, Steinbeck G. Decreased sexual capacity after external radiation therapy for prostate cancer impairs quality of life. *Int J Radiat Oncol Biol Phys* 1995;32:33–39.

89. Roach M, Chinn DM, Holland J, Clark M. A pilot survey of sexual function and quality of life following 3D conformal radiotherapy for clinically localized prostate cancer. *Int J Radiat Oncol Biol Phys* 1996;35:869–874.

90. Caffo O, Fellin G, Graffer U, Luciani L. Assessment of quality of life after radical radiotherapy for prostate cancer. *Br J Urol* 1996;78:557–563.

91. Beard CJ, Propert KJ, Rieker PP, et al. Complications after treatment with external-beam irradiation in early-stage prostate cancer patients: A prospective multiinstitutional outcomes study. *J Clin Oncol* 1997;15:223–229.

92. Leandri P, Rossignol G, Gautier J, Ramon J. Radical retropubic prostatectomy: Morbidity and quality of life. Experience with 620 consecutive cases. *J Urol* 1992;147:883–887.

93. Hall MC. Management of erectile dysfunction after radical prostatectomy. *Semin Urol Oncol* 1995; 13:215–223.

94. Turner L, Althof S, Levine S, et al. Treating erectile dysfunction with external vacuum devices: Impact upon sexual, psychological and marital functioning. *J Urol* 1990;144:79–82.

95. Ganem J, Lucey D, Janosko E, Carson C. Unusual complication of the vacuum erectile device. *Urology* 1998;51:627–631.

96. Nadig P. Vacuum devices for erectile dysfunction. *Probl Urol* 1991;5:559–565.

97. Althof S, Turner L, Levine S, et al. Through the eyes of women: The sexual and psychological responses of women to their partner's treatment with self-injection or external vacuum therapy. *J Urol* 1992;147:1024–1027.

98. Sidi A, Becher E, Zhang G, Lewis J. Patient acceptance of and satisfaction with an external negative pressure device for impotence. *J Urol* 1990;144: 1154–1156.

99. Burnett A. Erectile dysfunction: A practical approach for primary care. *Geriatrics* 1998;53: 34–48.

100. Lewis R. The pharmacologic erection. *Prob Urol* 1991;5:541–558.

101. Godschalk M, Chen J, Katz P, Mulligan T. Treatment of erectile failure with prostaglandin E1: A double-blind, placebo-controlled, dose-response study. *J Urol* 1994;151:1530–1532.

102. Mulhall J, Daller M, Traish A, et al. Intracavernosal forskolin: Role in the management of vasculogenic impotence resistant to standard 3–agent pharmacotherapy. *J Urol* 1997;158:1752–1759.

103. Lakin MM, Montague DK, Medendorp SV, et al. Intracavernous injection therapy: Analysis of results and complications. *J Urol* 1990;143:1138–1141.

104. Mulchay J. Treatment options for erectile dysfunction in the post-prostatectomy patient. *Contemp Urol* 1997;9:4–22.

105. Costabile R, Spevak M, Fishman I, et al. Efficacy and safety of transurethral alprostadil in patients with erectile dysfunction following radical prostatectomy. *J Urol* 1998;160:1325–1328.

106. Goldstein I, Lue T, Padma-Nathan H, et al. Oral sildenafil in the treatment of erectile dysfunction. *N Engl J Med* 1998;338:1397–1404.

107. Licht M. Sildenafil for treating male erectile dysfunction. *Cleve Clin J Med* 1998;65:301–304.

108. Boolell M, Gepi-Attee S, Gingell J, Allen M. Sildenafil, a novel effective oral therapy for male erectile dysfunction. *Br J Urol* 1996;78:257–261.

109. Zippe CD, Kedia AW, Kedia K, et al. Treatment of erectile dysfunction after radical prostatectomy with sildenafil citrate (Viagra). *Urology* 1998;52:963–966.

110. Rosen R. Sildenafil: Medical advance or media event? *Lancet* 1998;351:1599–1600.

111. Lewis R. Long-term results of penile prosthetic implants. *Urol Clin North Am* 1995;22:847–856.

112. Yarbro CH, Ferrans C. Quality of life with prostate cancer treated with surgery or radiation therapy. *Oncol Nurs Forum* 1998;25:685–693.

113. Soffen E, Hanks G, Hunt M, Epstein B. Conformal static field radiation therapy of early prostate cancer versus non-conformal techniques: A reduction in acute morbidity. *Int J Radiat Oncol Biol Phys* 1992;24:485–488.

114. Kroser JA, Metz DC. Evaluation of the adult patient with diarrhea. *Gastroenterology* 1996;23:629–647.

115. Wright P, Thomas S. Constipation and diarrhea: The neglected symptoms. *Semin Oncol Nurs* 1995;11:289–297.

116. Johnson J, Fieler V, Wlasowicz G, et al. The effects of nursing care guided by self-regulation theory on coping with radiation therapy. *Oncol Nurs Forum* 1997;4:1041–1050.

117. Lawton CA, Won MM, Pilepich MV, et al. Long-term treatment sequelae following external beam irradiation for adenocarcinoma of the prostate: Analysis of RTOG studies 7506 and 7706. *Int J Radiat Oncol Biol Phys* 1991;21:935–939.

118. Swaroop VS, Gostout C. Endoscopic treatment of chronic radiation proctopathy. *J Clin Gastroenterol* 1998;27:36–40.

119. Chapius P, Dent O, Bokey E, et al. The development of a treatment protocol for patients with chronic radiation-induced rectal bleeding. *Aust N Z J Surg* 1996;66:680–685.

120. Cho KH, Lee CK, Levitt SH. Proctitis after conventional external radiation therapy for prostate cancer: Importance of minimizing posterior rectal dose. *Radiology* 1995;195:699–703.

121. Woo TC, Joseph D, Oxer H. Hyperbaric oxygen treatment for radiation proctitis. *Int J Radiat Oncol Biol Phys* 1997;38:619–622.

122. Warren DC, Feehan P, Slade JB, Cianci PE. Chronic radiation proctitis treated with hyperbaric oxygen. *Undersea Hyperb Med* 1997;24:181–184.

123. Hogan C. The nurse's role in diarrhea management. *Oncol Nurs Forum* 1998;25:879–886.

124. Waselenko JK, Dawson NA. Management of progressive metastatic prostate cancer. *Oncology* 1997;11:1551–1568.

125. Walsh D. Palliative care: Management of the patient with advanced cancer. *Semin Oncol* 1994;21(4, Suppl 7):100–106.

126. Stockler MR, Osoba D, Goodwin P, et al. Responsiveness to change in health-related quality of life in a randomized clinical trial: A comparison of the prostate cancer specific quality of life instrument (PROSQOLI) with analogous scales from the EORTC QLQ-30 and a trial specific module. *J Clin Epidemiol* 1998;51:137–145.

127. Kornblith AB, Herr HW, Ofman US, et al. Quality of life of patients with prostate cancer and their spouses: The value of a data base in clinical care. *Cancer* 1994;73:2791–2802.

128. Garnick MB. Prostate cancer: Screening, diagnosis, and management. *Ann Intern Med* 1993;118:804–818.

Chapter 14

ADVANCED PROSTATE CANCER: SYMPTOM MANAGEMENT

JEANNE HELD-WARMKESSEL

OVERVIEW

BLADDER OUTLET OBSTRUCTION
URETERAL OBSTRUCTION
LEG EDEMA
 Deep Vein Thrombosis
 Lymphedema
 Scrotal Edema

DISSEMINATED INTRAVASCULAR
 COAGULATION
BONE PAIN
 Nursing Management
SPINAL CORD COMPRESSION
 Nursing Management
CONCLUSION

Advanced prostate cancer may produce distressing symptoms that require prompt and appropriate nursing assessment, planning, intervention, and evaluation to enhance the patient's quality of life (QOL). Among problems common to patients with advanced prostate cancer are bone pain, spinal cord compression, leg and scrotal edema, coagulation disorders, and bladder outlet or ureteral obstruction. This chapter describes the assessment and management of these problems, along with the nursing implications.

BLADDER OUTLET OBSTRUCTION

Bladder outlet obstruction occurs when the prostatic urethra is obstructed by an enlarging tumor mass or lymph nodes that compress and obliterate the urethral lumen. (See Assessment and Diagnosis, Chapter 4, Figure 4-1.) Symptoms present before complete bladder outlet obstruction include frequency, urgency, nocturia, and slow urinary stream.[1] Urine accumulates in the bladder, producing distressing symptoms, including the inability to void and lower abdominal pain and pressure from the distended bladder. When outlet obstruction remains untreated, urine will continue to accumulate and distend the bladder. Chronic obstruction results in the backup of urine into the ureters, and hydronephrosis ensues. Renal failure may then develop.

Bladder outlet obstruction may be acute or chronic in onset. The type of presentation helps guide the treatment. The acute onset of bladder outlet obstruction requires the insertion of an indwelling urinary drainage catheter, such as a Foley catheter. Because of the tumor compressing the urethra, catheter insertion may be difficult and may require placement by the physician. A local topical anesthetic gel may be used to reduce the discomfort of catheter placement. Complications associated with an indwelling urinary catheter include infection, urinary tract bacterial colonization, and discomfort from the presence of the catheter. Bladder spasms may produce urine leakage around the catheter.[1] Chronic problems associated with indwelling urinary catheters include calcification of the catheter or balloon, urosepsis, urethra structure, and inflammation of the urethra or epididymis.[1] To reduce the risk of complications associated with an indwelling urinary catheter, a suprapubic catheter may be inserted instead. A suprapubic catheter is inserted percutaneously into the bladder and sutured in place. Infections may still occur with these catheters. Nurses must change the suprapubic catheter dressing each day and when wet or soiled as well as monitor the catheter exit site for drainage, which may indicate an infection. Infection may also be present in the urine if it is cloudy or malodorous or if the patient has a fever. If an infection is suspected, a urine specimen is sent for urine analysis and culture and sensitivity.

Clean, intermittent self-catheterization may be an option in some patients. Highly motivated patients can be taught to perform this procedure to avoid an indwelling catheter and its associated problems. Using clean technique, a straight red rubber catheter is inserted via the urethra to empty the bladder at a predetermined time, usually every 3 to 4 hours. To sleep well during the night, self-catheterization is performed at bedtime, and fluids are restricted for 3 hours before retiring.[2] Otherwise, 2 L of fluid should be consumed each day. The fluid should be consumed in small, frequent amounts so that small volumes of fluid are consumed regularly throughout the day and excess amounts that could over distend the bladder are avoided.[3] Juices that acidify the urine, such as cranberry and blueberry juices, should be consumed as part of the diet to reduce bacterial adherence to the urethra lining. Residual urine is monitored at regular intervals to reduce the risk of infection.[1] Home care nursing follow-up may help with the patient's adjustment to home self-catheterization and enables one to monitor the patient for use of correct technique to reduce the risk of infection. See Table 14-1 for nursing care standard.[2–4]

Historically, hormonal manipulation has been a common method of managing bladder outlet obstruction resulting from advanced prostate cancer.[5] Testosterone castration levels may be achieved by orchiectomy, the use of estrogens, or luteinizing hormone-releasing hormone (LHRH) agonists. These approaches are most useful in patients who have not previously experienced hormonal manipulation. Flutamide, an

TABLE 14-1. Standard of Care for the Patient with Advanced Prostate Cancer

NURSING DIAGNOSIS: *Knowledge deficit related to performance of intermittent self-catheterization*

PATIENT OUTCOME: Pt-family will be able to perform intermittent self-catheterization.

NURSING INTERVENTIONS:

1. Assess pt's understanding of urinary tract anatomy and how to perform self-catheterization.
2. Use anatomic pictures or 3-D models of urinary tract to teach pt location of bladder and urethra.
3. Instruct pt-family in clean technique of self-catheterization.
   - Wash hands well with soap and running water and dry.
   - Gather equipment.
   - Wash penis with soap and water, rinse and dry.
   - Set up supplies.
   - A lubricant may be used to ease catheter insertion.
   - Grasp and straighten penis and lift upward while inserting catheter.
   - Completely empty bladder.
   - Wash and dry catheter and store in a clean plastic self-closing bag.
4. Teach pt to balance fluid consumption throughout day and not consume large amounts of fluid at one time. Total fluid volume consumed each day should be about 2 Ls. Fluids consumed should include cranberry juice.
5. Self-catheterization must be performed on a routine schedule of every 3–4 hours. About 350–400 mL urine should be obtained with each catheterization.
6. Symptoms of urosepsis, such as fever, chills, or change in appearance of urine, must be reported to nurse or physician.

NURSING DIAGNOSIS: *Knowledge deficit related to care of PNT*

PATIENT OUTCOME: The pt-SO will be able to demonstrate care of PNT.

NURSING INTERVENTIONS:

1. Assess pt-SO understanding of purpose of PNT.
2. Teach pt-SO in care of PNT. Cleanse around tube exit site with saline or soap and water according to policy. Pat dry. Cover exit site with dry gauze and tape securely in place.
3. Tubes must be securely taped in place at all times to avoid dislodgment.
4. Inspect exit site with each dressing change for infection: redness, change in color, or amount of drainage. Report changes to nurse or physician.
5. Empty PNT drainage bag when 1/2 to 2/3 full to avoid overfilling of bag.
6. Use clean technique when emptying bags to avoid contamination.
7. Monitor pt for other complications of PNT: reduced urine output from dislodgment or blockage and bleeding. Notify physician.
8. Teach pt about importance of maintaining schedule of appointments for routine catheter changes, usually every 3 months or as prescribed by physician.
9. Tubing must not be kinked, which would block urine flow. It must be taped to be maintained in a straight position.
10. Flush PNT with NSS as ordered. Teach pt to prepare NSS flush and how to flush PNT.

NURSING DIAGNOSIS: *Potential for infection related to catheters in urinary tract*

PATIENT OUTCOME: Pt will have prompt recognition of s-s of UTI.

NURSING INTERVENTIONS:

1. Assess urine and catheters for sign of infection: odor, color, purulent drainage, change in clarity, pain.
2. Monitor vital signs for infection: ↑T, ↑HR, ↑respiratory rate, ↓BP.
3. Obtain urine culture and blood culture as ordered.
4. Administer antipyretics, antibiotics as ordered.
5. Teach pt s-s of UTI and to notify nurse or physician when s-s present.
6. Use clean technique when emptying drainage bags and doing catheter care.
7. Never raise drainage bag above level of bladder.
8. Empty drainage bag when 1/2 to 2/3 full.
9. Keep drainage bags off floor. Hang from bed frame.
10. Keep tubing straight to allow for drainage.
11. Teach pt to perform meatal care with soap and water and to perform twice a day when indwelling urinary catheter in place.
12. Teach pt/SO to change to straight urinary drainage bag at night and to use leg bag during day.

NURSING DIAGNOSIS: *Potential for fluid and electrolyte imbalance from postrenal obstruction*
PATIENT OUTCOME: Pt will have prompt recognition of fluid and electrolyte abnormalities.
NURSING INTERVENTIONS:

1. Assess I&O; daily weights.
2. Monitor fluid balance closely after placement of catheters because diuresis often occurs after obstruction relieved.
3. Monitor lab results—BUN, creatinine, electrolytes—and notify physician of abnormal results.
4. Administer IV fluids and electrolytes as ordered.
5. Monitor amount of peripheral edema.

NURSING DIAGNOSIS: *Alteration in comfort related to scrotal edema*
PATIENT OUTCOME: Pt will verbalize increased comfort level.
NURSING INTERVENTIONS:

1. Assess amount of edema.
2. Assess level of discomfort using scale ranging from 0 to 10.
3. Elevate scrotum on folded towels placed between thighs or use towel as a supportive device by laying towel across legs and placing scrotum on top of towel. Change towel at least daily and when wet or soiled.
4. Monitor for signs of infection such as redness, drainage, pain.
5. Provide good skin care: Wash skin well and thoroughly dry twice a day and when wet.

NURSING DIAGNOSIS: *Altered comfort related to leg edema*
PATIENT OUTCOME: Pt will verbalize increased comfort.
NURSING INTERVENTIONS:

1. Assess severity of leg edema. Measure legs daily and record measurements. Daily weight.
2. Assess level of discomfort using a scale ranging from 0 to 10.
3. Elevate legs above heart.
4. Consider consultation to multidisciplinary lymphedema program after discussion with physician.
5. Educate pt to avoid injury to feet and skin on legs. Pt should wear clean socks and shoes at all times. Nail care should be done by a podiatrist. Skin must be inspected daily for breakage. After washing skin, lubricate with lotion.
6. Consider use of gentle exercise to reduce edema. Consult physical therapist after discussion with physician.
7. Avoid tight constrictive garments on affected leg other than compression garment.
8. Teach pt/SO to apply compression devices, garments.

NURSING DIAGNOSIS: *Risk for injury related to anticoagulation therapy for DVT*
PATIENT OUTCOME: Pt will not sustain an injury from anticoagulation therapy.
NURSING INTERVENTIONS:

1. Educate pt as to bleeding precautions.
2. Obtain baseline PT/INR, PTT, platelet counts as ordered and monitor results throughout therapy.
3. Obtain specimens from peripheral vein or from central venous catheter according to institutional policy.
4. Initiate heparin therapy with heparin bolus and follow with continuous infusion of heparin.
5. Institute bleeding precautions. Educate pt to avoid injury, use an electric razor, use a toothette for oral care.
6. Repeat PTT in 6 hours after start of heparin therapy, adjust rate as ordered, and check PTT after each infusion rate change. Report results to physician.
7. Start warfarin after heparin drip initiated.
8. Monitor pt for bleeding.
9. Monitor platelet count. If platelet count falls < 100,000, notify physician and interrupt heparin infusion. Pt may be developing HITT.
10. After heparin level therapeutic, monitor daily PTT.
11. Educate pt as to use of warfarin at home and need for ongoing monitoring of PT/INR while on therapy.
12. Consult home health nurse to monitor PT/INR at home and assess pt.

NURSING DIAGNOSIS: *Risk for injury related to DIC-induced bleeding*
PATIENT OUTCOME: Pt will have reduced bleeding.
NURSING INTERVENTIONS:

1. Assess body system for bleeding:
   - Skin: oozing, petechiae, ecchymoses
   - Mucous membranes of nose and mouth, rectum for bleeding
   - CNS: neurologic checks, level of consciousness, vision changes, headache, confusion

Continued on next page

TABLE 14-1. Continued

- Lungs: pulse oximetry, chest pain, hemoptysis, abnormal breath sounds, cyanosis, mottling, tachypnea
- Cardiovascular: tachycardia, hypotension, vital sign changes, arrhythmias
- Renal: hematuria, oliguria, I&O, BUN, creatinine
- Extremities: pulses, color sensation, motor activity
- GI tract: bowel sounds, abdominal distention, melena, hematemesis, hematochezia
- Any prior venipuncture site or site of injury
- Pain level

2. Institute bleeding precautions: no IM injections, no enemas or suppositories, no aspirin or NSAIDs, no razors.
3. Use sponge toothettes for oral care.
4. Obtain and monitor lab work.
5. Administer prescribed blood products, heparin, antibiotics, volume expanders, IV fluids, oxygen.
6. Avoid invasive procedures and venipunctures.
7. Monitor vital signs, I&O, neurologic checks q4h.
8. Elevate HOB to improve ventilation. Encourage coughing and deep breathing.
9. Turn q2h to reduce pressure.
10. Monitor amount of blood loss.
11. Test urine, stool, and emesis for blood. Monitor sputum for blood.
12. Apply direct pressure to bleeding sites.
13. Consult dentist to pack bleeding gums. Provide gentle oral care, saline mouth rinses.
14. Offer pain medication.
15. Institute safety precautions, prone to fall precautions.
16. Keep pt warm: Use blankets, change wet linens and gown.
17. Perform gentle range of motion.

NURSING DIAGNOSIS: *Anxiety related to bleeding*
PATIENT OUTCOME: Pt will have reduced anxiety.
NURSING INTERVENTIONS:
1. Assess level of anxiety.
2. Consult with social worker to assist with helping pt manage anxiety.
3. Use distraction and relaxation exercises, such as music therapy and guided imagery.
4. Encourage pt verbalization. Offer support.

NURSING DIAGNOSIS: *Altered comfort related to pain in bones*
PATIENT OUTCOME: Pt will verbalize adequate level of analgesia.
NURSING INTERVENTIONS:
1. Assess pain using scale ranging from 0 to 10. Identify location, onset, duration, precipitating and alleviating factors. Document data on a pain assessment form. Encourage pt to keep a pain diary.
2. Administer routine and rescue analgesics, NSAIDs, and other medications for pain.
3. Administer stool softeners and laxatives to prevent narcotic-induced constipation. Educate pt to increase fluid consumption.
4. Reevaluate analgesic regimen on routine basis and titrate doses as needed.
5. Reduce dose as needed after administration of bone-seeking radionuclide.
6. Educate pt as to management of pain at home.
7. Educate pt to use of heat and cold, distraction, music therapy, and other forms of pain control
8. Consult pain management team as needed.
9. Consult with PT-OT to enhance mobility.
10. Use therapeutic mattress to reduce pain.

Data compiled from Weber-Jones,[2] Black and Matassarin-Jacobs,[3] Parker-Berding,[4] Parke,[15] Humble,[16] Galindo-Ciocon,[19] Lechner,[23] Majoros and Moccia,[27] Simko and Lockhart,[25] Elzer and Houdek,[26] Schafer,[32] Nakashima et al,[35] Luckmann,[38] Thompson et al,[39] Forest,[72] Mayer et al,[73] Struthers et al,[75] Papanicolaou.[93]

Pt, patient; 3-D, three dimensional; PNT, percutaneous nephrostomy tube; SO, significant other; NSS, normal saline solution; s-s, signs-symptoms; UTI, urinary tract infection; T, temperature; HR, heart rate; BP, blood pressure; I&O, intake and output; BUN, blood urea nitrogen; IV, intravenous; PT/INR, prothrombin time/international normalized ratio; PTT, partial thromboplastin time; HITT, heparin-induced thrombocytopenia and thrombosis; DIC, disseminated intravascular coagulation; CNS, central nervous system; GI, gastrointestinal; IM, intramuscular; NSAIDS, nonsteroidal antiinflammatory drugs; HOB, head of bed; PT, physical therapy; OT, occupational therapy.

antiandrogen, should be initiated 1 week before an LHRH agonist to avoid the testosterone level increase ("flare"), which occurs with the initiation of LHRH agents. (See Chapter 11 for details on hormonal therapy.) In this way, the symptoms of outlet obstruction will not increase with the start of the LHRH agent. The patient should be able to void in 2 to 3 weeks after hormone levels fall to castrate levels.[1] If this does not occur, catheterization or surgery is required.

Surgical resection of the malignant prostate tissue may be performed by transurethral resection of the prostate (TURP). Using electrocautery, chips of cancerous tissue are removed. Incontinence may occur after surgery from cancer cells invading the external urethra sphincter.[1] An alternative surgical procedure is a channel TURP, which removes less tissue than a traditional TURP. The goal is to remove enough tumor to reduce the patient's symptoms and allow for voiding. Radiation therapy may also be administered after TURP.[5]

Radiation therapy may be used as the primary form of palliative treatment for patients with bladder outlet obstruction requiring an indwelling urinary catheter.[6] In a study of 19 patients with an indwelling urinary catheter, radiation in doses ranging from 21 to 55 Gy was administered. Seventeen of the patients were able to void and did not require a catheter after the completion of radiation therapy. After completing treatment, 2 patients needed recatheterization (3 months and 64 months later, respectively) and TURP, and another patient underwent TURP but did not need a catheter. Side effects included mild to moderate bowel toxicity and mild to moderate dysuria. (See Chapter 10 on radiation therapy for nursing management.) The patients with large tumors (T4) were less likely to have a palliative response.

Urethra stents were developed for use in men with benign prostatic hyperplasia (BPH) and have been used in patients with prostate cancer to avoid TURP or catheterization. Stents work by enlarging the diameter of the obstructed urethra to allow for normal voiding. The stents are placed under local anesthesia. Several types are available, including woven mesh made of a heat-sensitive self-expanding material,[7] nickel-titanium self-expanding coil,[8] and a superalloy woven mesh.[9] A suprapubic cystostomy tube may be placed before stent placement. Use of this tube improves visibility during stent placement and may be left open to drain for the first 24 hours after surgery. A cystoureteroscopy is done to measure for the correct length of the stent to be placed. The devices are inserted into the prostatic urethra using the provided insertion applicator. After correct placement, 88 to 100% of patients have been able to void.[7-9] Postoperative problems include dysuria, blood clots related to traumatic insertion, frequency, nocturia, urgency, transient hematuria, and perineal pain. These problems resolved in 2 weeks to 1 month in most patients. Urinary tract infections were managed with antibiotics. Stents may remain patent for several years. For patients who are not candidates for other forms of treatment, stents are a viable option to avoid an indwelling urinary catheter. Patients are discharged usually after 24 hours of observation to monitor voiding. Oral antibiotics may be continued at home.

URETERAL OBSTRUCTION

Advanced prostate cancer may also produce upper urinary tract or ureteral obstruction. Enlarged pelvic and paraaortic lymph nodes may compress the ureters.[10] Spread of cancer to the bladder trigone may prevent the outflow of urine into the bladder.[5, 11] Compression of the ureterovesical junction is the most common cause of ureteral obstruction.[5] The obstruction often occurs bilaterally and may be present for months before the development of symptoms.[5] Hydronephrosis, renal failure, and uremia develop as urine is unable to leave the kidney. Death will follow without treatment. Symptoms of uremia include fluid and electrolyte imbalance, acidosis, nausea, vomiting, anorexia, fatigue, and changes in mental status such as memory changes.[1, 3]

The insertion of ureteral stents or the placement of a nephrostomy tube are common methods of managing hydronephrosis. Radiation therapy and hormonal therapy have also been used. In a patient who can undergo anesthesia, ureteral stents are placed using a cystoscope to visualize the ureteral orifices directly and to pass a ureteral catheter into the kidney to allow urine to drain to the bladder. If this procedure is unsuccessful, percutaneous nephrostomy tubes (PNTs) will be required. Under fluoroscopic guidance, PNTs are placed into the renal pelvis to drain urine into an external urinary drainage bag.[3] Complications related to PNT include urinary tract infection, sepsis, dislodgment, obstruction, and bleeding. Frequent catheter changes are required to maintain tube patency. Indications that the PNT may require replacement include reduced urine output, leakage of urine, blockage, and encrustation. Occasionally, external PNT can be internalized to reduce these problems and improve the patient's QOL.[1] Ureteral stents may occlude with time and require replacement. Stents are available in polyurethane and metal. Perioperative antibiotics are used to reduce the risk of infection.[12]

Patients who have not previously received hormonal manipulation may live longer after placement of ureteral stents than those patients previously treated with hormones. In a research study, 12 patients without prior hormonal treatment lived 646 days compared with 80 days in 24 patients who had prior hormonal treatment ($P < .01$).[13] Of the 24 patients with prior hormonal treatment, 8 had catheters inserted and lived an average of 92 days. The other 16 patients did not have catheters placed and lived an average of 74 days ($P =$ ns).[13] The patients receiving catheters spent less time in the hospital than those not decompressed with catheters. The authors concluded that bilateral ureteral decompression would be of most use in patients who had not previously received hormonal therapy.

Medical management of ureteral obstruction may be an option for patients who want to avoid tube placement. Dexamethasone has been administered to patients with ureteral obstruction to improve urinary flow.[14] Included in the research study were 11 men with ureteral obstruction from advanced prostate cancer. Of the 11 men, 7 had not been previously diagnosed and 4 had received prior therapy with hormones or radiation therapy. All patients received 8 mg intravenous (IV) bolus dexamethasone and then were subsequently treated with a wide range of dexamethasone doses and frequencies. Five of the newly diagnosed patients underwent bilateral orchiectomy. Two of the newly diagnosed patients died soon after hospital admission from heart failure. Of the 11 patients, 10 responded with improved renal function and underwent diuresis within 72 hours of receiving dexamethasone.[14] Six of the responding 10 patients were newly diagnosed and demonstrated an ongoing response to hormonal manipulation. Dexamethasone may be useful in patients with ureteral obstruction who have not previously received hormonal therapy. The patients who had failed prior therapy also had improved renal function but did not respond to bilateral orchiectomy or radiation therapy. See Table 14-1 for nursing care standard.[3, 4, 15]

LEG EDEMA

Leg edema in advanced prostate cancer may be related to lymphatic or venous obstruction, inguinofemoral node dissection, or other medical problems.[16] Lymphatic fluid is high in protein. When lymphatic flow is blocked by metastatic disease-bearing pelvic lymph nodes, the lymphatic fluid backs up in the lymphatic vessels of the legs. This backup of lymph fluid allows protein and fluids to accumulate in the tissues. The protein in the tissues increases tissue oncotic pressure and promotes the accumulation of more fluid and increases lymphedema.[16]

Clots from deep vein thromboses (DVTs) may cause impaired venous return and increased venous pressure and may promote leg edema.[17] Low serum albumin levels also cause leg edema. When serum albumin levels are low, oncotic pressure within the blood vessel is reduced. Fluid that has left the blood vessel from hydrostatic pressure and entered the tissues is unable to leave the tissues to return to the blood because oncotic pressure produced by albumin in the vessels is not sufficient enough to pull fluids from the tissues, and edema results.

Medical conditions such as congestive heart failure and venous insufficiency also cause leg edema.[18] In elderly cancer patients, the aging process itself predisposes patients to leg edema.[19] Additional risk factors for edema in the elderly include reduced renal function and reduced cardiac function.

Diagnostic studies useful in evaluating patients with leg edema include serum albumin level and bilateral venous Doppler studies to evaluate for the presence of DVT, which may be unilateral or bilateral. A magnetic resonance imaging (MRI) scan of the abdomen and pelvis may be useful in identifying lymph node metastases, which may obstruct lymphatic drainage, resulting in lymphedema.

Assessment of the extremity will assist in identifying the cause of the leg edema. When the cause of leg edema is a DVT, there is often unilateral swelling, pain, dilated veins, redness, and increased warmth in the area affected.[3] The patient may have a history of reduced mobility and the leg changes usually have developed over a short period of time. DVTs can occur in both legs, however, and both legs should always be assessed. In this way, comparison can be made between the affected leg and the unaffected leg. Lymphedema often develops slowly, beginning in the foot and eventually involving the

TABLE 14-2. Assessment of Leg Edema

Venous Cause

Is the edema unilateral or bilateral?
Has the patient been spending more time in bed?
Are the leg(s) warm, painful, or red?
Does the patient have a low-grade temperature?
Are the leg veins dilated?
Does the patient have symptoms of pulmonary embolus, such as chest pain, anxiety, shortness of breath?
Is a positive Homans' sign present?

Lymphatic Cause

Has the patient had a pelvic lymphadenectomy?
Has an injury occurred to the affected extremity?
Do(es) the leg(s) feel heavy?
Has the patient received large doses of radiation therapy to the affected extremity?
Does elevation of the extremity reduce the swelling?
Are the toes square in appearance?
Is leg tissue woody, fibrotic, or indurated?

Data compiled from Black and Matassarin-Jacobs,[3] Humble,[16] and Creager and Dzau.[20]

TABLE 14-3. Severity of Lymphedema

Difference in Leg Measurements (cm)	Severity of Lymphedema
1–1.5	Diagnosable
1.5–3	Mild
3–5	Moderate
> 5	Severe

Source: From Humble CA. Lymphedema: Incidence, pathophysiology, management and nursing care. Oncology Nursing Forum 1995;22:1503–1509. Used with permission.

entire leg. The tissue is soft and, with thumb pressure, produces an indentation.[20] As the edema becomes chronic, the tissues feel woody and are fibrotic and indurated, and the toes look square[20] (Table 14-2).

The severity of the edema must be evaluated. Edema is evaluated on a scale ranging from 0 to 4, with 0 indicating no edema and 4 indicating edema deeper than 1 cm when the tissues are depressed with the thumb. Edema should be evaluated daily and findings documented. Also the nurse should weigh the patient to monitor the amount of fluid reduction.

The nurse must measure the legs at specific areas and then document the measurements daily on a flow chart to assess the effectiveness of nursing interventions or medical treatment. Using a flexible tape measure, the nurse measures the legs at the following landmarks: metatarsophalangeal joint, instep, ankle, lower calf, calf, knee, lower thigh, upper thigh, and gluteal fold[16, 21] (see Figure 14-1 for measurement landmarks). The severity of the lymphedema can then be determined by comparing one leg with the other (Table 14-3).

As part of the assessment, the nurse should check the pulse in both extremities[22] and perform sensory and motor evaluations on the legs. The nurse also must evaluate the

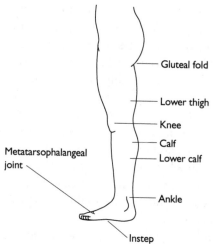

Gluteal fold

Lower thigh

Knee

Calf

Metatarsophalangeal
joint

Lower calf

Ankle

Instep

FIGURE 14-1. Measurement landmarks

impact of leg edema on the patient's QOL. The nurse should identify the impact of edema on walking, self-care, and self-esteem and assess the severity of pain using a scale ranging from 0-10. The nurse needs to know the extent of the deleterious effect of the edema on the patient's functioning and lifestyle. If severe, depression may be present secondary to changes in the ability to perform activities of daily living.[22] Referral to a social worker or other appropriate healthcare provider can then be made.

After the cause of the leg edema has been identified, appropriate treatment can be instituted.

DEEP VEIN THROMBOSIS

A diagnosis of DVT requires prompt heparinization and the initiation of warfarin in anticipation of discharge home after adequate anticoagulation has been achieved. Before initiation of therapy, coagulation blood studies are performed. Evaluation includes measurement of the prothrombin time (PT)–international normalized ratio (INR) and activated partial thromboplastin time (PTT). The platelet count is also checked. Afterward, an IV bolus of heparin is administered, followed by a continuous infusion of heparin. Heparin interferes with clotting factor IX and thrombin and new clot formation.[23] The PTT is checked in 6 hours, and the heparin rate is adjusted based on the results. PTT values are checked after each manipulation of the heparin infusion until the PTT reaches the therapeutic range (1.5–2.0 times control); when the patient reaches the therapeutic range, the PTT is checked daily. The nurse monitors the patient for bleeding from the nose, from the mouth, and in the urine or stool. The patient is placed on bleeding precautions (see Table 14-1) while receiving anticoagulation therapy. After the patient has been adequately anticoagulated with an INR of 2.0 to 3.0 for 2 days,[3] heparin can be discontinued.

A newer method of heparin anticoagulation involves the use of weight-based heparinization.[23] On the basis of the patient's weight, heparin is administered. The goal is to reduce the amount of time that the patient is overanticoagulated and underanticoagulated. Weight-based low-molecular-weight heparin (LMWH) is also used to manage DVT. The patient receives twice-daily subcutaneous injections of LMWH with warfarin initiated on Day 2 of LMWH therapy.[24] The injections are continued until the PT-INR is therapeutic (INR, 2.0–3.0), and then the injections are discontinued. This type of anticoagulation may be done at home; however, the patient or family needs to be able to perform the injections, and home care is needed to monitor the patient and blood work after discharge. A potential complication associated with the use of heparin therapy is heparin-induced thrombocytopenia and thrombosis (HITT).[25–26] The nurse monitors all patients undergoing heparin therapy for a falling platelet count which may indicate the condition has developed.

While undergoing anticoagulation, the patient is kept on bed rest with the leg elevated. Warm soaks may be applied to the affected extremity. One must never massage the patient's calf, and the patient must be instructed never to massage his lower legs. Ambulation may be permitted in several days. The nurse monitors the patient's leg for changes, such as increase or decrease in edema or change in pain or warmth.

Warfarin is begun after initiation of heparin therapy. The anticoagulation action of warfarin is to interfere with the formation of vitamin K–dependent clotting factors produced in the liver.[3] Common starting dosages of warfarin range from 5 to 10 mg/day for 2 days followed by dosing dependent on daily INR results. Warfarin therapy is continued for about 3 to 6 months after DVT.[20] PT/INR is monitored while the patient is receiving warfarin therapy. The patient needs to understand the need to keep doctors' appointments and adhere to laboratory blood work schedules and to report bleeding to the physician because over- or underanticoagulation can be life threatening. Home health nursing should be provided to draw laboratory specimens and to monitor the patient for bleeding or other complications associated with anticoagulant therapy. The patient who is not a candidate for anticoagulation therapy may benefit from the placement of an inferior vena cava filter. A serious life-threatening complication of DVT is pulmonary embolus.[27] Symptoms of pulmonary embolus include chest pain, dyspnea, shortness of breath, tachycardia, and tachypnea. See Table 14-1 for nursing care standard.

LYMPHEDEMA

When leg edema is caused by the lymphatic system, a different approach to edema management is taken. Management of lymphedema is multidisciplinary, involving skin care, education, massage, exercise, and supportive hose.[22] The multidisciplinary team may consist of members from nursing, medicine, and physical therapy. The patient needs to understand that lymphedema management requires the patient's commitment to a daily prescribed regimen that will control the edema. Management is a lifelong process, and the patient is responsible for performing self-care after proper instruction is completed.

Skin care consists of daily cleansing, lubricating, and inspecting. During inspection, the patient looks for breaks in the skin that could result in infection. Every effort must be made to avoid injury to the affected extremities.[28]

Massage or manual lymphatic drainage is used to move lymphatic fluid from the extremities toward the trunk. Only light touch is used to move the fluid manually. The therapist or nurse begins massage with unobstructed lymph vessels in the trunk and unaffected extremity and then works on the affected limb, proximal to distal. [22, 28] External compression devices are also part of therapy. Leg garments, intermittent compression devices, and sequential compression devices are available to assist with lymphedema management.[29] These are applied after massage and skin care.[22] Additional components of lymphedema management include exercise and elevating the extremity above the heart. These are done wearing the compression sleeve. Because lymphedema management requires time commitment on the part of the patient and the lymphedema management team before results are seen, the patient should have a prognosis that is going to allow the palliative effects of this treatment to be evident. Equipment is expensive, and all costs may not be covered by insurance. Some of the devices are difficult to apply, may require the assistance of another person for application, and may be heavy or uncomfortable. For patients with a limited prognosis, leg elevation alone may be the best option to help manage leg edema.

Medications have been used to manage lymphedema. Antibiotics are used when infection is present.[16, 22] Diuretics, if used, result only in depleting the intravascular volume.[30] If used, the patient must be monitored for fluid volume deficit by checking the blood pressure and assessing the patient for lightheadedness or dizziness. Benzopyrones reduce edema through proteolysis.[31] One agent, coumarin, has been tested in patients with arm and leg edema. In a randomized, placebo-controlled trial, patients received a placebo or 400 mg of coumarin daily. No other treatment was administered during the trial. Twenty-one of the 52 patients included in the study had leg edema. In the group of patients receiving coumarin, edema was reduced, tissue was softer, and the patients had fewer symptoms resulting from lymphedema such as tightness and improved mobility. Side effects were limited to mild nausea and diarrhea, which resolved after the first month. Additional research is needed using this drug before recommending its use.

SCROTAL EDEMA

Scrotal edema may occur from advanced prostate cancer. Additional causes of scrotal edema include infection, irritation, surgery, and allergic reactions.[3] Scrotal skin is thin and contains many folds, which make the skin prone to injury. Good hygiene is necessary to reduce the risk of infection. (See Table 14-1 for nursing management of the patient with scrotal edema.)

DISSEMINATED INTRAVASCULAR COAGULATION

Disseminated intravascular coagulation (DIC) occurs in patients with prostate cancer. The process may be acute (fulminant), chronic (compensated), or intermediate.[32] DIC is overstimulation of the normal clotting process precipitated by a triggering event. In the body, there is a natural ongoing process of clotting and clot dissolution. Normally, the process of clot formation and clot dissolution is kept in balance. An injury to a body tissue causes the release of materials that promote clotting. The process is initiated by the release of serotonin by the injured blood vessel.[32] Platelets adhere to the injured site and form a plug. Additional factors are released by the platelets and the injured blood vessel. These factors stimulate the clotting cascade and a fibrin clot forms. [33] The body has two clotting mechanisms: intrinsic and extrinsic. The intrinsic system is stimulated by endothelial damage, and the extrinsic system is stimulated by tissue damage.[3] These pathways culminate in a common pathway in which prothrombin is converted to thrombin, which converts fibrinogen to fibrin, and then a fibrin clot develops.[3, 32] After clotting occurs, clot breakdown or fibrinolysis begins. The fibrinolytic process produces products known as fibrin split products (FSPs) or fibrin degradation products (FDPs), which, in excess amounts, have an anticoagulant activity.

The triggering event in DIC causes rapid development of fibrin thrombi, clotting factor consumption, and fibrinolysis.[33, 34] The result is the formation of clots in small blood vessels, the use of platelets and clotting factors, and subsequent bleeding. The incidence of DIC in prostate cancer is not well known. A study was done using blood samples from 101 men with prostate cancer with the following stages of disease: Stage A, n=4; Stage B, n=22; Stage C, n=23; and Stage D, n=52.[35] Tumor necrosis factor (TNF), a cytokine with a wide range of biologic activity, was found in 19.2% of the samples. When broken down by stage, Stage A patients had 0% serum specimens positive for TNF, Stage B patients, 9.1%; Stage C, 4.3%; and Stage D, 30.9%. In Stage D patients with relapsed disease, 82.4% of the patients had elevated TNF levels. D-dimer is a test used to evaluate for the presence of DIC and is considered the most reliable test for this disease process.[36] In patients with elevated TNF, the D-dimer levels were also elevated and were higher than in patients without elevated TNF levels. FDP levels were also higher in patients with elevated TNF levels. Therefore, the authors concluded that TNF may be involved in the pathogenesis of DIC in prostate cancer.[36] Other factors may be involved in the pathogenesis of DIC in prostate cancer, including the release of procoagulant material into the bloodstream.[33]

Signs of acute DIC include bleeding from multiple body sites (e.g., orifices and sites of skin or mucous membrane trauma such as venipuncture sites). The severity of DIC may vary from oozing to hemorrhage. Multiple body organs may be involved, including the brain, kidneys, liver, lungs, and gastrointestinal (GI) tract. A complete and thorough nursing assessment is needed to identify all the affected body areas. Mottling resulting from small blood vessel occlusion may be present in the skin.[36] There may also be petechiae, ecchymoses, or purpura of the skin and mucous membranes.[3] Pulses may be weak as a result of poor tissue perfusion.[36] Frequent assessment of the patient's mental status and neurologic checks must be done. There may be confusion, headache, or changes in the level of consciousness from intracranial bleeding.[36] The presence of bleeding in the lungs may produce hemoptysis and shortness of breath. GI bleeding may produce melena, hematochezia, hematemesis, abdominal distention, and tenderness. Renal involvement may produce hematuria, oliguria, and renal failure.

TABLE 14-4. Laboratory Studies Used in the Diagnosis and Monitoring of DIC

Test	Normal result	Value	Diagnostic of DIC
D-dimer	<10 μcg/mL	↑	> 500 μcg/mL
FDP	10 μcg/mL	↑	> 45 μcg/mL
Antithrombin III	89–120%	↓	< 80%
Fibrinogen	200–400 mg/dL	↓	< 150–195 mg/dL
PT	12–15 seconds	↑	4–5 s above normal
Platelet count	150,000–400,000/mm³	↓	< 100,000–100,000/mm³
PTT	25–39 seconds	↑	> 60 seconds
Clotting factors		↓	

Data compiled from Black and Matassarin-Jacobs,[3] Schafer,[32] Murphy-Ende,[33] Gobel,[34] Finley,[36] Luckmann,[38] and Thompson et al.[39]
DIC, disseminated intravascular coagulation; FDP, fibrin degradation product; PT, prothrombin time; PTT, partial thromboplastin time.

Unlike acute DIC, chronic (compensated) DIC produces few signs or symptoms.[34] The patient may have problems with bleeding from the mucous membranes, GI tract, or skin, but the bleeding is minor.[34] Complications from chronic DIC include venous thrombosis and endocarditis.[37]

DIC may also present as abnormal blood work results without clinical evidence of disease.[34] Diagnostic studies used in the diagnosis and monitoring of DIC are listed in Table 14-4.[3, 32, 34, 36, 38, 39]

Treatment of DIC involves the identification of the triggering event such as infection or previously untreated prostate cancer. Antibiotics are used to treat infection. Previously untreated prostate cancer responds to the removal of androgens.[5] IV or subcutaneous heparin is used to interfere with clot formation.[40] The patient with acute DIC is a critical care nursing challenge. The goal is to maintain homeostasis while correcting or eliminating the causative factor. Frequent nursing assessment of body systems is needed to identify new sites of bleeding or improvement in the patient's status. Assessments should be done every 4 hours or more often as needed. Close monitoring of all body systems is required to maintain their functioning. The patient requires blood product replacement of platelets, washed red blood cells, volume expanders such as albumin, and antithrombin concentrates.[40] Products containing fibrinogen are avoided because they may worsen DIC.[40] Thromboses of the small vessels of the body organs are the major cause of patient morbidity and mortality.[40]

Patients with abnormal blood work or chronic DIC will require monitoring for worsening of their blood work or the development of signs of acute DIC. A home health nurse should be consulted to monitor the patient at home and obtain required blood specimens. See Table 14-1 for nursing care standard.[32–40]

BONE PAIN

Pain is a common problem in men with advanced prostate cancer, and multiple causes of pain have been identified. Pain may be local from the spread of cancer to adjacent organs; referred to the back, legs, or abdomen; or emanate from bone.[41] Bone pain is the most important of the pain problems in this population; the majority of patients require bone pain management at some time during the disease process.[5, 41, 42] Bone pain is produced by the presence of metastatic lesions, most often located in the pelvis and spine.[41] It has been hypothesized for the last 50 years that prostate cancer cells spread to the vertebral spine via Batson's plexus of vertebral veins.[43] This system of vertebral veins is associated with the spine locally and also with the intercoastal veins.

The development of bone metastases is not a random process; rather, the bones provide a rich environment for the growth of metastatic lesions. Prostate cancer cells probably possess factors that promote the spread of cancer to this area.[43] These factors include proteolytic enzymes that allow tumor cell detachment, loss of adhesive capabilities, movement of cells into the circulation, and the ability of cancer cells to evade the immune system.[43] Cells important in bone metastases from prostate cancer are the osteoclast and osteoblast. The osteoclast is stimulated by the presence of the tumor cells and tumor-related factors and also probably causes bone loss.[43] Osteoclast stimulation may also be a step in the development of osteoblastic bone tumors, which are the primary metastatic bone tumors in prostate cancer.[44] Osteoblasts are stimulated to lay down new bone, thus producing osteoblastic lesions.

The exact mechanism producing bone pain is not known. Pain may be produced by the destruction and development of new bone.[45] Prostaglandins appear to play a role in the bone metastatic process.[46] Receptors that may play a role in bone pain include peripheral opioid receptors, nociceptors, and N-methyl-D-aspartate receptors.[45] Patients with spinal metastases that compress nerve roots or the spinal cord often have both bone pain and neuropathic pain.[45]

Complaints of bone pain are evaluated with a bone scan and plain radiographs. The pain is diffuse, is increased at night, and may be located around the joints.[47] The patient describes the pain in a variety of terms, including ache, burn, or stab.[47] There may be a neurogenic component to the pain as a result of periosteal involvement.[47] Lying down does not improve the patient's comfort level. Pain may be constant, intermittent, or constant with episodes of breakthrough pain or incidental pain.

Pain has the ability to affect significantly the patient's QOL. The medications used for pain management also produce side effects that impact on the patient and need to be managed in an aggressive manner so as to detract no further from the patient's well-being.[47]

Multiple methods of metastatic bone pain management are available. Treatment includes the use of analgesics, radiation therapy, strontium 89 (SR-89), and bisphosphonates. In patients who have not previously received hormonal manipulation, this is the initial treatment of choice.[48] Orchiectomy produces pain relief in 24 hours.[5] Antiandrogens are initiated before starting luteinizing hormone-releasing hormone (LHRH) agonists to avoid an increase in bone pain, which can occur when LHRH agonists are given as single agents. Analgesics useful in the management of bone pain are the opioids and the nonopioids. Nonopioids include the group of nonsteroidal antiinflammatory drugs (NSAIDs) and acetaminophen. NSAIDs are the first step in the World Health Organization (WHO) pain ladder.[49, 50] This type of agent is useful for managing mild to moderate pain and is frequently used for bone pain. These drugs may be given alone or with an opioid for moderate to severe pain. Dosing the NSAIDs above their usual dosage range for each drug does not increase analgesia but will increase the risk of drug-related side effects.[51] Side effects commonly associated with NSAIDs include interference with platelet aggregation, gastric ulcers, impaired renal function, dizziness, and drowsiness.[52] Acetaminophen and NSAIDs must be used with caution in patients who use alcohol or have a history of liver disease. NSAIDs that are useful in oncology patients include choline magnesium trisalicylate and nabumetone because they do not affect platelet function.

Opioids are useful in patients with moderate to severe pain. Codeine and hydrocodone may be useful for moderate pain but are frequently prescribed with acetaminophen, as is oxycodone. These combination products cannot be titrated beyond the maximum daily dose of the acetaminophen or other nonopioid analgesic in the product. This ceiling on dose escalation limits their usefulness, and patients may need to be switched to a short-acting opioid. Opiates useful in patients with severe advanced cancer pain include morphine, hydromorphone, oxycodone, and fentanyl.[53] Meperidine is a poor choice of analgesic for use in cancer pain.

Morphine is a frequently prescribed analgesic used in the management of cancer pain. It is available in a variety of formulations, including parenteral, rectal, short-acting oral, and long-acting (controlled-release) oral preparations. Frequently, patients are started on a short-acting dose of morphine. The dose is given frequently enough to relieve pain and yet not produce distressing side effects that interfere with the patient's QOL. After the patient has achieved good analgesia with a short-acting formulation, conversion is made to a controlled-release form that can be given every 12 hours (or 8 hours if needed). (See Table 14-5 for equianalgesic conversions.) If a patient does not tolerate morphine, another short-acting opioid should be tried. Long-acting opioids with long half-lives such as a methadone are difficult to titrate because of the need to balance analgesia with sedation and other toxicities that develop as the drug accumulates in the blood. Often the toxicities interfere with the ability to achieve satisfactory pain control. Opioids are continued for as long as required. The development of tolerance will allow for dose increments if pain severity increases.

Narcotics are most often administered by mouth because this is an effective, inexpensive, and normal way of administering medications. Other routes that are useful for cancer pain are transdermal and occasionally rectal. Parenteral and epidural routes may be useful in patients who cannot achieve a balance of satisfactory pain relief and side effects with other routes.

The dose of drugs administered is individualized to meet the patient's needs. A frequent method of initiating therapy for a patient with continuous pain is to start with a set dose of opioid administered routinely around the clock with an as-needed rescue dose of the same drug. The frequency of routine doses is based on the drug's duration of action and route of administration. Rescue oral doses are available every 1 to 2 hours, and the dose should be 5 to 15% of the total routine 24-hour dose.[53] The

TABLE 14-5. Equianalgesic Doses of Opioid Analgesics Used for the Control of Chronic Pain

Analgesic	Oral Dose (mg)	Dose Interval	Subcutaneous Dose (mg)	Comments
Meperidine (Demerol)	150	q2–3h	50	Toxic metabolite. Not recommended for severe chronic pain.
Codeine (3 tablets Tylenol No. 3)	100	q4h	60	Of limited value in severe chronic pain. Each Tylenol No. 3 tablet contains 30 mg codeine plus 325 mg acetaminophen.
Pentazocine (Talwin)	90	q4h	30	Not recommended for severe chronic pain.
Hydrocodone (3 tablets/capsules Vicodin/Lortab)	15	q4h	NA	Of limited value in severe chronic pain. Each Vicodin or Lortab tablet contains 5 mg hydrocodone plus 500 mg acetaminophen.
Morphine (MSIR, Roxanol)	15	q4h	5	SC dose essentially equal to IM dose. Equianalgesic IV dose equal to 75–80% of SC dose.
Morphine (MS Contin, Oramorph SR)	45	q12h	NA	Rectal suppositories available. PR dose is equal to PO dose.
Morphine (Kadian)	90	q24h	NA	
Oxycodone (2 tablets Percodan, Percocet, Roxicodone) OxyFast, OxyIR, Roxicodone Intensol 20 mg/mL, Roxicodone Intensol 20 mg/mL	10	q4h	NA	Each Percodan or Percocet tablet contains 5 mg oxycodone plus 325 mg aspirin (Percodan), 325 mg acetaminophen (Percocet). Roxicodone tablets and OxyIR capsules contain 5 mg oxycodone alone.
Oxycodone (OxyContin)	30	q12h	NA	Caution: Risk of toxicity from delayed accumulation.
Methadone (Dolophine)	10	q8–12h	5	SC dose essentially equal to IM dose. Equianalgesic IV dose equal to 75–80% of SC dose. Rectal suppositories available. PR dose is equal to PO dose.
Hydromorphone (Dilaudid)	4	q4h	1.5	Caution: Risk of toxicity from delayed accumulation.
Levorphanol (Levo-Dromoran)	2	q4–6h	1	Durogesic fentanyl transdermal system: (micrograms/hour dose of transdermal fentanyl = ½ × milligram/day dose of oral morphine (one 100 μg/h patch q3 days = 100 mg MS Contin PO q12h).
Fentanyl (Durogesic) Oral transmucosal fentanyl citrate (Actiq)	NA	q72h q30 min x 2 units, max. of 4 doses/day; begin dosage at 200 μg for all patients, for use only with narcotic-tolerant patients	NA	

DRUG, COMPANY, AND LOCATION LIST: Actiq, Anesta, Salt Lake City, UT and Abbot, North Chicago, IL; **Demerol,** **Talwin,** Sanofi Pharmaceuticals, New York; **Tylenol No. 3,** Ortho-McNeil Pharmaceutical, Raritan, NJ; **Vicodin,** Knoll Laboratories, Mt. Olive, NJ; **Lortab,** UCB Pharma, Inc., Smyrna, GA; **MSIR, MS Contin, OxyContin, OxyFast,** Purdue Frederick, Norwalk, VA and Purdue Pharma, Norwalk, CT; **Kadian,** Faulding, Raleigh, NC; **Roxanol, Oramorph, Roxicet, Roxicodone Intensol, Dolophine,** Roxane Laboratories, Columbus, OH; **Percodan, Percocet,** Endo Pharmaceuticals, Inc., Chadds Ford, PA; **Levo-Dromoran,** ICN Pharmaceuticals, Costa Mesa, CA; **Durogesic,** Janssen Pharmaceuticals, Titusville, NJ.

Equianalgesic doses listed were obtained from a variety of sometimes conflicting studies and experiences and are meant only as guidelines for around-the-clock, standing order, analgesic therapy of chronic pain. Developed and written by M. Levy, MD, PhD. Permission to adapt format and reprint granted by M. Levy, MD. Table adapted from data published in Levy M. Pharmacologic treatment of cancer pain. *N Eng J Med* 1996;335:1124–1132. Used with permission.

NA, not available; SC, subcutaneous; IM, intramuscular; IV, intravenous; PR, per rectum; PO, orally; h, hour.

baseline 24-hour dose should be increased based on the total milligrams of the patient's rescue doses plus baseline dose and then divided by the number of doses to be administered over 24 hours. Another method is to increase the dose by 30 to 50% in patients with inadequate pain relief.[53] Should intolerable side effects develop before acceptable analgesia, another opioid should be tried. The starting dose of the new drug needs to be reduced, administered at 50 to 66% of the equianalgesic dose of the prior drug.[54] The dose of the new drug is increased as needed. (See Table 14-5 for equianalgesic conversions.)

The most common opioid side effect, constipation, is best managed by anticipatory and preventive interventions designed to reduce or eliminate this problem for the patient. Beginning on Day 1 of narcotic dosing, a prophylactic stool softener and laxative are also administered (Figure 14-2). A useful combination medication of these two drugs is senna and docusate. Initial dosing is two tablets daily and titrated as needed so the patient has a soft, yet formed stool at least every other day. Increasing fluid intake is also important when managing constipation. Lactulose, 30 mL, is useful if the patient has not moved his bowels in 3 days before starting senna and docusate or any time after if more than 2 days are experienced without a bowel movement. Lactulose is administered every 6 hours until the patient has a bowel movement. Suppositories and enemas may be needed if the patient has not had a bowel movement in 4 days (see Figure 14-2). It is important to check the patient's platelet count and white blood cell count before proceeding with the administration of anything per rectum to avoid bleeding or the risk of infection if the patient is neutropenic or thrombocytopenic.

Nausea should also be anticipated because it occurs in 10 to 40% of patients receiving narcotics.[55] An antiemetic is not usually needed because tolerance to nausea develops quickly.[53] However, an antiemetic order should be available in case nausea is intolerable. Other side effects to which the patient develops a tolerance include sedation and respiratory depression. If sedation is a problem, one should first be certain that other sedating or unnecessary drugs are eliminated. Otherwise, the narcotic dose should be reduced by 25%.[53] Another option is to try a different opioid or add methylphenidate.

Bone metastases may be limited to one or a few sites or may be widely metastatic throughout the skeleton. When limited to a few sites of metastases, radiation therapy is effective in reducing pain and narcotic usage and improving the patient's activity level.[56] Radiation doses delivered to palliate bone pain vary widely, and the best dose and schedule of dose delivery have yet to be determined.[57] Partial or complete pain relief is produced in 75% of patients who receive radiation.[58] Doses delivered range from 1 to 50 Gy.[57] Lower doses (4 Gy) delivered as a single fraction appear to be less effective in reducing pain. Treatment of patients with a limited prognosis should be delivered as quickly as can be delivered safely.[56] In a large research trial, regimens that delivered 4,050 cGy over 15 treatments or 3,000 cGy over 10 treatments produced the best outcome.[59] Delivering the total dose of radiation in one fraction may also be useful in some patients. A study of a single fraction of radiation (10 Gy) produced a similar overall response rate as 5 fractions (22.5 Gy).[60] Nausea, vomiting, tiredness, and lassitude were the major side effects.

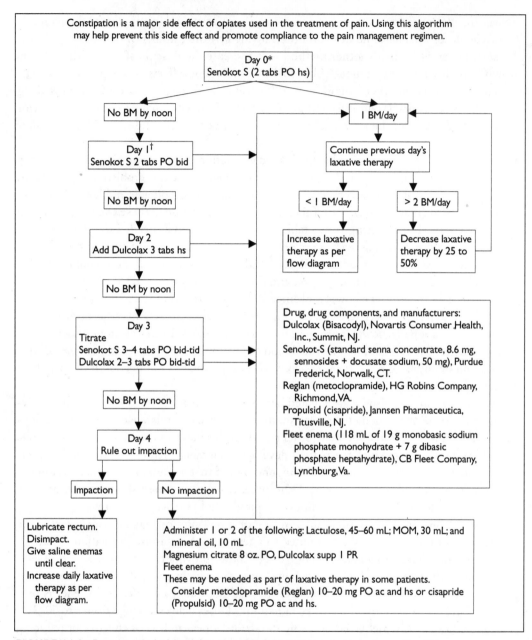

FIGURE 14-2. Recommended laxative therapy for cancer-associated constipation

Source: Adapted from data published in Levy MH. Constipation and diarrhea in cancer patients. *Cancer Bulletin* 1991;43:417. Adapted by M. Levy, P. Kedziera, and J. Koss. Used with permission of M. Levy, MD, PhD, and *Cancer Bulletin*.

tabs, tablets; PO, per os; PR, per rectum; hs, bedtime; BM, bowel movement; ac, before meals; AM, morning; bid, twice a day; tid, three times a day; supp, suppository.

* First day of opioid analgesia, no preexisting constipation.

† Start here if daily oral morphine equivalent ≥ 120 mg.

Systemic radionuclides such as SR-89 deliver radiation to areas of new bone formation such as metastatic bone tumors.[61] SR-89 is a pure β-emitting radioisotope that is quickly taken up by bone.[62] Radionuclides are particularly useful in patients who have widespread painful bone metastases that preclude the use of external beam radiation therapy. With SR-89, each metastatic site receives a dose of radioisotope. Small tumors are more responsive to SR-89 than large tumors.[56] SR-89 is administered by IV bolus at a dose of 40 to 60 μCi/kg in the radiation therapy or nuclear medicine department.[61] Side effects include facial flushing during drug administration; thrombocytopenia and leukopenia are the major drug-related toxicities.[61] Blood counts are monitored twice a week or more often if needed. Responses are seen in 80% of patients, and approximately 10% of these patients have complete pain relief, which may last 3 to 6 months.[63] Retreatment may be appropriate for increased pain if the platelet count and white blood cell (WBC) count have recovered.[63] The platelet count should be greater than 60,000/mm^3 and the WBC count greater than 2,400/mm^3 before treatment or retreatment.[64] Pain relief begins 2 weeks after treatment. An initial bone pain flare may precede pain relief, and patients may require additional analgesia during this time. Afterward, it may be possible to reduce narcotic doses, and a schedule should be set up to monitor and titrate narcotic doses. Samarium-153 is a newer systemic radionuclide with bone-seeking behavior. It is also effective in reducing bone pain and produces mild bone marrow depression.[65]

Bisphosphonates are a group of drugs that interfere with osteoclast activity.[66] Even though prostate cancer bone metastases are 95% osteoblastic in nature, there is some degree of bone resorption in these metastatic lesions.[66] This osteoclast activity in osteoblastic lesions may help explain the symptomatic improvement observed in patients with metastatic prostate cancer when bisphosphonates have been administered.[66, 67] Several prospective, randomized placebo-controlled studies using bisphosphonates in the treatment of prostate cancer have been published[68–70] (Table 14-6). The number of prostate patients in these trials is small, but these studies do demonstrate the potential ability of bisphosphonates to reduce pain with limited toxicity. However, until additional trials identify the best schedule, dose, and agent useful in these patients, the routine use of bisphosphonates outside a research setting cannot be recommended.[67]

NURSING MANAGEMENT

Patients with pain require an in-depth pain assessment to identify all components of the patient's pain experience. A tool (Figure 14-3) should allow for documentation of the data collected in the pain assessment. The nurse needs to understand clearly the patient's perception of the pain and the impact it has on his QOL. Other areas to be explored during pain assessment include the meaning of pain, self-image, pain beliefs, and how the patient and family believe pain should be managed.[71] Patient and family education begins during the assessment, when the nurse clarifies myths and misperceptions about pain. The patient needs to know the name of the drugs being administered, both generic and trade, the dose and frequency of analgesics, and how to manage drug-

TABLE 14-6. Bisphosphonate Trials in Advanced Prostate Cancer

Study	N	Endpoints	Drugs-Treatment Administered	Major Findings	Major Toxicities
Ernst et al [68]	24 13 breast 5 lung 4 prostate 2 other	Pain measured on a 10-cm linear analogue scale	Clodronate, 600 mg in 500 mL NSS IV vs. placebo	Reduced pain by 0.89 cm in patients receiving clo-dronate ($P < .01$); no difference in analgesic use	Increased creatinine
Robertson et al [69]	55 13 breast 2 lung 2 prostate 7 other	Pain measured on a 10 cm linear analogue scale	Oral clodronate, 1,600 mg/day vs. placebo	Reduced pain by 0.9 cm in clodronate group ($P = .03$); increase in placebo group by 0.4 cm; no difference in anal-gesic use	Difficulty swallowing tablets
Coleman et al [70]	52	Pain intensity + analgesic consumption + performance status = overall pain score	Pamidronate, 120 mg in 1,000 mL NSS IV over 2 h vs. placebo; 4 weeks later, all patients received pamidronate	24% symptomatic response in first 4 wk; 53% overall response rate in 8 weeks	

NSS, normal saline solution; IV, intravenous.

related side effects, such as constipation. Ongoing assessment and monitoring of pain and communication of pain to nurse and physician are enhanced with the use of a pain diary.[72] The patient with bone pain often benefits from the use of the NSAIDs, narcotics, and adjuvant analgesics.[73] Analgesics should be administered according to the WHO pain ladder, beginning with nonopioids and adding opioids as needed.[49, 50] NSAIDs interfere with the synthesis of prostaglandins.[52] These substances play a role in the breakdown and development of new bone, which results in pain.[46] Therefore, it is reasonable that these agents would be useful in the patient with advanced prostate cancer. Opioids relieve pain by binding with opiate receptors in the central nervous system and GI tract.[74] When combined, the drugs potentiate each other and enhance analgesia. A useful nonpharmacologic method of pain relief is the application of heat to painful areas for 20 minutes every 4 to 6 hours. In the patient with bone pain, therapeutic mattresses may enhance pain relief by supporting the affected area.[73] Using devices that aid in transferring the patient from bed to stretcher will also enhance comfort. The patient should be moved without adding pressure to painful areas. Movement should be in one smooth motion without jerking, which will increase pain. Physical and occupational therapies will assist the patient in avoiding injury and falls, which may result in fractures.[75] A comprehensive multidisciplinary approach to managing the patient with bone metastases will improve the patient's QOL, reduce pain, and enhance functioning.

FIGURE 14-3. Initial pain assessment tool

Date______________

Patient's Name: ______________________________ Age:________ Room: __________

Diagnosis: ______________________________ Physician: ______________________________

Nurse: ______________________________

1. LOCATION: Patient or nurse mark drawing.

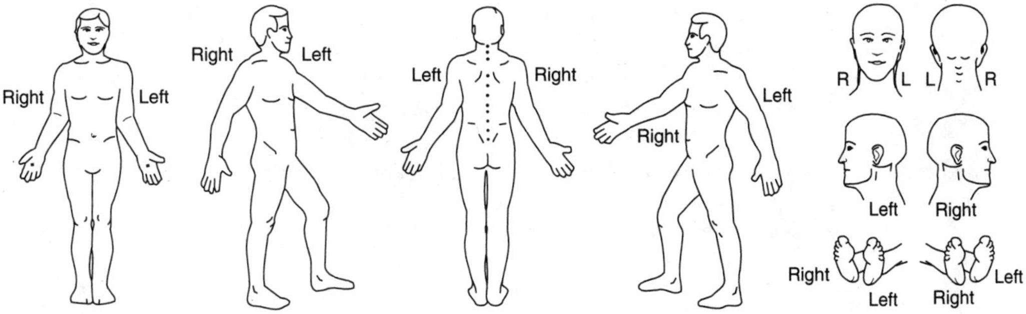

2. INTENSITY: Patient rates the pain. Scale used. ______________________________
   Present: ______________________________
   Worst pain gets: ______________________________
   Best pain gets: ______________________________
   Acceptable level of pain: ______________________________
3. QUALITY: (Use patient's own words, e.g., prick, ache, burn, throb, pull, sharp) ______________________________
4. ONSET, DURATION, VARIATIONS, RHYTHMS: ______________________________
5. MANNER OF EXPRESSING PAIN: ______________________________
6. WHAT RELIEVES THE PAIN? ______________________________
7. WHAT CAUSES OR INCREASES THE PAIN? ______________________________
8. EFFECTS OF PAIN: (Note decreased function, decreased quality of life.)
   Accompanying symptoms (e.g., nausea): ______________________________
   Sleep: ______________________________
   Appetite: ______________________________
   Physical activity: ______________________________
   Relationship with others (e.g., irritability): ______________________________
   Emotions (e.g., anger, suicidal, crying): ______________________________
   Concentration: ______________________________
   Other: ______________________________
9. OTHER COMMENTS: ______________________________
10. PLAN: ______________________________

Source: From McCaffery M, Pasero C. *Pain: Clinical Manual,* p. 60. Copyright © 1999, Mosby, Inc. Used with permission.

TABLE 14-7. Types of Pain Associated With Spinal Cord Compression

Location	Description
Local	Tenderness at site of tumor
	Progresses from mild to severe
	Present in 95% of patients
	Constant
	Increases with recumbent position, leg raising
	Increases with coughing and sneezing
	Increases at night
Radicular	Tight band around area of body at level of cord compression
	Spreads to legs
	Dermatomal distribution
	Increases with coughing, sneezing
	Unilateral with cervical or lumbar lesions
Referred	Poorly localized
	Described as burning, shooting; paresthesias

Data compiled from Surya and Provent,[5] Osborn et al,[76] Wilkes,[79] Weinstein,[80] Faul and Flickinger.[89]

SPINAL CORD COMPRESSION

Spinal cord compression (SCC) is the most devastating of all the complications associated with advanced prostate cancer. Approximately 10% of men with hormone-refractory prostate cancer will develop SCC.[42] Metastatic prostate cancer cells gain access to the venous system and travel to the spine, where they proliferate.[76] The most common area in the spine for tumor growth is the vertebral body; the neural arch is the second most common area.[76] The thoracic spine is the most frequent location in the spinal column for tumor growth followed by the lumbosacral region.[77]

Patients with SCC present with back pain, weakness, or sensory loss in the extremities below the level of the SCC. In patients with back pain and prostate cancer, a presumptive diagnosis of SCC can be made. In patients with a history of benign back pain, it is important to avoid assuming that the current back pain is related to the old pain process. Pain resulting from SCC may radiate to the lower extremities. Pain is caused by the pressure of a tumor or collapsed bone fragments on the spinal cord or cauda equina.[78] Pain may be present for weeks to months before a diagnosis of SCC.[5] Patients may feel as though they are being squeezed by a tight band around the area of the body at the level of the cord lesion. The area of the back where the tumor is located may be tender. (See Table 14-7 for types of pain associated with SCC.) Neurologic symptoms include muscle weakness. Sensory losses include paresthesias and changes in sensation such as inability to feel pinpricks and loss of heat and cold sensation. Autonomic nervous system (ANS) changes include bowel and bladder retention. Late ANS changes are loss of bowel and bladder control.

Diagnostic studies must be performed in a timely manner on presentation of any signs and symptoms of SCC. Loss of time in obtaining diagnostic studies may result in the progression of symptoms and resultant disability. Plain radiographs diagnose spinal metastases in 85% of patients.[79] A bone scan is also a useful diagnostic study. However, MRI is considered the most definitive diagnostic test for this problem.[80] If an MRI scan is not available or cannot be performed, a computed tomography scan with myelogram is a useful diagnostic tool.

After diagnosis of SCC, prompt intervention is required to prevent further progression of SCC. Left untreated, paralysis will develop, along with continued pain, incontinence, and loss of sensation.[81] The severity of functional disability at the time of SCC diagnosis will help predict the outcome of treatment. Of patients able to ambulate at the time of diagnosis, 75% will be able to ambulate after treatment, but only 28% of paraplegic patients will become ambulatory after treatment.[82]

Treatment of SCC may involve the use of dexamethasone, radiation therapy, or surgery. Dexamethasone is frequently used to manage SCC. Patients with symptoms and a clinical examination highly suggestive of SCC may receive dexamethasone before the completion of diagnostic imaging. It reduces pain and improves neurologic functioning. The recommended dose to be administered is controversial; doses as low as 16 mg/day and as high as 96 mg/day are administered.[81, 83, 84] Ambulatory outcome is improved in patients given high doses of dexamethasone compared with those given no dexamethasone (81% vs. 63%).[85] Side effects developed in 11% of the group receiving steroids and included perforated gastric ulcer, hypomania and psychoses. Initially, dexamethasone is given IV. A loading dose is administered followed by dosing every 6 hours. A frequently used regimen is a loading dose of 10-20 mg of IV dexamethasone followed by 4 mg every 6 hours.[5, 78, 81] Higher doses may be administered. After the patient is stable, he can be switched to the oral route and then the dose reduced by tapering. Should neurologic symptoms return with tapering, the dose will need to be increased and tapering attempted again. Histamine-$_2$ blockers and monitoring of blood glucose levels are required when initiating dexamethasone therapy. Patients who are ambulatory with radiologic evidence of SCC and who receive radiation therapy for their SCC may not require dexamethasone to prevent SCC progression.[86] Radiation therapy alone is probably effective in ambulatory patients.[87] Early diagnosis is critical for a good outcome to treatment.[88]

Radiation therapy is administered to two vertebrae above and below the area of compression. Doses of radiation administered are usually 30 Gy given in 10 fractions or 20 Gy given in 5 fractions.[89] The treatment is well tolerated. If there are multiple areas of SCC in a patient, then larger fields are used.[89] Treatment with radiation should begin within 24 hours of the diagnosis of SCC.

Surgery is indicated in patients who have no prior cancer diagnosis, in patients in whom the area of compression has already been irradiated, when neurologic deterioration continues while the patient is receiving radiation therapy, and when spinal instability is present.[81] The surgical procedure and method of approach are determined by tumor location and severity of bone destruction.[90] Thoracic spine lesions approached posteriorly with a laminectomy may produce spinal cord herniation or a worsened neurologic status. Anterior lesions are approached through the chest, and this incision allows for good visualization of the thoracic spine area.[90] Because the chest has been opened, pulmonary complications may occur in the postoperative period. After surgery, radiation therapy may be administered to ambulatory patients.[81]

NURSING MANAGEMENT

The patient with SCC may present with a wide range of signs and symptoms requiring nursing care. The ambulatory patient may only require pain management and education, whereas the patient with paralysis requires nursing management of a wide variety of problems. All patients with prostate cancer must be taught the signs and symptoms of early SCC. Prompt recognition of SCC and emergent treatment are crucial to maintaining good neurologic function. Patients who have previously been treated for SCC need to understand that SCC recurrence is possible. Approximately 45% of patients treated for SCC develop another SCC at the same site or a new one in the 2 years after initial presentation.[82] Therefore, the nurse must be ever vigilant in assessing for the presence of new back pain onset. The patient with back pain should be assumed to have SCC until proven otherwise.

Safety is a major concern in patients with SCC. The nurse should assume that the spine is unstable in a patient with SCC. Bed rest needs to be maintained until diagnostic studies have been completed and evaluated. Afterward, the patient's ambulatory status can be reevaluated and ambulatory privileges reinstated, if appropriate. Weak patients must not be allowed to ambulate unassisted. Cervical spine lesions are immobilized with a cervical collar.[91] Other braces or corsets may be used with noncervical lesions in the management of SCC. Braces provide stability and support to the spine.[90]

Pain management is critical in allowing patients to undergo and tolerate simulation and radiation treatment planning for treatment of SCC. Good pain management eases the promotion of ambulation, if appropriate, performance of activities of daily living, and participation in physical therapy for conditioning and strengthening. Pain management also improves QOL. The nurse must document the location and severity of pain and any precipitating and alleviating factors and reassess pain at least once a shift or more often as needed.

Ongoing neurologic assessment is essential. The baseline neurologic assessment is done at the first indication of SCC. Repeat assessments are performed at least every 8 hours and more often if the patient is experiencing a change in neurologic functioning. The assessment includes sensory and motor function (e.g., strength, sphincter function, and gait and stability, if appropriate). If the SCC is above C5, respiratory assessments are also necessary.[91]

SCC significantly impacts on the patient's QOL. The nurse should encourage the patient to verbalize his fears and concerns. The nurse should also provide supportive education and promote independence as appropriate for the individual. Social services or a psychiatric clinical nurse specialist should be consulted for counseling and support. Helping the patient with SCC to cope is a major component of the nurse's role and needs to be a priority when the nurse is planning to meet the needs of the patient.[92] (See Table 14-8 for a nursing care standard.)

TABLE 14-8. Nursing Care Standard for Patients With SCC

NURSING DIAGNOSIS: *Knowledge deficit regarding the etiology and treatment of SCC*
DESIRED PATIENT OUTCOME: Pt will verbalize understanding of the etiology, diagnosis, and treatment of SCC. Pt immediately will notify the physician of any symptoms of SCC.
NURSING INTERVENTIONS:
  1. Assess pt-SO understanding of etiology, diagnosis, and treatment of SCC.
  2. Educate pt-SO about cause, diagnostic workup, treatment goals, and treatment of SCC.
  3. Educate high-risk patients (e.g., with myeloma, sarcoma, prostate cancer, breast cancer, lymphoma, lung cancer) about s-s of SCC and need for prompt medical intervention.
     • Back pain (early sign)
     • Pain produced by percussion over spine
     • Pain radiating from back along dermatome to chest, abdomen, groin, legs, or buttock
     • Change in motor functioning and ability to walk
     • Decreased sensation in extremities
     • Loss of muscle tone
     • Constipation
     • Urinary retention
     • Loss of bowel-bladder continence (late sign)

DESIRED PATIENT OUTCOME: Pt-SO will verbalize understanding of methods used to prevent pressure sores, maintain bowel-bladder continence, prevent injury, reduce steroid-related side effects, and perform self-care management to reduce other therapy-related side effects.
NURSING INTERVENTIONS:
  1. Educate pt-SO about self-care management of SCC-related complications and treatment-related side effects.
     • Radiation therapy—skin care (with high doses of radiation), bone marrow depression, diarrhea (L-spine), esophagitis (cervical, thoracic spine), nausea
     • Pressure sores and their prevention
     • Bowel-bladder continence regimen
     • Safety
     • Weakness-fatigue; rest intervals between periods of activity; afternoon naps
     • Care of bowel-bladder continence devices and use of appropriate medications and procedures
     • Surgery: routine pre- and postop care (e.g., pulmonary hygiene, pain management, log rolling) and possible complications (e.g., infection, bleeding, pneumonia, deep vein thrombosis)
     • Steroids: take with food or antacids; monitor for s-s of side effects.

NURSING DIAGNOSIS: *Impaired physical mobility related to SCC*
DESIRED PATIENT OUTCOME: Pt will be free from further deterioration of motor or sensory function.
NURSING INTERVENTIONS:
  1. Assess pt's neurologic status, sensory perception, ability to walk or bear weight on legs, and ability to move around in bed and from side to side.
  2. Document neurologic status every shift or as prescribed; may be as frequent as every 2 h for first 3 days; continued until stable and then as needed. Notify physician of changes in patient's neurologic status.
  3. Consult physical therapy personnel to initiate rehabilitation program as soon as medical condition stabilizes.
  4. Encourage pt to change position at least every 2 h, if appropriate.
  5. Perform range-of-motion exercises on affected extremities; encourage pt to practice exercises, as prescribed by physical therapist, while listening to radio or watching television.
  6. Consult occupational therapist to initiate program for assisting pt in resuming independent activities of daily living.
  7. Consider pt's spine to be unstable until diagnostic studies are completed and pt is allowed out of bed.
  8. Have pt use brace when out of bed to stabilize spine.
  9. Have patient with a cervical lesion wear cervical collar at all times; avoid turning neck and neck rotation.
 10. Use footdrop protection devices.

NURSING DIAGNOSIS: *High risk for impaired skin integrity related to altered bowel or urinary elimination or impaired immobility*

(Continued on next page)

TABLE 14-8. Continued

DESIRED PATIENT OUTCOME: Pt will be free from pressure sores. Pt will have a bowel movement only after administration of suppository. Pt will not become constipated or experience impaction. Pt will be continent of bowel all other times. Pt will not experience bladder incontinence.

NURSING INTERVENTIONS:
1. Assess integrity of skin every shift and as needed; pay particular attention to skin under braces and cervical collar.
2. Assess bowel-bladder continence, abdominal-bladder distend, and bowel sounds.
3. Turn pt on routine schedule; use over-bed trapeze to allow for use of upper motor muscles; use special mattress to reduce risk of pressure sores, if appropriate.
4. Initiate bowel training regimen if pt is incontinent of bowel; give stool softener daily; start bisacodyl suppository M-W-F in morning after breakfast. If pt is constipated, begin routine laxatives and stool softeners at bedtime. Titrate dose to achieve goal of easy bowel movement every other day.
5. If pt experiences urinary incontinence, apply condom catheter (male) or insert Foley-type catheter (female). If pt experiences urinary retention, insert Foley-type catheter or initiate program of intermittent straight catheterization.
6. Encourage intake of oral fluids (for pts on intermittent straight catheterization regimens; hold fluids after 8 PM)
7. Monitor pt for signs of paralytic ileus and impaction.
8. Encourage high-fiber diet and consumption of prunes, prune juice, and large volumes of fluids (3 L/day).

NURSING DIAGNOSIS: *High risk for infection related to surgical wound*

DESIRED PATIENT OUTCOME: Pt's incision will be clean and intact. Pt's wounds will heal promptly. Pt will be free from wound infection.

NURSING INTERVENTIONS:
1. Assess wound for signs of infection daily.
2. Assess wound for delayed healing or dehiscence resulting from radiation therapy (radiation part usually will include most of wound.)
3. Change dressing at least daily.
4. Monitor pt for cerebrospinal fluid leak and signs of meningitis.
5. Take vital signs every 4 h for 24 h and then every shift and as needed.
6. Culture wound if signs of infection are present.
7. Encourage high-protein, high-calorie diet.

NURSING DIAGNOSIS: *Pain related to tumor growth*

DESIRED PATIENT OUTCOME: Pt will experience minimal pain.

NURSING INTERVENTIONS:
1. Assess quantity and quality of pain, and reassess at least every shift.
2. Administer narcotics with NSAIDs, if appropriate, on a routine and PRN basis.
3. Consult with physician if pt is receiving inadequate analgesia from prescribed medication(s).
4. Administer dexamethasone, as prescribed.
5. Turn pt using log-rolling technique.
6. Keep pt's body in proper alignment.
7. Encourage use of relaxation, imagery, and diversional activity.
8. Premedicate before radiation therapy treatments and before other painful activities.

NURSING DIAGNOSIS: *High risk for ineffective breathing pattern related to general anesthesia or to high cervical spine lesions*

DESIRED PATIENT OUTCOME: Pt will maintain normal breathing pattern.

NURSING INTERVENTIONS:
1. Assess respiration (including rate and depth), cough, presence of rales or wheezing at least daily.
2. Encourage pt to cough, deep breathe, and move around in bed every hour.
3. Get pt out of bed every shift, if not contraindicated by medical condition or unstable spine.
4. Monitor for systemic signs and symptoms of infection; culture sputum, if appropriate, and notify physician.
5. Suction as needed.
6. Take routine postoperative vital signs.
7. Consult respiratory therapy personnel for chest physical therapy and incentive spirometry.

NURSING DIAGNOSIS: *High risk for altered peripheral circulation related to deep vein thrombosis*
DESIRED PATIENT OUTCOME: Pt will be free from deep vein thrombosis.
NURSING INTERVENTIONS:
1. Assess pt for presence of Homans' sign, calf pain, tenderness, redness, and edema at least once a shift and before performing range-of-motion exercises.
2. Perform range-of-motion exercises with morning and evening care and with turning.
3. Notify physician of presence of signs and symptoms of deep vein thrombosis.
4. Apply antiembolic stockings or intermittent compression boots as prescribed.

NURSING DIAGNOSIS: *High risk for injury related to sensory and motor deficits*
DESIRED PATIENT OUTCOME: Pt will be free from injury.
NURSING INTERVENTIONS:
1. Assess pt for loss of pain and temperature sensation and for sensory deficits, paresthesias, impaired motor status (gait, coordination, range of motion), and impaired ability to perform activities of daily living.
2. Assess pt's environment for hazards that obstruct mobility (e.g., furniture obstructing pathways, loose objects, wet spots on floor).
3. Protect pt from thermal and other types of injury.
4. Keep pt on bed rest if spine is unstable.
5. Keep cervical collar intact if pt has cervical lesion.
6. Have pt use brace when out of bed.
7. Log roll to avoid twisting spine.
8. Avoid stress or pressure to bones at risk of fracture.
9. Use towels, pillows, and blankets to position pt every 2 hours.
10. Keep head of postop pt's bed at 30° angle.
11. Keep side rails elevated and call bell light and personal items in reach.

NURSING DIAGNOSIS: *High risk for ineffective coping related to living with the risk of an oncologic emergency and with anxiety, depression, residual disability, loss of control, or threat of loss of life*
DESIRED PATIENT OUTCOME: Pt will be helped to adapt to diagnosis of SCC, its accompanying self-care deficits, and potential loss of life.
NURSING INTERVENTIONS:
1. Assess pt's type and level of altered coping.
2. Include family-SO in assessment, planning, and implementation of care plan.
3. Assist pt in developing realistic and achievable short-term goals.
4. Offer support and active listening.
5. Consult with oncology social worker to assist with counseling and discharge planning and referrals to hospice, visiting nurse, or rehabilitation center.
6. Consult with psychiatry or psychiatric liaison nurse, if appropriate.
7. Consider use of antianxiety or antidepressant medications PRN.

NURSING DIAGNOSIS: *High risk for altered sexuality patterns related to motor deficits, psychological distress, or family disruption.*
DESIRED PATIENT OUTCOME: Pt will be helped to adapt to altered sexuality.
NURSING INTERVENTIONS:
1. Assess importance of sexual activity to pt's quality of life.
2. Assess changes in sexual function caused by SCC and cancer diagnosis.
3. Educate pt about relationship between SCC and altered sexual functioning.
4. Discuss intimacy concerns and alternate forms of sexual expression (e.g., holding, touching, kissing, cuddling).
5. Consult with or refer to sexual rehabilitation counselor, if appropriate.

Based on information from Baldwin, 1983; Carnevali and Reiner, 1990; Chernecky et al, 1984; Couillard-Getreuer, 1985; Dietz and Flaherty, 1990; Dyck, 1991; Gentzsch, 1991; Raney, 1991; Synder, 1986. Adapted from Held JL and Peahota A. Nursing care of the patient with spinal cord compression. *Oncology Nursing Forum* 1993;20(10):1507–1516. Used with permission.

SCC, spinal cord compression; pt, patient; SO, significant other; s-s, signs-symptoms; preop, preoperative; postop, postoperative; M-W-F, Monday-Wednesday-Friday; NSAIDs, nonsteroidal antiinflammatory drugs; PRN, as occasion requires.

CONCLUSION

The nursing care of patients with advanced prostate cancer is challenging and rewarding. Helping the patient to adapt and adjust to the symptoms produced by advanced disease allows the nurse to use many nursing skills and interventions based on a thorough nursing assessment. Some of the problems associated with advanced disease include pain, SCC, leg edema, DVT, scrotal edema, lymphedema, and DIC. More than one complication may occur simultaneously, such as pain and SCC, and compounds the complexity of patient care. Prompt assessment and management of each problem will enhance the patient's QOL.

REFERENCES

1. Hirshberg SJ, Greenberg RE. Urologic issues of palliative care. In: Berger A, Portenoy RK, Weissman DE (eds.) *Principles and Practice of Supportive Oncology*. Philadelphia: Lippincott-Raven, 1998: 371–383.
2. Weber-Jones JE. Performing clean intermittent self-catheterization. *Nursing '91*. 1991;21(8):56–59.
3. Black JM, Matassarin-Jacobs E. *Medical-Surgical Nursing: Clinical Management for Continuity of Care,* 5th ed. Philadelphia: WB Saunders, 1997: 1377–1386, 1397–1443, 1447–1579, 2343–2385.
4. Parker KP, Berding C. Nursing assessment and common urinary interventions. In: Burrell LO, Gerlach MJM, Pless BS (eds). *Adult Nursing: Acute and Community Care,* 2nd ed. Stamford, CT: Appleton & Lange, 1997:1198–1238.
5. Surya BV, Provent JA. Manifestations of advanced prostate cancer: Prognosis and treatment. *J Urol* 1989;142:921–928.
6. Wells P, Hoskin PJ, Towler J, et al. The effect of radiotherapy on ureteral obstruction from carcinoma of the prostate. *Br J Urol* 1996;78:752–755.
7. Gottfried HW, Gnann R, Brandle E, et al. Treatment of high-risk patients with subvesical obstruction from advanced prostate cancer using a thermosensitive mesh stent. *Br J Urol* 1997;80:623–627.
8. Yachia D, Aridogan IA. The use of a removable stent in patients with prostate cancer and obstruction. *J Urol* 1996;155:1956–1958.
9. Guazzoni G, Montorsi F, Beramaschi F, et al. Prostatic urolume wallstent for urinary retention due to advanced prostate cancer: A 1-year follow up study. *J Urol* 1994;152:1530–1532.
10. Saitoh H, Yoshida K, Uchijima Y, et al. Two different lymph node metastatic patterns of a prostatic cancer. *Cancer* 1990;65:1843–1846.
11. O'Reilly PH. The effect of prostatic obstruction on the upper urinary tract. In: Fitzpatrick JM, Krane RJ (eds). *The Prostate*. Edinburgh: Churchill Livingstone, 1989:111–118.
12. Lopez-Martinez RA, Singireddy S, Lang EK. The use of metallic stents to bypass ureteral stricture secondary to metastatic prostate cancer: Experience with 8 patients. *J Urol* 1997;158:50–53.
13. Paul AB, Love C, Chrisolm GD. The management of bilateral ureteric obstruction and renal failure in advanced prostate cancer. *Br J Urol* 1994;74:642–645.
14. Hamdy FC, Williams JL. Use of dexamethasone for ureteric obstruction in advanced prostate cancer: Percutaneous nephrostomies can be avoided. *Br J Urol* 1995;75:782–785.
15. Parke KP. Disorders of the kidneys. In: Burrell LO, Gerlach MJM, Pless BS (eds). *Adult Nursing: Acute and Community Care,* 2nd ed. Stamford, CT: Appleton & Lange, 1997:1239–1290.
16. Humble CA. Lymphedema: Incidence, pathophysiology, management and nursing care. *Oncol Nurs Forum* 1995;22:1503–1509.
17. Ruschhaupt WF III. The swollen limb. In: Young JR, Graor RA, Olin JW, Bartholomew JR (eds). *Peripheral Vascular Diseases*. St. Louis, MO: Mosby-Yearbook, 1991:639–650.
18. Ciocon J, Fernandez B, Ciocon DG. Leg edema: Clinical clues to the differential diagnosis. *Geriatrics* 1993;48(5);34–45.

19. Galindo-Ciocon D. Nursing care of elders with leg edema. *J Gerontol Nurs* 1995;21(7):7–11.

20. Creager MA, Dzau VJ. Vascular diseases of the extremities. In: Fauci AS, Braunwald E, Isselbacher KJ, et al (eds). *Harrison's Principles of Internal Medicine,* 14th ed. New York: McGraw-Hill, 1998: 1389–1406.

21. Pappas CJ, O'Donell TF. Long term results of compression treatment for lymphedema. *J Vasc Surg* 1992; 16:555–564.

22. Farncombe ML. Lymphedema. In: Berger A, Portenoy RK, Weissman DE (eds). *Principles and Practice of Supportive Oncology.* Philadelphia: Lippincott-Raven, 1998:275–283.

23. Lechner DL. Sizing up your patients for heparin therapy. *Nursing '98* 1998;28(8):36–41.

24. Levine M, Gent M, Hirsh J, et al. A comparison of low-molecular-weight heparin administration primarily at home with unfractionated heparin administered in the hospital for proximal deep vein thrombosis. *N Engl J Med* 1996;334:677–681.

25. Simko LC, Lockhart JS. Heparin-induced thrombocytopenia and thrombosis. *Nursing '96* 1996;26 (3):33.

26. Elzer R, Houdek DL. Case managing heparin-induced thrombocytopenia. *Clin Nurse Spec* 1998; 12:238–243.

27. Majoros KA, Moccia, JM. Pulmonary embolus. *Nursing '96* 1996;26(4):27–31.

28. Smith JK. Oncology nursing in lymphedema management. *Innov Breast Cancer Care* 1998;3:82–87.

29. Rymal C. Compression modalities in lymphedema therapy. *Innov Breast Cancer Care* 1998;3:88–92.

30. Hardy JR. Lymphedema—prevention rather than cure. *Ann Oncol* 1991;2:532–533.

31. Casley-Smith JR, Morgan RG, Piller NB. Treatment of lymphedema of the arms and legs with 5,6-benzo-[α]-pyrone. *N Engl J Med* 1993;329:1158–1163.

32. Schafer SL. Oncologic complications. In: Otto SE (ed). *Oncology Nursing* (3rd ed.). St. Louis, MO: Mosby Year-Book, 1997:406–474.

33. Murphy-Ende K. Disseminated intravascular coagulation. In: Chernecky CC, Berger BJ (eds). *Advanced and Critical Care Oncology Nursing.* Philadelphia: WB Saunders, 1998:119–139.

34. Gobel BH. Bleeding disorders. In: Groenwald SL, Frogge MH, Goodman M, Yarbro CH (eds). *Cancer Nursing: Principles and Practice,* 4th ed. Sudbury, MA: Jones and Bartlett, 1997:604–639.

35. Nakashima J, Tachibana M, Veno M, et al. Tumor necrosis factor and coagulopathy in patients with prostate cancer. *Cancer Res* 1995;55:4881–4885.

36. Finley JP. Disseminated intravascular coagulation (DIC). In: Ziegfeld CR, Lubejko BG, Shelton BK (eds). *Oncology Fact Finder: Manual of Cancer Nursing.* Philadelphia: Lippincott-Raven, 1998:436–440.

37. Shuey KM. Platelet associated bleeding disorders. *Semin Oncol Nurs* 1996;12:15–27.

38. Luckmann J (ed). *Saunders Manual of Nursing Care.* Philadelphia: WB Saunders, 1997:1167–1168.

39. Thompson JM, McFarland GK, Hirsch JE, Tucker, SM. *Mosby's Clinical Nursing.* St. Louis, MO: Mosby-Year Book, 1997:1268–1270.

40. Bick RL. Disseminated intravascular coagulation. *Med Clin North Am* 1994;78:511–543.

41. Payne R. Pain management in the patient with prostate cancer. *Cancer* 1993;71:1131–1137.

42. Esper PS, Pienta, KJ. Supportive care in the patient with hormone refractory prostate cancer. *Semin Urol Oncol* 1997;15:56–64.

43. Mundy GR. Mechanisms of bone metastases. *Cancer* 1997;80:1546–1556.

44. Goltzman D. Mechanisms of the development of osteoblastic metastases. *Cancer* 1997;80:1581–1587.

45. Payne R. Mechanisms and management of bone pain. *Cancer* 1997;80:1608–1613.

46. Fulfaro F, Casuccio A, Ticozzi C, Ripamonti C. The role of bisphosphonates in the treatment of painful metastatic bone disease: A review of phase III trials. *Pain* 1998;78:157–169.

47. Coleman RE. Skeletal complications of malignancy. *Cancer* 1997;80:1588–1594.

48. Taub M, Begas A, Love, N. Advanced prostate cancer: Endocrine therapies and palliative measures. *Postgrad Med* 1996;100:139–154.

49. Eisenberg E, Berkey CS, Carr DB, et al. Efficacy and safety of nonsteroidal antiinflammatory drugs for cancer pain: A meta-analysis. *J Clin Oncol* 1994; 12:2756–2765.

50. World Health Organization. *Cancer Pain Relief.* Geneva, Switzerland: World Health Organization, 1986.

51. World Health Organization Expert Committee. *Cancer Pain Relief and Palliative Care.* Geneva, Switzerland: World Health Organization, 1992.

52. McCaffery M, Portenoy RK. Nonopioids: Acetaminophen and nonsteroidal antiinflammatory drugs (NSAIDs). In: McCaffery M, Pasero C (eds).

Pain: Clinical Manual, 2nd ed. St. Louis, MO: CV Mosby, 1999:129–160.

53. Cherney NI, Foley KM. Management of pain associated with prostate cancer. In: Raghavan D, Leibel SA, Scher HI, Lange P (eds). *Principles and Practice of Genitourinary Oncology.* Philadelphia: Lippincott-Raven, 1997:613–627.

54. Coyle N, Cherny N, Portenoy RK. Pharmacologic management of cancer pain. In: McGuire D, Yarbro C, Ferrell BR (eds). *Cancer Pain Management,* 2nd ed. Sudbury, MA: Jones and Bartlett, 1995:89–130.

55. Campora E, Merlini L, Pace M, et al. The incidence of narcotic induced emesis. *J Pain Symptom Manage* 1991;6:428–430

56. Healey JH. Metastatic cancer to the bone. In: DeVita V, Hellman S, Rosenberg SA (eds). *Cancer: Principles and Practice of Oncology,* 5th ed. Philadelphia: Lippincott-Raven, 1996:2570–2586.

57. Catton CN, Gospodarowicz MK. Palliative radiotherapy in prostate cancer. *Semin Urol Oncol* 1997; 15:65–72.

58. Porter AT, Fontanesi, J. Palliative irradiation for bone metastases: A new paradigm [editorial]. *Int J Radiat Oncol Biol Phys* 1994;29:1199–1200.

59. Blitzer PH. Reanalysis of the RTOG study of the palliation of symptomatic osseous metastases. *Cancer* 1985;55:1468–1472.

60. Gaze MN, Kelly CG, Kerr GR, et al. Pain relief and quality of life following radiotherapy for bone metastases: A randomised trial of 2 fraction schedules. *Radiother Oncol* 1997;45:109–116.

61. Altman GB, Lee CA. Strontium-89 for treatment of painful bone metastases from prostate cancer. *Oncol Nurs Forum* 1996;23:523–527.

62. Mertens WC, Filipczak LA, Ben-Josef E, et al. Systemic bone-seeking radionuclides for palliation of painful osseous metastases: Current concepts. *CA Ca J Clin* 1988;48:361–374.

63. Robinson RG, Preston DF, Schiefelbein M, Baxter KG. Strontium-89 therapy for the palliation of pain due to osseous metastases. *JAMA* 1995;274: 420–424.

64. Patel BR, Flowers, WM. Systemic radionuclide therapy with strontium chloride Sr89 for painful skeletal metastases in prostate and breast cancer. *So Med J* 1997;90:506–508.

65. Serafini AN, Houston SJ, Resche I, et al. Palliation of pain associated with metastatic bone cancer using samarium-153 lexidronam: A double-blind placebo-controlled clinical trial. *J Clin Oncol* 1998; 16:1574–1581.

66. Adami S. Bisphosphonates in prostate carcinoma. *Cancer* 1997;80:1674–1679.

67. Body JJ, Bartl R, Burckhardt P, et al. Current use of bisphosphonates in oncology. *J Clin Oncol* 1998;12: 3890–3899.

68. Ernst SD, MacDonald N, Paterson AHG, et al. A double blind crossover trial of intravenous clodronate in metastatic bone pain. *J Pain Symptom Manage* 1992;7:4–11.

69. Robertson AG, Reed NS, Ralston SH. Effect of oral clodronate on metastatic bone pain: A double blind, placebo controlled study. *J Clin Oncol* 1995; 13:2427–2430.

70. Coleman RE, Purohit OP, Vinholes JJ, Zekri J. High dose pamidronate: Clinical and biochemical effects in metastatic bone disease. *Cancer* 1997;80: 1686–1690.

71. Iwamoto R. Men and pain. *Dev Supportive Cancer Care* 1997;1:66–68.

72. Forest P. The use of a pain diary in patients with advanced cancer of the prostate. *Urologic Nursing* 1993;13:17–19.

73. Mayer DK, Struthers C, Fisher G. Bone metastases: Part II: Nursing management. *Clin J Oncol Nurs* 1997;1:37–44.

74. Pasero C, Portenoy RK, McCaffery M. Opioid analgesics. In: McCaffery M, Pasero C. *Pain: Clinical Manual,* 2nd ed. St. Louis, MO: CV Mosby:1999, 161–299.

75. Struthers C, Mayer D, Fisher G. Nursing management of the patient with bone metastases. *Semin Oncol Nurs* 1998;14:199–209.

76. Osborn JL, Getzenberg RH, Trump DL. Spinal cord compression in prostate cancer. *J Neurol Oncol* 1995;23:135–147.

77. Rosenthal MA, Raghavan RD, Leicester J, et al. Spinal cord compression in prostate cancer. A 10-year experience. *Br J Urol* 1992;69:530–533.

78. Grossman SA, Lossignol D. Diagnosis and treatment of epidural metastases. *Oncology* 1990;4(4): 47–52.

79. Wilkes GM. Neurological disturbances. In: Groenwald SL, Frogge MH, Goodman M, Yarbro CH (eds). *Cancer Symptom Management.* Sudbury, MA: Jones and Bartlett, 1996:324–355.

80. Weinstein SM. Management of spinal neoplasm and its complications. In: Berger A, Portenoy RK,

Weissman, DE (eds). *Principles and Practice of Supportive Oncology.* Philadelphia: Lippincott-Raven, 1998:449–475.

81. Loblaw DA, Laperrier NJ. Emergent treatment of malignant extradural spinal cord compression: An evidence-based guide. *J Clin Oncol* 1998;16:1613–1624.

82. Huddart RA, Rajan B, Law M, et al. Spinal cord compression in prostate cancer: Treatment outcome and prognostic factors. *Radiother Oncol* 1997;44:229–236.

83. Byrne TN. Spinal cord compression from epidural metastases. *N Engl J Med* 1992;327:614–619.

84. Kim RY, Smith JW, Spencer SA, et al. Malignant epidural spinal cord compression associated with paravertebral mass: Its radiotherapeutic outcome on radiosensitivity. *Int J Radiat Oncol Biol Phys* 1993;27:1079–1083.

85. Sorensen S, Helweg-Larsen S, Mouridsen H, et al. Effect of high-dose dexamethasone in carcinomatous metastatic spinal cord compression treated with radiotherapy: A randomised trial. *Eur J Cancer* 1994;1:22–27.

86. Maranzano E, Latini P, Beneventi S, et al. Radiotherapy without steroids in selected metastatic spinal cord compression patients. A phase II trial. *Am J Clin Oncol* 1996;19:179–183.

87. Smith EM, Hampel N, Ruff RL, et al. Spinal cord compression secondary to prostate carcinoma: Treatment and prognosis. *J Urol* 1993;149:330–333.

88. Maranzano E, Latini P. Effectiveness of radiation therapy without surgery in metastatic spinal cord compression: Final results from a prospective trial. *Int J Radiat Oncol Biol Phys* 1995;32:959–967.

89. Faul CM, Flickinger JC. The use of radiation in the management of spinal metastases. *J Neurol Oncol* 1995;23:149–161.

90. Welch WC, Jacobs GB. Surgery for metastatic spinal disease. *J Neurol Oncol* 1995;23:163–170.

91. Sitton E. Central nervous system metastases. *Semin Oncol Nurs* 1998;14:210–219.

92. Held JL, Peahota A. Nursing care of the patient with spinal cord compression. *Oncol Nurs Forum* 1993;20:1507–1516.

93. Papanicolaou N. Urinary tract imaging and intervention: Basic principles. In: Walsh PC, Retik AS, Vaughan ED Jr, Wein AJ (eds). *Campbell's Urology,* 7th ed. Philadelphia: WB Saunders, 1998:170–260.

94. Baldwin P. Epidural spinal cord compression secondary to metastatic disease: A review of the literature. *Cancer Nurs* 1983;6:441–446.

95. Carnevali D, Reiner A. *The cancer experience: Nursing diagnosis and management.* Philadelphia: Lippincott, 1990.

96. Chernecky C, Ramsey P, Klein P. *Critical nursing care of the client with cancer.* Norwalk, CT: Appleton-Century-Crofts, 1984.

97. Couillard-Getreuer D. Spinal cord compression. In: Johnson B, Gross J (eds), *Handbook of oncology nursing.* New York: John Wiley and Sons, 1985:412–429.

98. Dietz K, Flaherty A. Oncologic emergencies. In: Groenwald S, Frogge M, Goodman M, Yarbro C (eds). *Cancer nursing: Principles and practice,* 2nd ed. Sudbury, MA: Jones and Bartlett, 1990:662–665.

99. Dyck S. Surgical instrumentation as a palliative treatment for spinal cord compression. *Oncol Nurs Forum* 1991;18:515–521.

100. Gentzsch P. Mobility, impaired physical, related to spinal cord compression. In: McNally J, Somerville E, Miaskowski C, Rostad M (eds), *Guidelines for oncology nursing practice,* 2nd ed. Philadelphia: WB Saunders 1991:267–272.

101. Raney D. Malignant spinal cord tumors: A review and case presentation. *J Neurosci Nurs* 1991;23:44–49.

102. Snyder C. *Oncology nursing.* Boston: Little, Brown and Company, 1986.

Chapter 15

PROSTATE CANCER RESOURCES FOR PATIENTS, FAMILIES, AND PROFESSIONALS

CAROL BLECHER

OVERVIEW

EARLY DETECTION AND SCREENING
  INFORMATION

INFORMATION REGARDING PROSTATE
  CANCER DIAGNOSIS AND TREATMENT
  OPTIONS

MATERIALS DEALING WITH ADVANCED
  PROSTATE CANCER

PSYCHOSOCIAL AND SUPPORT RESOURCES

AUDIOVISUAL MATERIALS

RESOURCES FOR PROSTATE CANCER
  INFORMATION

BOOKS REGARDING PROSTATE CANCER

PERSONAL ACCOUNTS

WORLDWIDE WEB RESOURCES

This chapter has been designed to present a variety of resources available for use by patients, families, and professionals. It is not an exhaustive listing but presents an initial set of options, available through a variety of sources. Some of the materials are obtainable free of charge, whereas others vary in cost anywhere from $4 to several hundred. All of the resources presented in this chapter have been reviewed for content and readability.

EARLY DETECTION AND SCREENING INFORMATION

An important patient education issue in prostate cancer is early detection and screening information. A large amount of material is available on this topic. The information may be presented to patients as health promotion behaviors in primary physician, urologist, and oncologist offices. Resources are included in Table 15-1.

TABLE 15-1. Early Detection and Screening

TITLE: *Real Men Get It Checked*[1]
SOURCE: American Cancer Society
CONTENT:

- Self-test
- Statistics
- Anatomy and physiology of prostate
- Testing
- Overview of prostate cancer
- Support services
- Signs and symptoms of prostate cancer
- Treatment options

CHARGE: Free

TITLE: *American Cancer Society's New Guidelines for the Early Detection of Prostate Cancer*[2]
SOURCE: American Cancer Society
CONTENT:

- 1997 Updated guidelines for screening and early detection

CHARGE: Free

TITLE: *The PSA Blood Test and Prostate Cancer*[3]
SOURCE: American Cancer Society
CONTENT:

- Information about the prostate
- Testing once PSA is elevated
- PSA testing and its meaning
- Screening recommendations

CHARGE: Free

TITLE: *Understanding Prostate Changes: A Health Guide for All Men*[4]
SOURCE: National Institutes of Health, National Cancer Institute
CONTENT:

- Rationale for publication
- Listing of prostate problems
- Review of tests involved in prostate screening
- Prostate cancer, risk factors, symptoms, early detection, screening, diagnostic workup, questions to ask the physician
- Glossary
- Anatomy and physiology of prostate
- Review of prostate problems and potential treatment, including prostatitis and BPH
- Prostate cancer prevention trials information
- References
- Resource listing

CHARGE: Free

TITLE: *For Women Who Care: Information on Prostate Disease to Share With the Men in Your Life*[5]
SOURCE: American Foundation for Urologic Disease
CONTENT:

- Quiz on prostate disease with answers
- Prostate facts
- Risk groups
- BPH
- Prostate cancer
- Why address women
- Rationale for concern about prostate disease
- Physical exam of prostate
- Prostatitis
- Glossary of medical terminology

CHARGE: Free

TITLE: *Prostate Health, Screening for Prostate Cancer*[6]
SOURCE: Krames Communication
CONTENT:

- Basic facts re prostate cancer and the need for screening
- Additional diagnostic tests after positive initial evaluation
- Myths surrounding prostate cancer
- Anatomy and physiology of the prostate
- Description of screening visit and examination
- Importance of continued screening
- Healthy lifestyle information

CHARGE: Contact Krames Communication, 1-800-333-3032

TITLE: *Treating Prostate Problems: Options for Improving Your Health*[7] (available in both English and Spanish)
SOURCE: Krames Communication

(Continued on next page)

CONTENT:

- Facts re prostate conditions
- Diagnosis of problems, history, exam, and testing
- Further workup and development of treatment plan

- Explanation of common prostate problems
- Symptom checklist
- Treatment of BPH
- Good health practice review

CHARGE: Contact Krames Communication, 1-800-333-3032

PSA, prostate-specific antigen; BPH, benign prostatic hypertrophy; re, regarding.

INFORMATION REGARDING PROSTATE CANCER DIAGNOSIS AND TREATMENT OPTIONS

Once the diagnosis of prostate cancer has been made, the patient needs to be presented with information on treatment options, risks, and benefits of each option, as well as all potential side effects associated with each form of treatment. This information is generally provided in the urologist's and oncologist's offices. The nurses in these practice settings should provide the patient with information on an as-needed basis. The nurse needs to be available to discuss information with the patient and family as well as answer questions and provide guidance. These nurses are vital to the patient and family in their effort to understand the diagnosis and treatment options.

An enormous variety of resources are available to assist in providing education related to prostate cancer and its treatment options, as well as information that is drug or program specific. Included in Table 15-2 is a sampling of available resources.

TABLE 15-2. Information on Treatment Options

TITLE: *Cancer Treatments Your Insurance Should Cover*[8]
SOURCE: Association of Community Cancer Centers, cosponsored by Oncology Nursing Society and National Coalition for Cancer Survivorship
CONTENT:

- Why insurance companies deny payment
- Action steps for obtaining coverage
- Resources—ACCC

- Actions to take when payment is denied
- Minimum standards for cancer benefits in insurance policies

CHARGE: Free

TITLE: *Cancer Facts and Figures—1998*[9]
SOURCE: American Cancer Society

- Early detection
- Education-support services
- Sexuality issues

- Psychsocial issues
- Treatment options

CHARGE: Free

TITLE: *Prostate Cancer 1998 Fact Sheet*[10]
SOURCE: American Cancer Society
CONTENT:

- Incidence
- Risk factors
- Treatment options
- Listing of ACS local service centers, including addresses and telephone numbers

- Signs and symptoms of disease
- Early detection
- Survival statistics
- ACS education-psychosocial support programs

CHARGE: Free

TITLE: *For Men Only: What You Should Know About Prostate Cancer*[11]
SOURCE: American Cancer Society
CONTENT:
- Question and answer format
- Incidence
- Detection
- Survival
- Anatomy and physiology of the prostate
- Symptoms
- Treatment options

CHARGE: Free

TITLE: *Facts on Prostate Cancer in African Americans*[12]
SOURCE: American Cancer Society
CONTENT:
- Description of prostate
- Prevention-early detection
- Incidence in the African American population
- Signs and symptoms
- Treatment options
- Sources of additional information and a list of ACS publications and videotapes.
- Identification of African Americans as high-risk group
- Risk factors
- Diagnosis, staging-grading
- Survival statistics
- Prevention-early detection

CHARGE: Free

TITLE: *Prostate Cancer: Asking the Questions, Finding the Answers*[13]
SOURCE: American Cancer Society
CONTENT:
- Question and answer format
- Statistics
- Early detection
- Treatment options
- Prostate cancer information
- At-risk populations
- Warning signs
- Further research

CHARGE: Free

TITLE: *After Diagnosis: Prostate Cancer, Understanding Your Treatment Options*[14]
SOURCE: American Cancer Society
CONTENT:
- Diagnosis information
- Prostate cancer
- Diagnosis
- Grading-staging
- Clinical trials
- Recurrent disease
- Questions to ask the physician
- Resource listing
- Anatomy and physiology of prostate
- Risk factors
- Testing
- Treatment options with risks and benefits
- NCI's Cancer Information Service number
- Support services
- Glossary of medical terminology

CHARGE: Free

TITLE: *What to Do If Prostate Cancer Strikes: A Helpbook for Patients*[15]
SOURCE: American Cancer Society and Cancer Research Institute of NJ
CONTENT:
- Condensed version of prior publication with same information
- Identifies books, support groups, Internet Web sites

CHARGE: Free

TITLE: *Sexuality & Cancer: For the Man Who Has Cancer and His Partner*[16]
SOURCE: American Cancer Society
CONTENT:
- General information regarding sexuality during cancer treatment
- Does not focus specifically on prostate-related issues
- Resources for further information

CHARGE: Free

(Continued on next page)

TITLE: *Prostate Cancer and You*[17]
SOURCE: ICI Pharma/Zeneca Pharmaceuticals
CONTENT:
- Initial presentation for prostate cancer patients
- Anatomy and physiology of the prostate
- BPH versus cancer
- Symptoms
- Workup
- Treatment options with common side effects

- Contains a slide kit for use by the health care professional and a brochure of patient-family information
- Diagnosis
- Staging

CHARGE: Free

TITLE: *Prostate Cancer: What It Is and How It Is Treated*[18]
SOURCE: ICI Pharma/Zeneca Pharmaceuticals
CONTENT:
- General cancer information
- Diagnosis of prostate cancer
- Treatment options based on staging
- Coping strategies
- Definition of medical terms

- Prostate information
- Workup
- Risks and benefits
- Resources for information and support services

CHARGE: Free

TITLE: *El Cáncer Prostático: ¿Qué es y cómo se trata?*[19]
SOURCE: ICI Pharma/Zeneca Pharmaceuticals
CONTENT:
- Same as prior booklet presented for Spanish speaking population

CHARGE: Free

TITLE: *The Cancer Information Service*[20]
SOURCE: National Cancer Institute
CONTENT:
- Bookmark that provides CIS 800 number (1-800-4-CANCER)

- Overview of information provided by service
- English and Spanish

CHARGE: Free

TITLE: *What You Need to Know About Cancer*[21]
SOURCE: National Cancer Institute
CONTENT:
- General cancer information
- Early warning signs
- Treatment options
- Questions to ask your physician
- Clinical trials
- Health promotion habits
- Resource listing

- Screening guidelines
- Diagnosis, staging, and testing
- Second opinions
- Side effects of treatment
- Psychosocial support issues
- Glossary of medical terms

CHARGE: Free

TITLE: *What You Need to Know About Prostate Cancer*[22]
SOURCE: National Cancer Institute
CONTENT:
- Overview plus anatomy and physiology of prostate
- Symptoms
- Prognosis data
- Psychosocial support issues
- Glossary of medical terms

- Definition of cancer
- Diagnosis, staging, and testing
- Treatment options-side effects
- Need for lifetime follow-up
- Research in prostate cancer
- Resource list includes related NCI patient education material

CHARGE: Free

TITLE: *A Patient's Guide for the Treatment of Impotence*[23]
SOURCE: Obson Medical Systems
CONTENT:

- Defines impotence
- Explanation of the erectile process
- What to expect when consulting a physician
- Discussion of sex counseling and therapy
- Discussion of processes that might be used in selecting appropriate treatment option

- Explores the desire to resolve this issue
- Identification of causes of impotence
- Treatment options with risks, benefits, costs, and information regarding insurance coverage

CHARGE: Free

TITLE: *Male Impotence: A Woman's Perspective*[24]
SOURCE: Obson Medical Systems
CONTENT:

- Discusses erectile problems
- Case study presentation of effects of impotence on both partners
- Identification of behaviors and coping mechanisms

- Suggested actions to overcome obstacles
- Exploration of feelings, thoughts, and beliefs
- Review of medical diagnosis and treatment options

CHARGE: Free

TITLE: *Cancer Terms: A Guide for Your Patients With Cancer*[25]
SOURCE: Pharmacia Inc.
CONTENT:

- Terminology related to cancer and its diagnosis, staging, and treatment

CHARGE: Free

TITLE: *Tumor Markers: A Guide for Your Patients With Cancer*[26]
SOURCE: Pharmacia Inc.
CONTENT:

- What are tumor markers?
- Monitoring disease status

- Use in establishing prognosis
- Includes a chart for patient use in documenting following tumor marker

CHARGE: Free

TITLE: *It's the Most Common Cancer in Men: The Facts About Prostate Cancer*[27]
SOURCE: Schering Oncology Biotech
CONTENT:

- Prostate cancer statistics
- Benefits of early detection
- Signs and symptoms
- Staging and grading
- Information regarding support services with a focus on the Schering program

- At-risk population
- Basic information regarding prostate cancer
- Diagnostic workup
- Treatment options with potential side effects with a heavy emphasis on the use of Schering products

CHARGE: Free

TITLE: *Prostate Cancer: Some Good News Men Can Live With*[28]
SOURCE: Schering Oncology Biotech
CONTENT:

- Audience: men older than 40
- At-risk population
- Signs and symptoms of prostate cancer
- Treatment options-potential side effects
- Sources of information

- Myths regarding prostate cancer followed by factual information
- Screening, diagnosis, and staging
- Information regarding second opinions

CHARGE: Free

TITLE: *Living With Prostate Cancer*[29]
SOURCE: Krames Communication

(Continued on next page)

CONTENT:

- Concerns surrounding a diagnosis of cancer
- Diagnostic workup with grading and staging
- Treatments along with potential side effects, risk, and complications
- Health maintenance and follow-up discussed

- Prostate anatomy: normal and abnormal
- Treatment planning
- Psychosocial support services and information on finding these programs are presented

CHARGE: Contact Krames Communication, 1-800-333-3032

TITLE: *Questions and Answers About Zoladex (Goserelin AcetateImplant) Therapy for the Treatment of Prostate Cancer*[30]
SOURCE: ICI Pharma/Zeneca Pharmaceuticals
CONTENT:

- Questions and answers re Zoladex, its administration, function, risks, and benefits
- Psychosocial support and coping
- Where to obtain additional information

- Information regarding insurance coverage
- Comparison of hormonal therapies
- Definition of terms

CHARGE: Free

TITLE: *Words to Live By: The Information Resource for Prostate Cancer Patients*[31]
SOURCE: IMMUNEX
CONTENT:

- Grouping of four booklets covering various aspects of prostate cancer
- Definitions of medical terminology
- Area for patients to list members of the healthcare team and their phone numbers
- Risk factors
- Options for treatment of advanced disease
- Sexuality
- Chemotherapy as a treatment option with the focus on Novantrone (IMMUNEX Corporation, Seattle, WA 98101)

- Folder identifies informational sources and psychosocial support services
- Available resources
- Anatomy and physiology of the prostate
- Definition of cancer
- Staging-diagnostic workup
- Pain control
- Coping issues

CHARGE: Free

TITLE: *Living With Stage D2 Prostate Cancer and Eulexin (Flutamide) Therapy*[32]
SOURCE: Schering Oncology Biotech
CONTENT:

- Anatomy and physiology of the prostate
- At-risk population
- Review of hormonal treatment

- Prostate cancer
- Treatment options
- Questions and answers regarding Eulexin therapy

CHARGE: Free

ACCC, Association of Community Cancer Centers; ACS, American Cancer Society; NCI, National Cancer Institute; CIS, Cancer Information Service; BPH, benign prostatic hypertrophy; re, regarding.

MATERIALS DEALING WITH ADVANCED PROSTATE CANCER

Advanced prostate cancer carries with it an entire set of problems and issues. When the disease has progressed, the patient is generally seen in the oncologist's practice. Oncology nurses now deal with the patient who has advanced disease and a very unique set of educational needs. Educational needs include pain management and systemic treatments. Table 15-3 lists several resources that deal specifically with drugs used in treatment of advanced prostate cancer and managing the pain associated with advanced disease.

TABLE 15-3. Materials Dealing With Advanced Prostate Cancer

TITLE: *Why Your Doctor Has Prescribed Casodex for You: Important Information for Men With Advanced Prostate Cancer*[33]
SOURCE: ICI Pharma/Zeneca Pharmaceuticals
CONTENT:

- Question and answer format on use of Casodex
- Rationale for use of Casodex (bicalutamide)
- Information re administration, history of agent, drug interactions, and duration of treatment
- What is advanced prostate cancer?
- Identification of the drug and its actions
- Information re psychosocial issues and resources

CHARGE: Free

TITLE: *The EPIC Manual Empowered Patients in Control: A Guide to Pain Management in Advanced Prostate Cancer*[34]
SOURCE: IMMUNEX
CONTENT:

- Treatment information-options for disease and pain
- Coping with advanced disease and depression
- Resource listing with services provided and telephone numbers
- Information regarding hormone refractory prostate cancer
- Patient-family support and information resources
- Bibliography
- Glossary

CHARGE: Free

TITLE: *Treatment Options for Living Longer With Advanced Prostate Cancer*[35]
SOURCE: Schering Oncology Biotech
CONTENT:

- Prostate cancer
- Diagnosis of disease
- Data re flutamide (Eulexin) therapy
- References for support services
- Anatomy and physiology of the prostate
- Treatment options—all stages
- Reimbursement information

CHARGE: Free

TITLE: *The Only Antiandrogen Proven to Delay Progression in Advanced Prostate Cancer*[36]
SOURCE: Schering Oncology Biotech
Content:

- Rationale for castration plus antiandrogens discussed
- Medical versus surgical castration
- Antiandrogen drug comparison, rationale for selection of Schering product

CHARGE: Free

---

re, regarding.

PSYCHOSOCIAL AND SUPPORT RESOURCES

Much of the material listed in this chapter contains references to psychosocial issues and presents resources to be accessed in the area of psychosocial support. Psychosocial support is a vital issue in the care of the patient with cancer. Support has been identified as a major factor in reducing the stresses involved in coping with the diagnosis of cancer. This type of information may be available for distribution and discussion in both the urologist's and oncologist's offices. Table 15-4 presents resources that have been designed primarily to address psychosocial support issues.

TABLE 15-4. Psychosocial and Support Resources

TITLE: *Man to Man News: Prostate Cancer News and Information from the American Cancer Society's Man to Man Program*[37]
SOURCE: American Cancer Society
CONTENT:

- Prostate cancer information on line
- Pain management
- Question and answer column
- Metastasis and recurrence
- Other resources for the patient with prostate cancer
- Definitions of medical terminology

CHARGE: Free

TITLE: *Man to Man: Prostate Cancer Education and Support Program*[38]
SOURCE: American Cancer Society
CONTENT:

- Review of services, group education and support, one-to-one support, newsletters, and Web site.
- Program introduction

CHARGE: Free

TITLE: *US TOO Prostate Cancer Survivor Support Group*[39]
SOURCE: American Foundation for Urologic Disease
CONTENT:

- Has tear sheet with request for more information, contributions to the American Foundation for Urologic Disease, or information on beginning a support group or chapter
- What is US TOO?
- Why was it formed?
- Purpose of the organization
- Information regarding meetings

CHARGE: Free

TITLE: *Into the Light: A Guide for the Prostate Cancer Patient and Those Close to Him*[40]
SOURCE: ICI Pharma/Zeneca Pharmaceuticals
CONTENT:

- Brief description of prostate
- Treatment and side effects
- Resource listing
- Information on prostate cancer
- Primary focus on psychosocial support issues

CHARGE: Free

TITLE: *CareNection: Helping You Get the Most From Eulexin*[41]
SOURCE: Schering Oncology Biotech
CONTENT:

- Information regarding a research program developed by Schering
- Designed for patients receiving Eulexin (flutamide)
- Provides counseling, support, information, and monthly telephone contact
- Includes a consent form and application for participation in the program

CHARGE: Free; postage paid mailer required

AUDIOVISUAL MATERIALS

Audiovisual materials in the form of videotapes provide the patient with an alternative approach to patient education. These can be viewed either in the physician's office with a healthcare professional available to answer questions or in the privacy of the patient's home with questions addressed at a later date. The information provided is much the same as that found in the printed materials, but not everyone learns through reading; therefore, information must be offered using different formats to accommodate all learning styles. Table 15-5 contains a sample of the audiovisual materials available.

TABLE 15-5. Audiovisual Materials

TITLE: *Living and Loving: Sexuality and the Prostate Patient*[42]
SOURCE: ICI/Pharma Zeneca Pharmaceuticals
CONTENT:

- Signs and symptoms of prostate cancer
- Treatment options
- Devices used to resolve impotency
- Information regarding support groups-additional resources

- Anatomy and physiology of prostate
- Dealing with impotency, both male and female perspectives

CHARGE: Free

TITLE: *Keeping Healthy: Overcoming Prostate Cancer*[43]
SOURCE: Schering Oncology Biotech
CONTENT:

- Overview of prostate cancer
- Hormones and the prostate
- Treatment options-side effects
- Discussion of psychosocial aspects of disease and support services available

- Anatomy and physiology of prostate
- Prostate cancer as a family disease
- Educational resources identified

CHARGE: Free

TITLE: *Every Man Should Know About His Prostate: A Disease Awareness Video*[44]
SOURCE: Merck and Company, Inc.
CONTENT:

- Misconceptions re prostate
- Location and function
- Signs and symptoms of BPH
- Screening recommendations

- Factual information
- Prostate enlargement—BPH
- Examination

CHARGE: Free

TITLE: *Taking Charge: Managing Advanced Prostate Cancer*[45]
SOURCE: Schering Oncology Biotech
CONTENT:

- US TOO meeting
- Work with physician
- Cellular functioning of normal prostate cells, prostate cancer
- Treatment options

- Patient advocacy re treatment
- Anatomy and physiology of prostate
- Metastatic disease
- PSA as screening and monitoring tool
- Social service support services

CHARGE: Free

TITLE: *Male Call: Prostate Cancer Awareness Program Featuring Sidney Poitier*[46]
SOURCE: American Cancer Society
CONTENT:

- General risks
- Statistics
- Anatomy and physiology of prostate
- Early detection—screening
- Patient reports
- American Cancer Society telephone number at the end

- Identification of high risk groups
- Lack of public knowledge re prostate, prostate cancer
- Sexual issues
- American Cancer Society screening recommendations
- Health promotion practices

CHARGE: Free

TITLE: *Into the Light*[47]
SOURCE: ICI Pharma
CONTENT:

- Feelings regarding diagnosis
- Anatomy and physiology of prostate
- Support groups—US TOO
- Importance of self-education

- Rationale for lack of discussion re prostate cancer
- Treatment options, all stages
- Patient/patient and patient/physician closeness
- Resources

CHARGE: Free

(Continued on next page)

TITLE: *When Someone You Love Has Prostate Cancer*[48]
SOURCE: Zeneca Pharmaceuticals
CONTENT:

- Open discussion by patients and their significant others re feelings surrounding diagnosis, treatment, survival with prostate cancer
- Treatment and side effects, focus on incontinence and impotence
- Sources of information

- Anatomy and physiology of prostate
- Survival statistics
- Information sources
- Physician appointments
- Support groups, coping mechanisms
- Advanced prostate cancer

CHARGE: Free

TITLE: *An Alternative Therapy for Prostate Cancer Radioactive Seed Implantation*[49]
SOURCE: Amersham Healthcare
CONTENT:

- Basic information re prostate cancer
- Overview of treatment options
- Seed implants: risks, benefits, cost effectiveness
- Information re brochure and further information

- What are seed implants?
- Explanation of brachytherapy
- In-depth view of procedure
- Patient reports with physician explanation

CHARGE: Free

BPH, benign prostatic hypertrophy; PSA, prostate-specific antigen; re, regarding.

RESOURCES FOR PROSTATE CANCER INFORMATION

Many sources of prostate cancer patient information are available to the healthcare team, the patients, their families, and the general public. Table 15-6 is a listing of a few of the available resources with addresses and phone numbers.

TABLE 15-6. Resources for Prostate Cancer Information

American Cancer Society (ACS)
1-800-ACS-2345
Internet at www.cancer.org
Local chapters listed in telephone book

American Foundation for Urologic Disease
300 West Pratt Street, Suite 401
Baltimore, MD 21201
1-800-242-2383

Amersham Healthcare
Medi-Physics, Inc.
2636 South Clearbrook Drive
Arlington Heights, IL 60005
1-800-433-4215

Association of Community Cancer Centers (ACCC)
11600 Nebel Street, Suite 202
Rockville, MD 20852
1-301-984-9496
Internet at www.ASSOC-Cancer-Ctrs.org

Krames Communication
1100 Grundy Lane
San Bruno, CA 94066-3030
1-800-333-3032

National Cancer Institute
9000 Rockville Pike
Bethesda, MD 20892
1-800-4-CANCER (1-800-422-6237)

Obson Medical Systems
Geddings Obson Foundation
P.O. Box 1593
Augusta, GA 30903

Pharmacea Inc.
P.O. Box 16529
Columbus, OH 43216-6529

ICI Pharma/Zeneca Pharmaceuticals
Wilmington, DE 19850-5437
1-800-456-3669, extension 7862

IMMUNEX Corporation
Seattle, WA 98101
1-800-220-6302

Schering Oncology Biotech
Schering Corporation
2000 Galloping Hill Road
Kenilworth, NJ 07033
1-908-298-4000

BOOKS ABOUT PROSTATE CANCER

Hundreds of books are available about prostate cancer; some tout natural cures and others are very technical in nature. There are also numerous books written by cancer survivors regarding their experiences with prostate cancer. Table 15-7 presents a review of some of the selections available from this voluminous list.

TABLE 15-7. Books About Prostate Cancer

AUTHOR: Chaitow (1998)[50]
TITLE: *Prostate Problems: Safe Alternatives Without Drugs*
CONTENT-REVIEW:
- Emphasis on use of osteopathy, naturopathy, acupuncture
- Recommends consultation with a qualified healthcare professional
- Description of prostate and its function
- Information on prostate cancer along with warning signs and symptoms
- Advocates a preventive approach to dealing with prostate problems
- Complementary strategies for dealing with prostate problems

AUTHOR: Whitney (1994)[51]
TITLE: *50 Things You Need to Know About the Prostate*
CONTENT-REVIEW: Begins with case study discussion of why prostate cancer has become a major issue; prostate gland is described incorporating information about what can go wrong
- Risk factors and testing
- Prostate problems defined
- Review of information on prostate cancer, including causes, staging, testing, prognosis, treatment options
- Case studies used to highlight issues
- Living after treatment
- Incontinence, sexuality, and psychosocial support issues

AUTHOR: Loo and Bentancourt (1998)[52]
TITLE: *The Prostate Cancer Source Book: How to Make Informed Treatment Choices*
CONTENT-REVIEW:
- Basic information regarding prostate, where and what it is, its function
- Review of prostate diseases
- Cancer and its development, risk factors, diagnosis, and staging
- Treatment alternatives for all stages of disease, along with decision-making pointers
- Information on clinical trials
- Recovery and follow-up issues
- Valuable information on insurance issues and financial aid for screening and treatment
- Information regarding patient's rights and Americans with Disabilities Act
- Appendices provide resource material, NCI, CancerFAX, CancerNet, and ACS

AUTHOR: Urbaniak (1998)[53]
TITLE: *Healing Your Prostate: Natural Cures That Work*
CONTENT-REVIEW:

- Identifies potential prostate problems
- Supplements and herbal therapies
- Discussions of hydrotherapy, reflexology, mind-body medicine, health, and healing
- How to modify one's diet to prevent problems
- Three pages devoted to conventional therapy and use of medications as a last resort

AUTHOR: Baggish (1998)[54]
TITLE: *Making the Prostate Therapy Decision*
CONTENT-REVIEW:

- Review of prostate and definition of prostate cancer
- Treatment options identified and examined
- Prevention and psychosocial issues presented
- Diagnosis and staging are covered along with PSA testing
- Clinical trials mentioned as late treatment option
- Appendices include material on PAACT and AFUD

AUTHOR: Morra and Potts (1996)[55]
TITLE: *The Prostate Cancer Answer Book: An Unbiased Guide to Treatment Choices*
CONTENT-REVIEW:

- Information on PSA testing
- Discussion of prostate, diagnosis of cancer, testing, and diagnostic procedures
- Data on every potential side effect and solutions presented
- Detailed data on researching topic through computer searches via NCI, ACS, and the Prostate Cancer Home Page Internet Web sites
- Where to obtain psychosocial support
- Treatment choices identified with in-depth discussion of each option
- Obtaining a second opinion before making treatment decisions is examined
- Clinical trials and unproven treatments are discussed

AUTHOR: Bostwick (1996)[56]
TITLE: *Prostate Cancer: What Every Man—and His Family—Needs to Know*
CONTENT-REVIEW:

- Supportive foreword
- Thorough discussion of cancer
- Medically in-depth anatomy and physiology lesson
- Explanation of diagnostic workup and testing
- Discussion of development of action plan, including all treatment alternatives
- Issues of incontinence, impotence, and psychosocial support highlighted
- Introduction that outlines the book and introduces the concepts
- Feelings regarding diagnosis are discussed, focusing on question "Why Me?"
- Review of grading and staging
- Honest dialogue regarding recurrence and metastatic disease
- Resources are listed with telephone numbers, Internet Web sites, description of available services

AUTHOR: Marks (1995)[57]
TITLE: *Prostate and Cancer: A Family Guide to Diagnosis, Treatment and Survival*
CONTENT-REVIEW:

- Presented in question and answer format
- Screening physical, biopsy, staging workup, and treatment options
- Material is provided regarding living wills and issues of end-of-life decisions
- Covers anatomy-physiology, cancer and prostate, evaluation of symptoms
- Data is given regarding average costs of most procedures and treatments
- Support resources are presented, although no computer access information is provided

AUTHOR: Kantoff et al (1997)[58]
TITLE: *Prostate Cancer*
CONTENT-REVIEW:

- Heavily medically oriented reference
- Anatomy and physiology, prostate cancer, screening, testing, staging, prognosis, and treatment options
- Each chapter has extensive reference listing
- Little emphasis on psychosocial aspects or issues of impotence and incontinence

AUTHOR: Lewis and Berger (1997)[59]
TITLE: *New Guidelines for Surviving Prostate Cancer*
CONTENT-REVIEW:

- Presents information in complex, in-depth fashion
- Material on studies
- Focus on issue of pain

- Identifies differences between old and new guidelines for diagnosis and treatment of prostate cancer
- Good reference for medical community
- Highlights psychosocial issues, impotence, and incontinence

AUTHOR: Blaivas (1998)[60]
TITLE: *Conquering Bladder and Prostate Problems*
CONTENT-REVIEW:

- Has 13-page section on prostate cancer
- Reviews statistics, screening, questions, and answers re prostate cancer and diagnosis

- Discussion of metastatic disease
- Information on finding a physician

AUTHOR: Wainrib and Haber (1996)[61]
TITLE: *Prostate Cancer—A Guide for Women and the Men They Love*
CONTENT-REVIEW:

- Emphasis on psychosocial support
- Consideration of healing partnership and why and how to develop this
- Dealing with diagnosis; speaks primarily to support person
- Educational and supportive resources, NCI, US TOO, PAACT, and ACS are highlighted
- Recommends that treatment options be discussed and mutually agreed on by partners
- Discussion hinges on living through treatment phase and afterward

- Open communication emphasized
- Information on questions to ask regarding tests during detection
- Focus on family, how they can support by listing questions and taking notes during consultations
- Emotional issues for patient and caregivers are stressed
- Suggested use of journals
- Quality of life issues are identified as part of decision-making process

AUTHOR: Meyer and Nash (1994)[62]
TITLE: *Prostate Cancer: Making Survival Decisions*
CONTENT-REVIEW:

- Begins by relating Meyer's experience
- Screening examinations, symptoms, and staging are reviewed
- Grading and staging are discussed as indicators of degree of illness

- Discussion of BPH and potential for denial of a cancer diagnosis
- Information on what happens during examinations
- Treatment options, along with risks and benefits, are identified

AUTHOR: Walsh and Worthington (1995)[63]
TITLE: *The Prostate: A Guide for Men and the Women Who Love Them*
CONTENT-REVIEW:

- Introduces BPH, prostatitis, and prostate cancer
- Details regarding treatment options
- Advanced cancer and treatment options using hormones and/or castration are discussed

- Information about anatomy, cancer risk factors, screening, and diagnosis
- Action steps to take to find correct physician
- Pain management, and potential for cord compression and pathologic fractures are presented as potential events during course of disease

AUTHOR: Clapp (1997)[64]
TITLE: *Prostate Health in 90 Days Without Drugs or Surgery*
CONTENT-REVIEW:

- Information and advice regarding nutrition, massage, herbal therapy, homeopathy, and alternative healing

- These treatments are recommended for use before more standard treatment, with feeling that standard therapy is always there as backup

AUTHOR: Salmans (1996)[65]
TITLE: *Prostate: Questions You Have . . . Answers You Need*
CONTENT-REVIEW:

- Answers to basic questions about prostate
- Treatment options available

- Description of BPH, prostatitis, and cancer
- Additional sources of materials and support services

AUTHOR: Wallner (1996)[66]
TITLE: *Prostate Cancer: A Non-Surgical Perspective*

- Large-print book
- Prostate cancer reviewed
- Information on physicians who specialize in treatment of prostate cancer

- Overview of rationale for publication
- Workup is described
- Treatment options are presented with most side effects
- Issues of impotence and psychosocial support are addressed

NCI, National Cancer Institute; ACS, American Cancer Society; PSA, prostate-specific antigen; PAACT, Patient Advocates for Advanced Cancer Treatment; AFUD, American Foundation of Urologic Disease; BPH, benign prostatic hypertrophy.

PERSONAL ACCOUNTS

Table 15-8 contains a listing of some of the books available written by prostate cancer survivors. They are personal accounts and can be offered to patients as the author's diary regarding the diagnosis and treatment of their individual disease. It is also a description of the personal manner in which individuals handled the crisis of their disease.

TABLE 15-8. Personal Accounts

AUTHOR: Lewis and Berger (1994)[67]
TITLE: *How I Survived Prostate Cancer, and So Can You: A Guide for Diagnosing and Treating Prostate Cancer*

AUTHOR: Martin (1994)[68]
TITLE: *My Prostate and Me: Dealing With Prostate Cancer*

AUTHOR: Farmer (1995)[69]
TITLE: *What Can I Do? My Husband Has Prostate Cancer*

AUTHOR: Kaltenbach and Richards (1996)[70]
TITLE: *Prostate Cancer: A Survivor's Guide*

AUTHOR: Korda (1996)[71]
TITLE: *Man to Man: Surviving Prostate Cancer*

AUTHOR: Newton (1996)[72]
TITLE: *Living With Prostate Cancer: One Man's Story: What Everyone Should Know*

AUTHOR: Wheeler et al (1996)[73]
TITLE: *Affirming the Darkness: An Extended Conversation About Living With Prostate Cancer*

AUTHOR: Gardiner (1997)[74]
TITLE: *How I Conquered Cancer in 6 Months: A Naturopathic Alternative*

AUTHOR: Hitchcox and Wilson (1997)[75]
TITLE: *Love, Sex and PSA—Living and Loving With Prostate Cancer*

AUTHOR: Maddox and Dole (1997)[76]
TITLE: *Prostate Cancer: What I Found Out & What You Should Know*

WORLDWIDE WEB RESOURCES

Searching the Worldwide Web (WWW) for information has become a popular method of obtaining data on almost any topic. Individuals with access to a personal computer with a modem at home, in a physician's office, or in the local library can use the WWW and perform a search. The amount of information obtainable from the WWW is almost limitless and can be overwhelming, providing more data than any individual can comfortably digest.

There are numerous search engines, among them Yahoo, AltaVista, Lycos, Infoseek, and Excite. Regardless of which search engine is used, information obtained from the search may not always be accurate or up to date. Some sites are not as reliable as others or may be listed solely for propietary reasons. The best advice for anyone searching the Web is "Let the buyer beware." Numerous sites are reliable and provide accurate and timely information. Table 15-9 lists some recommended sites that furnish credible, factual data that are reviewed and updated continually.

TABLE 15-9. Internet Resources

SITE NAME: 4 Cancer
WEB SITE ADDRESS: www.4cancer.com
MATERIAL AVAILABLE:
- Cancer research
- Publications
- Organizations
- Cancer treatments
- Products
- Related sites such as 4 Prostate Cancer

SITE NAME: American Foundation for Urologic Disease
WEB SITE ADDRESS: www.access.digex.net/~afud
MATERIAL AVAILABLE:
- Complete information on prostate cancer with description
- Glossary of medical terminology
- Examination, testing, and treatment information provided
- Quiz is available at end of formal presentation

SITE NAME: Association of Community Cancer Centers
WEB SITE ADDRESS: www.ASSOC-Cancer-Centers.org
MATERIAL AVAILABLE:
- Information re cancer centers
- Basic insurance information
- Treatments and standards

SITE NAME: Cancer-Links Prostate
WEB SITE ADDRESS: www.cancernews.com/male.htm
MATERIAL AVAILABLE:
- News reports on prostate cancer
- Links to other home and information pages
- Literature search—link to National Library of Medicine
- Books on prostate cancer
- Listing of prostate cancer Web resources
- Clinical trial search—link to NCI

SITE NAME: CancerNet information
WEB SITE ADDRESS: www.ncc.go.jp/cnet
MATERIAL AVAILABLE:
- Information from PDQ
- CANCERLIT communication
- Access to information from NCI's Office of Cancer Communication

(Continued on next page)

SITE NAME: Center Watch
WEB SITE ADDRESS: www.centerwatch.com
MATERIAL AVAILABLE:
- Clinical trials listing service
- Listing of recently approved drugs
- Research center profiles
- International list of active clinical trials
- Health-related Web sites
- Industry provider profiles

SITE NAME: CoMed Communications Internet Health Forum
WEB SITE ADDRESS: www.comed.com/prostate
MATERIAL AVAILABLE:
- Current prostate news
- Question and answer page
- Risk factors, signs and symptoms, prevention issues
- Area provided for patients to share information, ask questions, exchange knowledge and experiences, share details regarding other prostate cancer sites that were useful, and identify other materials that have proven helpful
- Current clinical trials information
- Information on anatomy and physiology of prostate
- Content regarding support organizations is provided, along with addresses and telephone numbers

SITE NAME: National Institutes of Health
WEB SITE ADDRESS: www.nih.gov
MATERIAL AVAILABLE:
- Leads into NCI database
- Clinical trials data
- CancerNet
- Patient information
- Cancer information service

SITE NAME: NCI CancerNet Cancer Information Service
WEB SITE ADDRESS: www.icic.nci.nih.gov/icichome
MATERIAL AVAILABLE:
- For patients, healthcare professionals, and basic researchers
- Access to current articles via Cancerlit
- Information regarding treatment screening, prevention, supportive care, and clinical trials

SITE NAME: OncoLink
WEB SITE ADDRESS: oncolink.upenn.edu/disease/prostate
MATERIAL AVAILABLE:
- General information about cancer
- Questions and answers about prostate cancer included
- Treatment options viewed
- Newspaper items pertaining to prostate cancer and related topics available for viewing or reprinting
- Can focus on prostate cancer
- Recommendations for screening
- Risk factors, prevention, and genetics
- Information on support groups

SITE NAME: ONS Online
WEB SITE ADDRESS: www.ons.org
MATERIAL AVAILABLE:
- Access to journal articles, discussion forums, excerpts from new books, and materials on genetics
- Information regarding prevention and detection
- Resource for ONS members

SITE NAME: PDQ -NCI's Comprehensive Cancer Data Base
WEB SITE ADDRESS: www.cancernet.nci.gov/pdq
MATERIAL AVAILABLE:
- Information regarding screening, prevention, and supportive care
- Designed for lay people using nontechnical language
- PDQ can be accessed for professional use and information re current clinical trials

SITE NAME: PhRMA, America's Pharmaceutical Companies
WEB SITE ADDRESS: www.phrma.org
MATERIAL AVAILABLE:
- Information regarding prostate cancer
- View initial reference
- Risk factors
- Treatment options
- Obtain summary of document or view entire manuscript
- Material targeting African Americans
- Matching search word "prostate"
- Information about prostate
- Testing for prostate cancer
- New treatments being developed
- Account of individuals' experiences during diagnosis and treatment
- Information for women

SITE NAME: Prostate Cancer Education Network
WEB SITE ADDRESS: www.htinet.com/archive/pcenarch
MATERIAL AVAILABLE:
- Can be viewed as transcript or listened to as audio presentation
- Sponsored by IMMUNEX with assistance from the AFDU
- Goal of the Prostate Cancer Education Network: make this an ongoing service
- Archive of a pilot project in which patients participated on line and were able to ask question of urologist and/or oncologist as well as exchanging information with other patients

SITE NAME: Prostate Cancer Home Page
WEB SITE ADDRESS: www.cancer.med.umich.edu/prostcan/prostcan
MATERIAL AVAILABLE:
- Articles
- Staging information
- Resources
- Information regarding staff at University of Michigan Comprehensive Cancer Center
- Clinical trials information
- Treatment options
- Sources of information
- Descriptions of some projects
- Links to other useful sites

SITE NAME: Prostate Cancer Patient Information Center
WEB SITE ADDRESS: www.hmro.com/managingyourhealth/prostatecancer/nilanpat
MATERIAL AVAILABLE:
- Launched by Hoechst Marion Roussel
- Includes resource guide published by AFUD
- Prostate cancer from patient's perspective
- Resources available on Web
- Provides basic information about prostate cancer
- Addresses women's perspectives on dealing with a significant other who has prostate cancer
- Option of receiving e-mail notification of updates of site

SITE NAME: The Prostate Forum
WEB SITE ADDRESS: www.prostateforum.com
MATERIAL AVAILABLE:
- Newsletter for patients-families written by Charles E. Myers, MD
- Side effects
- References
- Treatment issues
- Mechanisms of action
- Research

SITE NAME: US TOO International, Inc. Prostate Cancer Support Groups
WEB SITE ADDRESS: www.ustoo.com
MATERIAL AVAILABLE:
- Information regarding organization
- Publications (updated monthly)
- Information on clinical trials
- Information can be requested
- Support groups
- Current treatment options
- Links provided to related sites

SITE NAME: WWW Cancernet
WEB SITE ADDRESS: www.arc.com/cancernet/cancenet
- Alternate way of accessing NCI's cancer data bases, OncoLink, and University of Pennsylvania Cancer Center Resource

---

NCI, National Cancer Institute; AFUD, American Foundation for Urologic Disease; re, regarding.

The Internet can also be accessed for chat groups via America On-Line or forums via Compuserve. In these areas, one can interact via computer with other individuals interested in prostate cancer. Here again, the issue is that these chat rooms may provide unreliable or biased information. A chat room is only as effective as the leader and participants. If they are not knowledgeable, the chat room has the potential for being a waste of time and energy.

In summary, there are multiple resources for patients, families, and members of the healthcare team regarding prostate cancer. Depending on preference, information can be found in books, journals, pamphlets, or on-line sources. The material is available for all to access. The references in this chapter are merely the tip of the iceberg, each leading the patient, family, or healthcare professional onward in the search for information.

REFERENCES

1. American Cancer Society. *Real Men Get It Checked.* Atlanta, GA: Author, 1997.
2. American Cancer Society. *American Cancer Society's New Guidelines for the Early Detection of Prostate Cancer.* Atlanta, GA: Author, 1997.
3. American Cancer Society. *The PSA Blood Test and Prostate Cancer.* Atlanta, GA: Author, 1998.
4. National Cancer Institute. *Understanding Prostate Changes: A Health Guide for All Men.* Bethesda, MD: Author, 1998.
5. American Foundation for Urologic Disease. *For Women Who Care: Information on Prostate Disease to Share With the Men in Your Life.* Baltimore, MD: Author, 1992.
6. KRAMES Communication. *Prostate Health, Screening for Prostate Cancer.* San Bruno, CA: Author, 1993.
7. KRAMES Communication. *Treating Prostate Problems: Options for Improving Your Health.* San Bruno, CA: Author, 1994.
8. Association of Community Cancer Centers. *Cancer Treatments Your Insurance Should Cover: Information for Patients and Their Families.* Rockville, MD: Author, 1998.
9. American Cancer Society. *Cancer Facts and Figures—1998.* Atlanta, GA: Author, 1998.
10. American Cancer Society. *Prostate Cancer 1998 Fact Sheet.* Atlanta, GA: Author, 1998.
11. American Cancer Society. *For Men Only: What You Should Know About Prostate Cancer.* Atlanta, GA: Author, 1997.
12. American Cancer Society. *Facts on Prostate Cancer in African Americans.* Atlanta, GA: Author, 1997.
13. American Cancer Society. *Prostate Cancer: Asking the Questions, Finding the Answers.* Atlanta, GA: Author, 1998.
14. American Cancer Society. *After Diagnosis: Prostate Cancer: Understanding Your Treatment Options.* Atlanta, GA: Author, 1996.
15. American Cancer Society. *What to Do If Prostate Cancer Strikes: A Helpbook for Patients.* Atlanta, GA: American Cancer Society and Cancer Research Institute, 1997.
16. American Cancer Society. *Sexuality & Cancer: For the Man Who Has Cancer and His Partner.* Atlanta, GA: Author, 1995.
17. ICI Pharma/Zeneca Pharmaceuticals. *Prostate Cancer and You.* Wilmington, DE: Author, 1996.
18. ICI Pharma/Zeneca Pharmaceuticals. Prostate Cancer: *What It Is and How It Is Treated.* Wilmington, DE: Author, 1996.
19. ICI Pharma/Zeneca Pharmaceuticals. *El Cáncer Prostático: ¿Qué es y cómo se trata?* Wilmington, DE: Author, 1996.
20. National Cancer Institute. *The Cancer Information Service.* Bethesda, MD: Author.
21. National Cancer Institute. *What You Need to Know About Cancer.* Bethesda, MD: Author, 1993.
22. National Cancer Institute. *What You Need To Know About Prostate Cancer.* Bethesda, MD: Author, 1992.
23. Obson Medical Systems. *A Patient's Guide for the Treatment of Impotence.* Atlanta, GA: The Geddings Obson Foundation, 1995.
24. Obson Medical Systems. *Male Impotence: A Woman's Perspective.* Atlanta, GA: The Geddings Obson Foundation, 1993.

25. Pharmacia Inc. *Cancer Terms: A Guide for Your Patients With Cancer.* Columbus, OH: Author, 1995.

26. Pharmacia Inc. *Tumor Markers: A Guide for Your Patients With Cancer.* Columbus, OH: Author, 1995.

27. Schering Oncology Biotech. *It's the Most Common Cancer in Men: The Facts About Prostate Cancer.* Kenilworth, NJ: Schering Corporation, 1998.

28. Schering Oncology Biotech. *Prostate Cancer: Some Good News Men Can Live With.* Kenilworth, NJ: Schering Corporation, 1991.

29. KRAMES Communication. *Living With Prostate Cancer.* San Bruno, CA: Author, 1996.

30. ICI Pharma/Zeneca Pharmaceuticals. *Questions and Answers About Zoladex (Goserelin Acetate Implant) Therapy for the Treatment of Prostate Cancer.* Wilmington, DE: Author, 1996.

31. IMMUNEX. *Words to Live By: The Information Resource for Prostate Cancer Patients.* Seattle, WA: Author, 1996.

32. Schering Oncology Biotech. *Living With Stage D2 Prostate Cancer and Eulexin (Flutamide) Therapy.* Kenilworth, NJ: Schering Corporation, 1994.

33. ICI Pharma/Zeneca Pharmaceuticals. *Why Your Doctor Has Prescribed Casodex for You: Important Information for Men With Advanced Prostate Cancer.* Wilmington, DE: Author, 1996.

34. IMMUNEX. *The EPIC Manual Empowered Patients in Control: A Guide to Pain Management in Advanced Prostate Cancer.* Seattle, WA: Author, 1996.

35. Schering Oncology Biotech. *Treatment Options for Living Longer With Advanced Prostate Cancer.* Kenilworth, NJ: Schering Corporation, 1996.

36. Schering Oncology Biotech. *The Only Antiandrogen Proven to Delay Progression in Advanced Prostate Cancer.* Kenilworth, NJ: Schering Corporation, 1996.

37. American Cancer Society. *Man to Man News: Prostate Cancer News and Information from the American Cancer Society's Man to Man Program.* Atlanta, GA: Author, 1998(winter).

38. American Cancer Society. *Man to Man: Prostate Cancer Education and Support Program.* Atlanta, GA: Author, 1996.

39. American Foundation for Urologic Disease. *US TOO Prostate Cancer Survivor Support Group.* Baltimore, MD: American Foundation for Urologic Disease and US TOO International Inc.

40. ICI Pharma/Zeneca Pharmaceuticals. *Into the Light: A Guide for the Prostate Cancer Patient and Those Close to Him.* Wilmington, DE: Author, 1993.

41. Schering Oncology Biotech: *CareNection: Helping You Get the Most From Eulexin.* Kenilworth, NJ: Schering Corporation, 1996.

42. ICI Pharma/Zeneca Pharmaceuticals. *Living and Loving: Sexuality and the Prostate Patient.* Wilmington, DE: Author, 1996.

43. Schering Oncology Biotech. *Keeping Healthy: Overcoming Prostate Cancer.* Kenilworth, NJ: Schering Corporation, 1993.

44. Merck & Co., Inc. *Every Man Should Know About His Prostate: A Disease Awareness Video* [video]. Whitehouse, NJ: Author, 1993

45. Schering Oncology Biotech. *Taking Charge: Managing Advanced Prostate Cancer* [video]. Kenilworth, NJ: Schering Corporation, 1993.

46. American Cancer Society. *Male Call: Prostate Cancer Awareness Program Featuring Sidney Poitier* [video]. Atlanta, GA: Author.

47. ICI Pharma. *Into the Light* [video]. Foresight Communications for ICI Pharma, 1993.

48. Zeneca Pharmaceuticals. *When Someone You Love Has Prostate Cancer* [video]. Cypres, CA: MEDCOM, Inc., 1995.

49. Amersham Healthcare. *An Alternative Therapy for Prostate Cancer Radioactive Seed Implantation* [video]. Arlington Heights, IL: Amersham Healthcare, Medi-Physics, Inc.

50. Chaitow L. *Prostate Problems: Safe Alternatives Without Drugs.* Wellingborough, England: Thorsons Publishers, 1998.

51. Whitney CA. *50 Things You Need to Know About the Prostate.* New York: St. Martin's Press, 1994.

52. Loo MH, Bentancourt M. *The Prostate Cancer Source Book: How to Make Informed Treatment Choices.* Chichester, England: Wiley, 1998.

53. Urbaniak E. *Healing Your Prostate: Natural Cures That Work.* Gig Harbor, WA: Harbor Press, 1998.

54. Baggish J. *Making the Prostate Therapy Decision.* Chicago: Contemporary Books, 1998.

55. Morra M, Potts E. *The Prostate Cancer Answer Book: An Unbiased Guide to Treatment Choices.* New York: Avon Books, 1996.

56. Bostwick D. *Prostate Cancer: What Every Man—and His Family—Needs to Know.* New York: Villard Books, 1996.

57. Marks S. *Prostate and Cancer: A Family Guide to Diagnosis, Treatment, and Survival.* Tucson, AZ: Fisher Books, 1995.

58. Kantoff P, Wishnow K, Louglin K. *Prostate Cancer.* Malden, MA: Blackwell Science, 1997.

59. Lewis J Jr, Berger ER. *New Guidelines for Surviving Prostate Cancer.* Westbury, NY: Health Education Literary Publishers, 1997.

60. Blaivas JG. *Conquering Bladder and Prostate Problems.* New York: Plenum, 1998.

61. Wainrib B, Haber S. *Prostate Cancer—A Guide for Women and the Men They Love.* New York: Dell, 1996.

62. Meyer S, Nash SC. *Prostate Cancer: Making Survival Decisions.* Chicago: University of Chicago Press, 1994.

63. Walsh P, Worthington JF. *The Prostate: A Guide for Men and the Women Who Love Them.* Baltimore, MD: Johns Hopkins University Press, 1995.

64. Clapp L. *Prostate Health in 90 Days Without Drugs or Surgery.* Carlsbad, CA: Hay House, 1997.

65. Salmans S. *Prostate: Questions You Have . . . Answers You Need.* Allentown, PA: Peoples Medical Society, 1996.

66. Wallner K. *Prostate Cancer: A Non-Surgical Perspective.* Canaan, NY: Smartmedicine Press, 1996.

67. Lewis J Jr, Berger ER. *How I Survived Prostate Cancer, and So Can You: A Guide for Diagnosing and Treating Prostate Cancer.* Westbury, NY: Health Education Literary Publisher, 1994.

68. Martin W. *My Prostate and Me: Dealing With Prostate Cancer.* New York: Soho Press, 1994.

69. Farmer B. *What Can I Do? My Husband Has Prostate Cancer.* Battle Ground, WA: Pathfinder Press, 1995.

70. Kaltenbach D, Richards T. *Prostate Cancer: A Survivor's Guide.* New Port Richey, FL: Prostate Cancer Guide, 1996.

71. Korda M. *Man to Man: Surviving Prostate Cancer.* New York: Random House, 1996.

72. Newton AC. *Living With Prostate Cancer: One Man's Story: What Everyone Should Know.* New York: St. Martin's Press, 1996.

73. Wheeler C. *Affirming the Darkness: An Extended Conversation About Living With Prostate Cancer.* Beverly, MA: Memoirs Unlimited, 1996.

74. Gardiner E. *How I Conquered Cancer in 6 Months: A Naturopathic Alternative.* Houston: Emerald Isle Publishers, 1997.

75. Hitchcox R, Wilson B. *Love, Sex and PSA—Living and Loving With Prostate Cancer.* San Diego: TMC Press, 1997.

76. Maddox RL, Dole R. *Prostate Cancer: What I Found Out & What You Should Know.* Wheaton, IL: Harold Shaw, 1997.

Index

Adenocarcinomas, 40
Adhesion molecules, E-cadherin expression in metastatic cancer, 58
Adjuvant hormonal therapy, 181
Advanced cancer
  bladder outlet obstruction in, 254–255, 259
  information resources available, 292–293
  quality of life in, 247–248
  radiation therapy in, 148
  standard of care in, 256–258
  symptom management in, 254–282
  ureteral obstruction in, 50, 260–261
Age
  and prostate-specific antigen levels, 31, 55–56
  as risk factor for prostate cancer, 3–4, 25, 51
  and treatment decisions, 82
Albumin levels, and risk for prostate cancer, 11–12
Alcohol intake as risk factor for prostate cancer, 9–10
Alendronate in osteoporosis, 185
Alprostadil in erectile dysfunction, 184, 245
Alternate treatment modalities, 112–113
American Cancer Society screening guidelines, 27–28
American Joint Committee on Cancer with International Union Against Cancer, TNM staging system of, 68, 70–71
Aminoglutethimide, 89, 188
  complications from, 92
  in prevention of prostate cancer, 17
Analgesia
  drugs in, 270
  postoperative, patient-controlled, 129
Anastrozole in prevention of prostate cancer, 17
Anatomic considerations in prostate cancer, 44
Androgens
  and antiandrogens. See Antiandrogens
  intermittent suppression of, 189–190
  sequential blockade of, 189
  serum levels of
    and risk for prostate cancer, 4, 16, 27
    and tumor progression, 44–45

suppression or ablation of. See Hormonal therapy
  total blockade of, 88–89, 177
    complications from, 92
    in metastatic cancer, 177–179
Androstenedione, 172
  and dihydrotestosterone synthesis, 45
  and risk for prostate cancer, 11–12
Angiogenesis
  inhibitors in prevention of cancer, 17
  and tumor progression, 43–44
Anthropometric variables, and risk for prostate cancer, 13–14
Antiandrogens
  luteinizing hormone releasing hormone agonists with, 179
  pure, 175–176
    monotherapy with, 190–191
    side effects of, 176
  steroidal, 176–177
  withdrawal response, 89, 186–187
α_1-Antichymotrypsin, prostate-specific antigen bound to, 56
Anticoagulants in deep vein thrombosis, 263–264
Apoptosis induction, 172
Aromatase inhibition, and prevention of prostate cancer, 17
Attitudes of patients and partners
  toward erectile dysfunction, 241
  toward treatment, 111–112, 113
    in expectant management, 108–109
    in radiation therapy, 135–136
Audiovisual materials available, 294–296

Benign prostatic hypertrophy compared to cancer, 50, 51
Bicalutamide, 175–176
  complications from, 92
  luteinizing hormone releasing hormone agonists with, 179
  as monotherapy, 191
Biofeedback therapy in urinary incontinence, 236–237

Biopsies, 61–63
and postbiopsy discharge instructions, 63
Bisphosphonates in bone pain, 273, 274
Bladder
function after radiation therapy, 153–154
outlet obstruction from cancer, 50, 254–255, 259
training in incontinence, 237
Bleeding in disseminated intravascular coagulation, 266
Body mass index, and risk for prostate cancer, 13–14
Bone pain, 267–273
bisphosphonates in, 273, 274
drug therapy in, 268–271
radiation therapy in, 271
radioisotope therapy in, 88, 273
Bone scans, radionuclide, 61
in staging of tumors, 72–73
Books regarding prostate cancer, 297–300
Bowel disorders
and quality of life, 246–247
from radiation therapy, 150
Brachytherapy, interstitial, 87–88, 158–165
and neoadjuvant androgen ablation, 180–181
nursing care in, 164
preparation for, 160
procedure in, 160–161
side effects of, 163
temporary implants in, 159
Buserelin, complications from, 92

Caloric intake, and risk for prostate cancer, 15
Carcinogenesis, 37–39
Carcinosarcoma, 40
Catheterization in bladder outlet obstruction
indwelling catheters in, 255
self-catheterization in, 255
CD44 expression in cancer, 59
Cellular changes
in apoptosis, 172
in cancer development, 2, 37
and radiosensitivity, 138
Chemical exposure, and risk for prostate cancer, 10–11
Chemotherapy, 89–90, 195–222
candidates for, 215
combinations of agents in, 201–215
complications of, 93
failure of, treatment options after, 215
in hormone-refractory cancer, 189, 195–222
nursing management in, 216–217

patient education in, 215–216
psychosocial issues in, 217
single-agent, 198–201
standard of care in, 218–222
Clonidine for hot flashes, 182–183
Coagulation, disseminated intravascular, 265–267
Codeine for pain control, 270
Coexisting medical problems, and treatment decisions, 82
Computed tomography, 61
in staging of tumors, 72–73
Constipation from opioids, 271
Corticosteroid therapy, 187–188
Coumarin in lymphedema, 265
Cryoablation of prostate, 86, 130–132
complications of, 132
suprapubic tube care in, 131–132
Cyclophosphamide, 200
doxorubicin with, 211
etoposide with, 211
Cyproterone acetate, 177
Cystitis after radiation therapy, 154
Cytoreduction before radiation therapy, 147

Dehydroepiandrosterone, 172
and dihydrotestosterone synthesis, 45
Dexamethasone therapy, 188
in spinal cord compression, 277
in ureteral obstruction, 260–261
Diabetes mellitus, and risk for prostate cancer, 12
Diagnosis of cancer, 49–63
biopsy in, 61–63
CD44 in, 59
clinical features in, 45–46, 50–51
E-cadherin in, 58
history-taking in, 51
imaging in, 59–61
laboratory studies in, 53–59
p27Kip1 in, 58
physical examination in, 51–53
prostate-specific antigen in, 53–57
membrane antigen, 57
psychosocial impact of, 94–95
symptoms compared to benign prostatic hypertrophy, 51
Diarrhea from radiation therapy, 150, 246
antidiarrheal agents in, 151
foods to avoid in, 152
Dicyclomine in incontinence, 238

Diet
    low-residue, 154–155
    and risk for prostate cancer, 14–16, 27
Diethylstilbestrol, 188
    complications from, 92
    with radiation therapy, 165–166
Digital rectal examination
    in screening for cancer, 24, 29, 45–46, 51–53
    in staging of tumors, 71
Dihydrotestosterone levels, 172
    and risk for prostate cancer, 4, 11–12, 27, 54
    and tumor progression, 44–45
Diphenoxylate hydrochloride with atropine sulfate, in
    diarrhea, 151, 246
Disseminated intravascular coagulation, 265–267
    bleeding in, 266
    laboratory studies in, 267
    treatment of, 267
Docetaxel, 90, 201
    with estramustine, 207, 211–213
Doxazosin mesylate for urinary symptoms after
    radiation, 154, 156
Doxepin in incontinence, 238
Doxorubicin, 200–201
    with cyclophosphamide, 211
    ketoconazole with, 213
Drug therapy
    in diarrhea, 151
    in erectile dysfunction, 184, 244–245
    in pain control, 268–271
    in ureteral obstruction, 260–261
    in urinary incontinence, 237–239
Drugs affecting bladder function, 51

E-cadherin expression in metastatic cancer, 58
Edema
    leg, 261–265
    scrotal, 265
Electrical stimulation in incontinence, 237
Emepronium bromide in incontinence, 238
Endocrine therapy. *See* Hormonal therapy
Enteritis, radiation, 150
Environmental exposures, as risk factor for prostate
    cancer, 10–11
Epidemiology of prostate cancer, 1–2
Erectile dysfunction, 239–246
    drug therapy in, 184, 244–245
    management of, 183–184, 241–246
    penile implants in, 184, 245–246

vacuum devices in, 184, 241–243
Estradiol levels, and risk for prostate cancer, 11–12
Estramustine, 90, 200
    docetaxel with, 207, 211–213
    etoposide with, 208–209
        with additional drugs, 209
    nausea from, 205, 208, 209
    paclitaxel with, 205–206
    vinblastine with, 207
Estrogens
    inhibitors in cancer prevention, 17
    protectve role of phytoestrogens, 12
    therapy with, 88, 188
        complications from, 92
Ethanol use, and risk for prostate cancer, 9–10
Ethnic background
    as risk factor for prostate cancer, 4–6
    and uncertainty experiences, 113
Etiology of prostate cancer, 2–3, 37–39
Etoposide, 90, 201
    with cyclophosphamide, 211
    with estramustine, 208–209
        additional drugs with, 209
Exercise, and risk for prostate cancer, 14
Expectant management, 84–85, 102–114
    and initiation of hormonal therapy, 110
    nursing care in, 111
    patient and partner views of, 108–109
    patient eligibility criteria for, 107–108
    protocol for, 109–110
    psychoeducational interventions in, 111–113
    and quality of life information, 233
    rationale against, 105–106
    rationale for, 103–105
    therapeutic goal of, 106–107

Familial occurrence of prostate cancer, 6, 8, 25–26, 43,
    51
Farmers, risk for prostate cancer in, 10–11
Fat intake, and risk for prostate cancer, 14–15
Fatigue
    after radiation therapy, 157
    treatment of, 183
Fenretinide in prevention of prostate cancer, 17
Fentanyl in bone pain, 269, 270
Finasteride
    affecting cancer detection, 54–55
    in prevention of prostate cancer, 16
    terazosin with, 54

Flutamide, 175–176
  complications from, 92
  goserelin with, as neoadjuvant therapy
    before radiation, 180
    before surgery, 180
  leuprolide with, 178, 179
    as neoadjuvant therapy before brachytherapy, 181
  as monotherapy, 190
  side effects of, 166
  withdrawal of, 196–197
    and decreased prostate-specific antigen levels,
      89, 186–187
Follicle-stimulating hormone levels, and risk for
  prostate cancer, 11–12

Genetic factors in prostate cancer, 6–9, 25–26, 43, 51
  in hormone-resistant cancer, 213
Genitourinary symptoms after radiation therapy,
  153–156
Germ cell tumors, 40
Gleason grading system, 40–41, 42, 75–76
  and expectant management, 107–108
  and treatment decisions, 84
Goserelin, 173, 175
  antiandrogens with, 179
  complications from, 92
  flutamide with, as neoadjuvant therapy
    before radiation, 180
    before surgery, 180
  with radiation therapy, 165, 166
Grading of cancer
  Gleason system in, 40–41, 42, 75–76
  and treatment decisions, 84
Granulocyte colony-stimulating factor, as support in
  combination chemotherapy, 211
Granulocyte-macrophage colony-stimulating factor, as
  support in combination chemotherapy, 204
Growth of tumors
  angiogenesis affecting, 43–44
  routes of, 44

Heparin therpy in deep vein thrombosis, 263–264
Hereditary factors in prostate cancer, 6–9, 25–26, 43, 51
Hormonal factors in prostate cancer, 11–12
Hormonal therapy, 88–89, 170–191
  adjuvant therapy, 181
  and antiandrogen withdrawal response, 89, 186–187
  benefits of, 45
  biochemical effects of, 177

  in bladder outlet obstruction, 255, 259
  in bone pain, 268
  complications of, 92
  and hormone-refractory disease, 185–189
  indications for, 177–181
  initiation in expectant management, 110
  intermittent androgen suppression in, 189–190
  medical castration in, 173
  monotherapy with pure antiandrogens, 190–191
  neoadjuvant therapy, 180–181
    before radiation, 180–181
    before surgery, 180
  phases of responsiveness in, 197
  pure antiandrogens in, 175–176, 190–191
  radiation therapy with, 87, 147, 158, 165–166
    side effects of, 166
  rationale for, 171
  secondary therapies, 187–188, 197
  sequential androgen blockade in, 189
  side effect management in, 181–185
  standard of care in, 174
  steroidal antiandrogens in, 176–177
  surgical castration in, 173
  total androgen blockade in, 88–89, 177
    complications from, 92
    in metastatic cancer, 177–179
Hormone-resistant cancer, chemotherapy in, 189,
  195–222
Hot flashes, treatment of, 182–183
HPC1 gene, 8, 51
Hydrocodone for pain control, 270
Hydrocortisone, 89, 188
  mitoxantrone with, 204
  with suramin, 210–211
Hydromorphone in bone pain, 269, 270
Hydronephrosis, 260
Hypertrophy of prostate, benign, compared to cancer,
  50, 51

Imipramine in incontinence, 238
Impotence. *See* Erectile dysfunction
Incidence of prostate cancer, 103
Incontinence
  fecal, postoperative, 130
  urinary, 234–239
    after radiation therapy, 156, 234
    artificial sphincters in, 239
    assessment of, 235–236
    drug therapy in, 237–239

external devices in, 239
nursing interventions in, 236–239
overflow, 235
pads and garments in, 239
penile clamps in, 239
postoperative, 129–130
stress, 234–235
types of, 234–235
urge, 235
Insulin-like growth factor-I, role in prostate cancer, 2–3
Internet information resources, 301–304
Intraepithelial neoplasia, prostatic
diagnostic criteria for, 38
as precursor of prostate cancer, 2, 37–39

Kallikrein, glandular, ratio to prostate-specific antigen, 57
Kaolin-pectin in diarrhea, 151, 246
Kegel exercises, 236
postoperative, 129
Ketoconazole, 89, 188
complications from, 92
with doxorubicin, 213
with radiation therapy, 165–166

Laboratory studies, 53–59
in disseminated intravascular coagulation, 267
Leg edema, 261–265
assessment of, 261–263
in deep vein thrombosis, 261, 263–264
lymphatic, 264–265
Letrozole in prevention of prostate cancer, 17
Leuprolide, 173, 175
complications from, 92
flutamide with, 178, 179
as neoadjuvant therapy before brachytherapy, 181
Levorphanol for pain control, 270
Liarozole hydrochloride in prevention of prostate cancer, 17
Loperamide in diarrhea, 151, 246
Luteinizing hormone, 172
releasing hormone, 171
releasing hormone agonists, 88–89, 173, 175
antiandrogens with, 179
in bladder outlet obstruction, 255, 259
complications from, 92
serum levels of, and risk for prostate cancer, 11–12
and testosterone production, 16

Lymph nodes, treatment in radiation therapy, 144, 146
Lymphadenectomy, pelvic, in staging of tumors, 74
Lymphedema, 264–265
Lymphomas, 40

Magnetic resonance imaging, 59–61
in staging of tumors, 73–74
Medroxyprogesterone acetate, 188
in hot flashes, 183
Megestrol acetate, 177, 188
complications from, 92
in hot flashes, 182
with radiation therapy, 165–166
Meperidine for pain control, 270
Mesenchymal tumors, 40
Metastasis of cancer, 44
bone pain in, 267–273
E-cadherin expression in, 58
and quality of life, 248
symptoms in, 45
management in, 254–282
total androgen blockade in, 177–179
Methadone for pain control, 270
Mitoxantrone, 90, 198–199
high-dose, 204
hydrocortisone with, 204
paclitaxel with, 204
prednisone with, 202–204
Morphine in bone pain, 269, 270
Multicentric origin of prostate cancer, 44
Myelosuppression from radiation therapy, 157–158
Narcotics in bone pain, 269–271

Nausea
from estramustine, 205, 208, 209
from opioids, 271
Neoadjuvant hormonal therapy, 180–181
Nephrostomy tubes, percutaneous, 260
Nilutamide, 175–176
with orchiectomy, 178–179
Nonsteroidal anti-inflammatory drugs
in bone pain, 268–269
in prevention of prostate cancer, 17
Nuclear scans, 61
in staging of tumors, 72–73
Nutrition
low-residue diet in, 154–155
and risk for prostate cancer, 14–16, 27

Obesity as risk factor for prostate cancer, 14
Occupational hazards as risk factor for prostate cancer,
10–11
Octreotide acetate in diarrhea, 246
Oncogenes in cancer development, 37, 43
Opioids
in bone pain, 269–271
side effects of, 271
Orchiectomy, bilateral, 88, 89, 132–133, 173
in bone pain, 268
complications from, 92, 133
nilutamide with, 178–179
with radiation therapy, 165–166
Osteoporosis management, 184–185
Oxybutynin in incontinence, 238
Oxycodone in bone pain, 269, 270
Oxygen, hyperbaric, for radiation-induced
proctopathy, 247

p27Kip1 expression in cancer, 58
p53 gene, and prostate cancer development, 43
Paclitaxel, 90, 201
with estramustine, 205–206
etoposide with, 209
mitoxantrone with, 204
Pain
assessment of, 273–275
in bone metastases, 267–273
perineal, from interstitial brachytherapy, 164
from spinal cord compression, 276–281
Papillomavirus infection, and risk for prostate cancer,
12–13
Paregoric in diarrhea, 151
Pathophysiology of prostate cancer, 40
Patient-controlled analgesia, postoperative, 129
Pelvic lymphadenectomy in staging of tumors, 74
Penis
implantable prostheses, 184, 245–246
intracavernosal injections for erectile dysfunction,
244–245
Pentazocine for pain control, 270
Personal accounts of cancer survivors, 300
Phenylpropanolamine in incontinence, 238
Physical examination, 51–53
Phytoestrogens, protective role of, 12
Pituitary hormone levels, and risk for prostate cancer,
11–12
Polymerase chain reaction, reverse transcriptase, as
assay for prostate-specific antigen, 57

Prednisone, 188
mitoxantrone with, 202–204
Prevention of prostate cancer, 16–18
clinical trials in, 17–18
nursing implications, 18
Proctitis from interstitial brachytherapy, 164
Proctopathy, radiation-induced, 247
Progesterone therapy, 89
Progestins, therapy with, 188
Prognostic indicators, 41
Propantheline in incontinence, 238
Prostaglandin E therapy in erectile dysfunction, 245
Prostate Intervention Versus Observation Trial
(PIVOT), 105, 109–110
Prostate-specific antigen, 53–57
assays for
approved by FDA, 30
reverse transcriptase-polymerase chain reaction
in, 57
chemoprevention agents affecting, 17
density of, 55
evaluating levels of, 196
and expectant management of cancer, 107–108
factors affecting, 30
as marker of disease activity, 110
membrane antigen, 57
molecular forms of, 56–57
posttreatment levels of, 147–148
ratio to human glandular kallikrein, 57
reference ranges for, 31, 55–56
in screening for cancer, 24, 30–32
in staging of tumors, 72
suramin affecting levels of, 196, 211
and treatment decisions, 82–83
Prostatectomy, radical, 85–86, 123–130
clinical pathway in, 127
complications of, 91–92, 128–130
fecal incontinence after, 130
and neoadjuvant hormonal therapy, 180
patient-family timeline in, 128
and quality of life information, 233
radiation therapy after, 147–148
sexual dysfunction after, 240
urinary incontinence after, 129–130, 234
Prostatic acid phosphatase levels, 196
in staging of tumors, 71–72
Prostatic intraepithelial neoplasia
diagnostic criteria for, 38
as precursor of prostate cancer, 2, 37–39

Psychosocial issues
  in cancer diagnosis, 94–95
  in chemotherapy, 217
  information resources available, 293–294
  in radiation therapy, 166–167

Quality of life, 227–249
  in advanced cancer, 247–248
  in bowel disturbances, 246–247
  definition of, 227–228
  in expectant management of cancer, 104, 106–107, 111
  in localized cancer, 233
    treatment options in, 233
  questionaires for assessment of, 231–232
  research in prostate cancer
    challenges to, 230–231
    credibility in, 230
    reasons for, 228–230
  in sexual dysfunction, 239–246
  in urinary incontinence, 234–239

Race
  and prostate-specific antigen levels, 31
  as risk factor for prostate cancer, 4–6, 26, 51, 103
Radiation therapy, 86–88, 137–167
  in advanced disease, 148
  after prostatectomy, 147–148
  in bladder outlet obstruction, 259
  in bone pain, 271
  bowel sequelae in, 150, 246–247
  compared to surgery, 138–138
  complications of, 91–92
  control rate in, 146
  external beam, 86–87, 143–158
  fatigue from, 157
  field size in, 144–145
  fractionation of, 138
  genitourinary symptoms from, 153–156, 234
  hormonal therapy with, 87, 147, 158, 165–166
    side effects of, 166
  interstitial brachytherapy in, 87–88, 158–165. *See also* Brachytherapy, interstitial
  low-residue diet in, 154–155
  lymph node treatment in, 144, 146
  myelosuppression from, 157–158
  and neoadjuvant androgen ablation, 180–181
  patient's perspective on, 135–135
  pretreatment workup in, 139
  psychosocial issues in, 166–167
  and quality of life information, 233
  sexual function after, 156–157, 240
  side effects of, 149–158
  simulation-treatment planning in, 139–143
  skin reactions in, 150, 153
  in spinal cord compression, 277
  in stage T1a or T1b, 145
  in stage T1c, 146
  in stage T3 or T4, 147
  three-dimensional, 148–149
  total androgen suppression with, 147
Radioisotope therapy, 88
  in bone pain, 273
  in interstitial brachytherapy, 158
Radionuclide bone scans, 61
  in staging of tumors, 72–73
Rectal exam, digital
  in screening for cancer, 24, 29, 45–46, 51–53
  in staging of tumors, 71
5α-Reductase
  and dihydrotestosterone formation, 4, 54
  inhibitors in prevention of prostate cancer, 16–17
Regional distribution of prostate cancer, 44
Resources available, 286–304
  on advanced cancer, 292–293
  audiovisual materials, 294–296
  early detection and screening information, 286–288
  in Internet, 301–304
  prostate cancer information in, 296–297
    in books, 297–300
    in personal accounts, 300
  on psychosocial and support services, 293–294
  on treatment options, 288–292
Risk factors for prostate cancer, 3–16, 25–27
  nursing implications of, 18

Screening for cancer, 24–34
  barriers to, 28–29
  controversy over, 25
  cost effectiveness of, 32
  digital rectal examination in, 24, 29
  factors affecting, 28
  guidelines of American Cancer Society, 27–28
  information resources available, 286–288
  program development in Philadelphia, 32–34
  prostate-specific antigen in, 24, 30–32
  transrectal ultrasonography in, 32
Scrotal edema, 265

Sex hormone-binding globulin levels, and risk for prostate cancer, 11–12, 27
Sexual activity as risk factor for prostate cancer, 12–13
Sexual function
    after radiation therapy, 156–157
    dysfunction affecting quality of life, 239–246. *See also* Erectile dysfunction
    postoperative, 130
Sildenafil in erectile dysfunction, 184, 245
Skin reactions in radiation therapy, 150, 153
    in interstitial brachytherapy, 164
Small cell tumors, 40
Smoking, as risk factor for prostate cancer, 9–10
Socioeconomic status, and risk for prostate cancer, 6
Spinal cord compression
    dexamethasone in, 277
    nursing management in, 278
    pain in, 276–281
    radiation therapy in, 277
    standard of care in, 279–281
    surgery in, 277–278
Spouses and partners. *See* Attitudes of patients and partners
Staging of cancer, 66–79
    bone scans in, 73
    digital rectal examination in, 71
    histologic grade in, 75–76
    imaging procedures in, 72–74
    pathologic stage in, 75, 76
        prediction of, 77–78
    pelvic lymphadenectomy in, 74
    serum tumor markers in, 71–72
    significance of, 74–75
    T1c tumors in, 70
    TNM system in, 67–68, 69
        1992 AJCC-UICC revision of, 68
    and treatment decisions, 83
    Whitmore-Jewett system in, 67, 69
Stents
    ureteral, in hydronephrosis, 260
    urethral, in bladder outlet obstruction, 259
Steroidal antiandrogens, 176–177
Support services, information resources available, 293–294
Suprapubic tube in cryosurgery, management of, 131–132
Suramin, 90, 210
    affecting prostate-specific antigen levels, 196, 211
    hydrocortisone with, 210–211

Surgical treatment, 85–86, 117–133
    bilateral orchiectomy in, 132–133, 173. *See also* Orchiectomy, bilateral
    in bladder outlet obstruction, 259
    compared to radiation, 138–139
    complications of, 91
    cryoablation in, 86, 130–132
    and neoadjuvant androgen ablation, 180
    radical prostatectomy in, 123–130. *See also* Prostatectomy, radical
    in spinal cord compression, 277–278
    standard of care in, 118–120
    transurethral resection of prostate, 117–123, 259
        complications of, 121, 123
Symptom management in advanced cancer, 254–282
    in bladder outlet obstruction, 254–255, 259
    in bone pain, 267–273
    in disseminated intravascular coagulation, 265–267
    in leg edema, 261–265
    in spinal cord compression, 276–281
    in ureteral obstruction, 260–261
Symptoms of cancer, 45–46, 50–51

Tamsulosin hydrochloride for urinary symptoms after radiation, 154, 156
Terazosin
    finasteride with, 54
    for urinary symptoms after radiation, 154, 156
Testosterone
    production by Leydig cells, 172
    serum levels of
        and risk for prostate cancer, 11–12, 27
        and tumor progression, 44–45
    suppression of. *See* Hormonal therapy
Thrombosis, deep vein, 263–264
    leg edema in, 261
TNM classification system, 67–68, 69
    1992 AJCC-UICC revision of, 68
        benefits of, 71
        limitations of, 70
    T1c tumors in, 70
Transitional cell carcinoma, 40
Transurethral resection of prostate, 117–123, 259
    clinical pathway in, 122
    complications of, 121, 123
    patient-family timeline in, 124
Treatment of cancer
    alternate modalities in, 112–113

attitudes of patients and partners toward, 111–112, 113

  in expectant management, 108–109

  in radiation therapy, 135–136

chemotherapy in, 89–90, 195–222

clinical trials in, 90

complications of, 91–93

cryosurgery in, 86, 130–132

decision-making in, 81–97

  and quality of life information, 229–230

hormonal therapy in, 88–89, 170–191

  radiotherapy with, 87

information resources available, 288–292

nursing issues and concerns in, 96–97

patient data collection in, 82–84

psychosocial issues in, 94–95

radiation therapy in, 86–88, 137–167

selection for individual patient, 93–94

surgery in, 85–86, 117–133

watchful waiting in, 84–85, 102–114

Tumor markers

  and staging of cancer, 71–72

  and treatment decisions, 84

Tumor necrosis factor levels in disseminated intravascular coagulation, 266

Twins, prostate cancer in, 9

Ultrasonography, transrectal, 59

  in screening for cancer, 32

  in staging of tumors, 72–73

Uncertainty in therapy, management of, 111–113

Ureters

  obstruction from cancer, 50, 260–261

  stents in hydronephrosis, 260

Urethral stents in bladder outlet obstruction, 259

Urinary incontinence, 234–239

  after radiation therapy, 156, 234

  postoperative, 129–130

Urinary symptoms after radiation therapy, 153–156

  in interstitial brachytherapy, 164

Vacuum devices in erectile dysfunction, 184, 241

Vascular endothelial growth factor, role in prostate cancer, 2

Vasectomy, and risk for prostate cancer, 13

Videotapes available, 294–296

Vinblastine, 200

  with estramustine, 207

Vinorelbine with estramustine and etoposide, 209

Vitamin A intake, and risk for prostate cancer, 15

Vitamin D intake, and risk for prostate cancer, 15–16

Vitamin E intake, and risk for prostate cancer, 15

Vorozole in prevention of prostate cancer, 17

Warfarin in deep vein thrombosis, 264

Watchful waiting as treatment option, 84–85, 102–114. *See also* Expectant management

Whitmore-Jewett classification system, 67, 69

Workplace exposures, and risk for prostate cancer, 10–11